Beyond Medicine

Włodzimierz Piątkowski

Beyond Medicine

Non-Medical Methods of Treatment in Poland

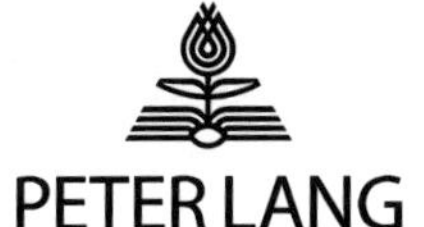

PETER LANG
Frankfurt am Main · Berlin · Bern · Bruxelles · New York · Oxford · Warszawa · Wien

Bibliographic Information published by the Deutsche Nationalbibliothek
The Deutsche Nationalbibliothek lists this publication in the Deutsche Nationalbibliografie; detailed bibliographic data is available in the internet at http://dnb.d-nb.de.

Cover Design:
© Olaf Gloeckler, Atelier Platen, Friedberg

The publication was financially supported
by the University of Lublin UMCS,
Department of Philosophy and Sociology

ISBN 978-3-631-62190-5

www.peterlang.de

For Alicja and Kajetan

Contents

Foreword

Non-medical therapies are gradually disappearing from among themes discussed in classic handbooks of sociology of health and medicine. Similarly, medical education programs usually omit the subject or mention it only in terms of its negative connotations, as falling outside of the scope of modern Evidence Based Medicine.

To many medical sociologists non-medical therapies are not attractive enough to become worthy of research interest – perhaps because the term itself is rather ambiguous and vague, the range of various behaviors to take into account quite large, and the practices used by proponents and representatives of this trend quite numerous. Another factor might be the connotations of traditional folk medicine, perceived primarily as a "cultural relict", often embarrassing in times of civilization progress, or superficially associated only with backward rural communities.

Non-medical therapies constitute a many-faceted problem – from harmless, and even health-promoting practices, to actions which may lead to health problems or even have life-threatening consequences. At the same time non-medical treatments are difficult to assess due to the fact that their use remains largely uncontrolled, and their true spread, for example in Poland, is unknown. There are few quantitative and qualitative studies on how often patients choose non-medical treatment or on the ways it affects the lives of different social groups. The problem is more often mentioned in research on illness behavior, when the "lay referral system" is disclosed. Another aspect missing from qualitative research is the experience of patients who undergo non-medical treatment or seek alternative health advice (mainly from healers), or people for whom alternative therapies are the reason to delay or forgo conventional medical treatment.

In the discussion of non-medical therapies, the author of the present work focuses on the growth of healer practices in Poland in connection with the period of political and economic transition, and considers non-medical practices as one of the strategies to cope with stress resulting from the ongoing changes and continuous unsuccessful reforms of the health care system, leading to inefficient health care services, lack of proper access to and low quality of medical care available. The patients' dissatisfaction with the system has always related to interactions with health professionals.

The period of economic and political transformation, different attitudes towards change, but also the anomie accompanying these changes, were juxtaposed with complex historical, political and religious considerations, demonstrating how people searching for a way out of difficult and crisis situation resorted first of all to folk religion, transcendental forces or to the belief in supernatural abilities attributed to various healers advertised in Poland. This exceptional susceptibility to healers' therapeutic practices, exemplified by seeking direct contact with them (and the belief that healing occurs through touch) and submitting to "distance healing" (through television screenings), was a response to specific social needs, a way to relieve social stress, and to express the need for support. Healers were expected to provide an immediately effective cure, to defuse tension, to heal.

The demand for this type of "healing actions" gave rise to new successful "business", whereby many people made considerable profits. In addition, the opening of borders brought about new ideas related to the promotion of health, such as return to nature and natural health care, effectively aided by multiple environmental movements.

Nevertheless, non-medical practices have a long-established tradition in Poland and have been the subject of interesting research. An overview of different types of attitudes, beliefs and convictions in relation to the general outlook of medical sociology, confronted with other non-medical treatment systems may provide a valuable contribution to the development of a new subdiscipline in the field of medical sociology.

For many readers, directly or indirectly involved in medicine, as well as for those who take little interest in it, this book can become an opportunity to think about and reflect on the place and significance of non-medical therapies in the era of modern scientific medicine, when almost every day brings new advances and practical solutions, and new hopes for recovery from diseases so far considered incurable. It is clear that such hopes cannot always be met because some diseases have not yet been effectively controlled and for many patients modern medicine does not provide effective treatment. Therefore, is the escape into the realm of unconventional treatment the search for the "last" or "unique" chance for successful recovery?

The question also arises as to which perspective should be chosen to assess non-medical therapies – the historical perspective, in which such treatments are primarily associated with distinctive cultural contexts, mainly with folk medicine, or perhaps the perspective which focuses on the relationships between non-medical and medical practices employed in various states of health or disease.

Will the author's presentation of non-medical treatment in Poland achieve its goal? The readers can judge for themselves.

Professor Beata Tobiasz-Adamczyk, PhD
Former Vice President of European Society for Health and Medical Sociology

Acknowledgments

This book was written owing to the support in the form of a publication grant, which I obtained in January 2011 from the American foundation that promotes science in East Central Europe. Further costs of publication have been covered by Maria Curie-Skłodowska University Faculty of Philosophy and Sociology in Lublin. At this point I would like to extend my special gratitude to the Dean of my Faculty, Professor Teresa Pękala, PhD for her personal commitment and kindness at all the stages of this project. Special thanks are due to the anthropologist Anna Witeska-Młynarczyk, PhD, of Adam Mickiewicz University in Poznań for her valuable substantive remarks and suggestions which allowed me to make this book better. I am also grateful to John R. Coast and Jerzy Adamko, MA for valuable language consultations. I would also like to extend cordial thanks to Professor Beata Tobiasz-Adamczyk, PhD Head of the Dept. of Epidemiology and Preventive Medicine, Jagiellonian University Medical College in Krakow, and former Vice President, European Society for Health and Medical Sociology (E.S.H.M.S) for writing the Foreword to this book and for her kind attitude to my project.

This book could not have been published had it not been for the assistance, patience and support offered by Łukasz Gałecki of Peter Lang International Academic Publishers, Frankfurt a. Main, which encouraged me to finalize my project, at the same time aiding me in overcoming obstacles and difficulties.

Finally, I would like to thank my doctoral student Michał Nowakowski for our editorial cooperation.

Włodzimierz Piątkowski

General introduction

The research interests of the author of this monograph stem from the awareness that medicine has a comparatively small impact on the state of health of human populations while the crucial role in this field is played by diverse ways of support and aid in illness which remain **outside of** the area of domination by medical institutions and professions. These systems of help make up the area of non-medical healthcare with its three fundamental pillars: **self-treatment, traditional folk healing systems, and healing practices of present-day healers.** This domain of popular knowledge and the system of practical activities are an important and constant element in the satisfaction of health needs in a large majority of modern-day European societies, which is also the case in Poland. It should be added that the often repeated thesis (voiced by prominent representatives of the medical community) that modernization processes occurring Poland (building of a democratic civil society, creating of a system of market economy, a progressing IT revolution, etc.) will eliminate or at least reduce the importance of health services provided by non-physicians (lay people) has not yet been confirmed. The systematic sociological studies (the first of this type in Poland and some of the first in Europe), which the author initiated, were aimed at the creation of scientific foundations for the "sociology of non-medical healing systems". They were also intended as an attempt to create a model of comprehensive and multifaceted description and interpretation of this important but insufficiently identified social problem. The complexity of the present approach consists *inter alia* in the introduction into "sociological narrative" of legislative themes (subchapter: Non-Medical Healing Systems – Legal Status), ethical issues (medical deontology vis-à-vis treatment methods offered by lay people), or historical themes (the presentation of Polish folk healthcare systems from the broad perspective of social changes from the late nineteenth century). The author's intention was also to emphasize multidisciplinarity as an effective research guideline which enables the presentation of the described and interpreted phenomena of practicing healing methods by non-professionals in their entire complexity; hence the book takes into account the standpoints of anthropology and history of medicine as well as clinical sciences (see the chapter dealing with the analysis of non-medical healing systems interpreted from the standpoint of the three aforementioned disciplines). This study was initially meant for the Polish reader, hence its *Bibliography* lists mainly Polish sources; however, strong and many-years-old ties of the Polish sociology of health and illness with its Western European and US versions, which go back to the pioneering period when the Professor Magdalena Sokołowska built the scientific foundations of our subdiscipline, prompted me to discuss the presented themes in the broader context of the achievements of European and US sociology (see the chapter *Complementary and Alternative Medicine (CAM) as Interpreted by American and European Sociology*). The methodological context of the research problems presented in this project is defined by qualitative techniques of gathering sociological data, especially the analysis of the unique and extensive collection of personal documents: 1311 letters sent to the Polish public television by mass viewers who systematically watched serial programs of the non-conventional therapist, A.M. Kashpirovsky. We might add that this TV series enjoyed immense popularity in Poland: this was one of the programs that attracted the largest audiences for two years (on average eight to nine million viewers). The author of the present study was one of the permanent commentators of the series; consequently, he was able to ask the viewers to send in their own accounts of TV programs concerned with non-conventional approaches to health and illness. The collected material was analyzed using qualitative and quantitative methods, the selected results having been presented and interpreted in Part III of this book, chapter: *The Kashpirovsky Phenomenon in the Context of the Changing Society*. We should add that a tangible effect of the analysis was an attempt to reconstruct the structure and character of everyday thinking about health problems. As a result of these studies, we managed to describe the elements of health culture of the viewers of the program, variants of behavior in health and in illness, opinions on the physician's social role, judgments on the systemic transformations which occurred in Poland after 1989, attitudes towards religious elements associated with healing, and finally, to characterize the viewers' attitudes to TV programs watched by mass audiences. We might expect that the present publication will also be more attractive to the English-speaking readers after they have read its Part II, which discusses Polish folk medical systems. A European Union member since 2004 (the largest among the new EU states), Poland has its own social specificity: it largely remains a society with its traditional social structure, with an important position of the peasant (farmer) class. More than one fifth of the population still live in the country and earn a living from agriculture. At the same time the majority of the large-city population has "peasant roots". These circumstances emphasize the importance of the guideline, which reads that if one wants to understand "Polish mentality" and "Polish specificity" well, it is necessary to get to know *inter alia* the shape or Polish culture, whose integral part is the peasant knowledge about health and illness (concerning everyday etiological conceptions, commonsense prevention, and diagnostic and treatment methods still applied by the countryside inhabitants). In Part II the author also presents in detail the state of research on folk medical (healing) systems, writes about methodological problems connected with the exploration of this form of treatment and the ways of solving them. The book also discusses the problem of "irrationality" of peasants' views on health and illness, and points to difficulties in working out a universal taxonomy in studies of this kind, etc. Furthermore, the book characterizes the social context of the functioning of rural self-treatment and folk healing systems, with a particular emphasis on the determinants of the presented phenomena and processes concerning collective life at the micro-, meso- and macrosocial levels. This approach shows *inter alia* the special role of women as "home therapists" and the significance of cultural (including religious) elements which make up the context in which folk healing systems are functioning today.

The Polish society is a good example that shows the origin, character, course and results of systemic modernization effected after the collapse of the totalitarian system in 1989 and accelerated by civilization changes consequent upon Poland's entry into the European Union. A sociologically interesting fact is that the type of society described here is becoming modernized in a specific and its own special way; on the one hand we witness speedy and thoroughgoing economic, cultural and morals transformations (the rise of the middle class, "educational revolution", the development of the information society, the spread of postmodern culture, etc.); on the other hand, we notice that which is Poland's *differentia specifica* (the persistent influence of religion on social life, the importance of the Church in public life, the size and importance of the peasant class, or the deepening social differences, etc.). All the aforementioned specific features of Polish society are also noticeable when we conduct a systematic sociological analysis of the "phenomenon of non-medical healing systems", then we can clearly see both "modern elements" typical of Western European societies (the use of the electronic media and the Internet by urban healers for information and advertising purposes, the institutionalization and commercialization of "other medicine", quick adaptation of "therapeutic fashions" coming from the West, etc), while at the same time we are witnessing and recording phenomena typical of Poland (the stable role of traditional village doctors, the high significance of religious elements in non-conventional therapies, reference to the "spiritual aid in illness" by blessed John Paul II, the occurrence of magic elements during the performance of acts of non-conventional treatment, and the generally positive attitude of Church institutions to spiritual healing etc). The persisting role of self-treatment popular in Polish society should also be emphasized; sociological surveys indicate that if they feel ill, most Poles practice this "home" form of treatment without utilizing institutional medicine: we should be reminded that according to the assumptions adopted in this book, self-treatment is one of three forms of non-medical healthcare.

The present book is concerned with the social aspects that create the context for the practice of non-conventional methods of treatment: it is part of the mainstream problems investigated by the Western sociology of health, illness and medicine; well-known scholars have recently recognized this research theme as so significant that for several years they have modified the titles of college handbooks in our subdiscipline, and have used the term "a sociology of health, **healing** and illness" (Weiss, Lonnquist 2006; Pescosolido et al. 2011).

Finally, we should express our hope that systematic sociological studies on the evolution of non-conventional healing methods will allow us to better investigate, become acquainted with and interpret such important social problems as health awareness, attitudes towards health and illness, health needs, and finally, behaviors around health and illness undertaken by so-called "ordinary people". We may expect that this direction of analyses will continue to develop fast in the European Union countries not only in the realm of the sociology of health, healing and illness but also within sociology-related disciplines such as psychology and anthropology because such studies supplement the general knowledge on present-day societies by significant sociomedical issues.

Włodzimierz Piątkowski,
November 5, 2011

Introduction

The decision to commence systematic studies on non-medical treatment systems is based on a number of significant reasons, primarily the lack of a monograph entirely concerned with this socially important subject in the Polish and European sociology of health and illness[1]. An additional argument for the implementation of this research project is the desire to describe a sector of changes in Polish society related to health and illness. These transformations taking place after 1989 laid and continue to lay the foundations of communal life. The differences between new and old forms of social life are qualitative: they are permanent and irreversible, having been the object of sociological interest for over two decades. We are witnessing, as Piotr Sztompka writes, changes in the 'composition of the system' (political and organizational transformations, migrations etc.), in 'the structure of the system' (changes in how interactions, interests, norms and ideas function etc.), in the 'functions exercised by various elements of society' (e.g. fundamental transformations in the structure of the family, in the scope of its autonomy and internal identity), and in the boundaries of the system and its environment (Sztompka, 2002: 437-438). These far-reaching structural changes cover such diverse spheres of communal life as demographic processes, social structure, living standards of citizens, religion and religiosity, ad the dynamics and course of pathological phenomena etc. (Marody 2004:11 et seq. See also Mariański 2005:359-360. On changes in religion see Libiszowska-Żółtkowska 2001:9-10). A paradoxical effect of this period, so rich in many new phenomena and processes, is the continual sense of inadequate and reliable knowledge of society because representatives of particular sociological subdisciplines '[...]find it difficult', M. Marody writes, 'to comprehend the multitude [...] of new processes and convert them into a comparatively coherent system of propositions' (M. Marody, op. cit.: 11). We might add incidentally that in recent years medical sociologists have tried to describe and interpret social changes that directly or indirectly concerned the sphere of health and illness. However, there

1 The term 'sociology of non-medical treatment methods' was introduced by the author in 1998 (cf. M. Libiszowska-Żółtkowska et al. (eds.) (1998), chapter by W. Piątkowski, (17-37). The term 'non-medical treatment' was characterized in W. Piątkowski's book *Spotkania z inną medycyną* (1990). A similar term was used by Philip Tovey and Jon Adams in their article in the sociomedical journal "Social Science and Medicine". See Tovey, J. Adams, 2003:1469-1480. They use the term 'a sociology of complementary and alternative medicine'. See also The Role In Complementary medicine in: Senior and Viveash, 1998: 290-293; The Emergence of Alternative Therapist in: Thomas 2003: 148-151; Cant and Sharma 2009: 221-227.

has been no monograph on the 'sociology of non-medical treatment'[2]. The present study is a response to the demands voiced by sociologists in general and tries to fill the gap in describing the mechanisms taking place in a society undergoing transformation in the area defined by these concepts: health – illness – medicine. The description of phenomena in this domain shows *inter alia* that the vitally important element of the 'old scheme', which was the centralized, formalized, bureaucratic, etatist and essentially inefficient system of the national health service, is losing its monopoly on providing medical services. New entities emerge, taking advantage of capitalist, free-market realities, in which everything that is not prohibited is allowed: the so-called 'healing business' is gaining ground. A good example of this type of situation is the rise and development of a private business offering unconventional psychotherapy on a mass scale. This successful business venture undertaken by a 'post-Soviet' (!) healer A. M. Kashpirovsky was made possible by the support of public television for his business – for almost two years it broadcast a series of 'healing programs'. That is why the present book contains a study of the 'Kashpirovsky case'. This unusual phenomenon could only have happened in the context of the first, turbulent period of Polish transformation. It was then, as A. Jawłowska observes, that '[…] a new kind of social relations began to be established, different from the relatively stable ones, based on known and accepted rules, which were replaced by incidental, impermanent relations that were not so much the result of a norm but of an individual choice' (Jawłowska 1995:17). At the time when the reliability of the system of long-standing institutions was being challenged or even defied, in this study we are mainly interested in medical institutions and 'medicine understood as a whole - '[…] "classical" values were criticized and […] increasingly large groups started to emerge, which tried to implement new types of values such as post-materialist […] especially **alternative values** [*my emphasis* W. P.] and minority group values.' (Ziółkowski 1995: 36). During the period in question the Poles started more and more frequently to seek new rules and priorities, which they gradually came to regard as attractive, treating them as an element of their redefined identity. In this book I intend to show that these strivings and actions also applied to the area of health and illness[3]. It appears that in the late 1990s a special transformational effect surfaced which also accelerated transformations in the attitudes to health and was conducive to the building of

2 I defined the key term 'non-medical treatment' in 1990. I use it throughout this study and describe it in detail in part I, 1.1.2. For stylistic reasons I also use equivalent expressions, e.g. 'unconventional treatment'.

3 For interesting examples of medical phenomena embedded in cultural transformation processes, see Mucha, (1995:112).

a 'new awareness'. We speak here of the rapidly growing popularity of the ecological movement and its accompanying ideas. One of the elements of the new thinking about the human natural environment was a critical view of 'techno-chemical medicine', and the parallel promotion of an 'alternative' approach. It is in this field that 'safe, natural methods of treatment' are preferred, with therapeutic means being drawn for example from phytotherapy, naturopathy, or homeopathy. P. Gliński stresses that there is a gradually growing fear of degradation of the natural environment and a sense of the adverse effects of this process on health in its individual and social dimension. All this has prompted better educated, well-off, city-dwelling [young urban professional] Poles to become interested in 'pure' and apparently complication-free 'alternative medicine'. Analogous processes were indicated in sociological studies describing a similar situation in wealthy Western countries in the 1970s and 1980s (this theme of 'new ecological awareness' overlapping with the growing acceptance of complementary and alternative medicine has been described in Part One). (Gliński 1998: 309). We will again return to Piotr Sztompka's reflections, this time on changes in the collective consciousness of the Poles and progressive 'cultural disorientation'. One the one hand, new patterns and norms connected with capitalism, the free market, pluralism and competition emerge, while on the other there is an ongoing struggle to defend and preserve traditional culture. We should add that the melting pot of new and old values realizable in postmodern societies now also embraces dilemmas concerning the choice of methods of treatment: traditional, related to clinical medicine, or unconventional[4] (Sztompka 2003:79).

Triggered and accelerated by a system transformation, the elements of disorganization and disorientation discussed by P. Sztompka have a broad and complex (as well as civilizational and cultural) context. The importance of culture and cultural phenomena stems from the fact that they cover knowledge, art, law and morality as well as various abilities and habits acquired by man in the course of social life (L. Dyczewski 1995: 36 et seq.). L. Dyczewski emphasizes that culture is a dynamic process, with new elements and new connections between existing elements incessantly arising and clashing with one another in the process of social transformations (Ibid:39). Culture as an integral part of changes in the society under transformation can undergo a crisis. As Z. Krasnodębski points out, 'Crisis does not consist in the incomplete or wrong realization of norms but in doubts about the validity of any norms and all ideals' (Krasnodębski 1996:13) The result of broader cultural transformations is most often not so much the decomposition or disregard of old values as the unre-

4 Observe that the term 'tradition/traditional' functions in different contexts.

stricted coexistence of their different forms. Various contradictions are possible here, there is a gradual individualization and (also alternative) interpenetration of meanings and communications. More and more often the society turns into a set of autonomous subjects who are looking for attractive (including health) choices offered by postmodernity and for opportunities to actualize them. An individual in the world of culture begins to be the designer of his/her life and the collector of subjective experiences, feelings and emotions. (Ibid: 123 et seq.). It is in this world of transformations, crisis and chaos that a cultural model of successful life can also include health understood as a complete feeling of wellness and wellbeing. Health is sometimes associated with another highly-regarded value - 'efficiency' - which comes down to 'absorbing a growing amount of sensations', 'creatively responding' to diverse stimuli, and to adaptive abilities to act in the rapidly changing society. (Bauman, 1995:55). Zygmunt Bauman writes, 'Every moment, therefore, of satisfaction with one's own efficiency is poisoned by the thought of "true" efficiency, never fully attained [...] No drug turns out to be entirely effective, each brings only momentary relief, the faith in its magic power will disappear the day after it has been used. Therefore we continually seek new wonder drugs and magic charms, pricking up our ears listening [...] to confidential instructions by folk doctors, only to be disappointed with their advice tomorrow and ashamed that we trusted them yesterday.' (Ibid:92). As the cultural sociologist M. MacLachlan emphasizes, postmodern society not only develops mass culture, which it uses, but it also creates a special sector of healthcare services, which he calls 'the popular sector'. The influence of this sector on health and illness is the largest and most important. It is made up of 'everyday ideas about health and illness [...]discussed by "lay" nonprofessional people.' (MacLachlan 1997:232). We may be witnessing the rise of 'pop medicine' as we once witnessed the making of 'pop culture'. This 'popular' ('folk') sector consists of a network of health advisers who do not have formal, professional qualifications. These are the family, friends, acquaintances, and neighbors etc. The sector's influence lies in its ability to shape the notions of 'an ordinary man' about health and illness and to directly or indirectly determine whether a person seeks help from medical institutions or practices self-treatment, or consults complementary and alternative medicine practitioners. (Ibid:232). As we can see, in different countries social transformations trigger and accelerate civilizational changes, which include transformations in health customs, resulting in health becoming increasingly relativistic and cultural. (Siciński 2002:107-123). Summing up the remarks on the relations between the two areas in question – culture and health – A. Siciński concludes, 'In present-day Europe [...] for treatment, people mostly turn to appropriate health service institutions or to formally qualified, individual physicians. Apart from those, however, patients frequently consult practitioners **outside official medicine** [*my emphasis*, W.P.] (this practice is now commonly and euphemistically referred to as "unconventional" methods of treatment or "alternative medicine"). There is no room here, however, for discussion of the now sensitive issue of relations between "official" and "alternative" medicine, although this is **unquestionably a cultural problem** [*my emphasis*, W.P.]' (Ibid:123). Anna E. Kubiak points out, in turn, that an element of mass (popular) culture, which grows stronger in Poland in its new forms during social transformations, is the New Age movement containing many guidelines and references to health. (Kubiak 1999:73-74). In this movement, treated as a phenomenon of postmodern culture, one of the priorities is to focus attention on health: the ability to individually shape and design one's body, and the ability to experience diverse emotions as well as the capacity to 'self-treat' is as important as 'self-religion' (Kubiak, 2005:42-43). In the New Age area, the patient seeking a healer's help can also be a self-healer. The emphasis on self-reliance and independence in the area of health prompts one to depart from medicine and take responsibility for one's own health wherever possible. The concepts of 'healing' and 'self-healing' are not simply methods and techniques of treatment, diagnosis, etiological theories and prevention principles, but also the state of mind and attitude to other people and the world at large[5] (Ibid: 44, 45-46). Because holism is one the central elements of the 'philosophy of healing' based on different New Age currents, the terms 'health' and 'healing' have a broader meaning than in biomedicine. The broadly understood 'alternative definition of health' is an element of a larger whole: its is the preferred lifestyle of New Age followers, which is to strive for general wellbeing. Definitions of lifestyle are constructed in opposition to the vision of capitalist, consumer society, whose pillar is commercial, 'techno-chemical' medicine. If we accepted the uncontroversial thesis that an element of general transformational changes is cultural transformations, including those with New Age characteristics, then, in turn, an element of the latter transformations are changes, clearly occurring after 1989, in the lifestyle of the Poles, especially observable among the social groups which are largely the 'products' of the aforementioned processes. We have in mind the growing group of young, educated, comparatively well-paid people living in large cities (young

5 New Age ideologists distinguish the following treatment techniques: sensory (diets , e.g. vegetarian, macrobiotic, touch healing, hydrotherapy, acupuncture, yoga, rebirthing, Alexander Technique), psychotherapeutic (Rogers therapy, hypnosis, psychodrama etc.), psychotronic (astrology, clairvoyance, bioenergy therapy) and religious (faith in the power of religious symbols and objects, etc.) (Kubiak, 2005:45-46) and Bradby 2009: 58-59.

urban professionals), who want to decide for themselves about their health and illness, to shape and design their own bodies, and to take into consideration ecological values; consequently, they prefer more 'natural' rather than 'technological' methods of treatment. The trends in question, also relating to health and illness, not only continue but are even becoming highly popular, as the latest surveys indicate. (Czy Polacy..., 2006).

The present book therefore points out that the syndrome of transformational changes contains many cultural themes, including those we are especially interested in because they are not only related to health and illness in general, but are also directly associated with the revival of unconventional methods of treatment. In the 1990s Poland witnessed the emergence of 'pro-health lifestyles', defined as permanent and consistent behaviors. A special element of these types of behaviors was 'lay' healthcare methods, consisting of elements of everyday knowledge that might take the form of popular self-treatment (Ostrowska 1999:29). Under these circumstances, as has been pointed out, there was an increase in the number of actors who played their roles **outside** the stage on which the doctor and medicine predominated; among them appeared ordinary people who also wanted to be doctors for themselves (self-treatment) or those who believed that despite having no formal medical education they could offer their healing abilities to others (healers and folk doctors). (Ibid: 193). A good illustration of the thesis that healing and its representatives are present even in the consciousness of the people not interested in medicine in everyday life can be found in an excerpt from Ryszard Kapuściński's *Lapidarium*, 'A miracle worker Harris is coming to Warsaw! This briskly moving young Englishman with a somewhat vacant look, as if somewhat dazed and surrounded by an invisible though perceptible cloud, walks among the rows of lying, sitting or standing people; he stops at each one for a moment – asks through the interpreter what he or she is suffering from, touches the indicated spot for a split second, and hurries on. Large crows are coming to see Harris! Tickets sell out many weeks before his arrival. These crowds [..] make us aware of one thing: how much suffering there is around us!' (Kapuściński, 1997).

General sociology, describing and characterizing changes occurring during transformations, also characterizes other than the previously described dimensions of these transformations, e.g. those concerning the social structure and its effect on the attitudes and behaviors of human communities. Satisfaction or dissatisfaction with the general direction and character of social transformations influence satisfaction and dissatisfaction with the system of healthcare services and with one's individual health condition. H. Domański observes that many results of opinion polls (by CBOS [Public Opinion Research Center], OBOP [Center for Public Opinion Polls], and PGSS [Polish

General Social Survey]) show that the medical system in question has become '[...] the object of as many unsuccessful experiments as reforms, adversely assessed by the public, political opposition and the successive governments' (Domański, 2005:12). It should be remembered that these persistent, negative appraisals of the effectiveness and quality of the healthcare system are articulated first of all by the growing category of people of higher social status (income, education, professional position and prestige). It is they who, on the one hand, criticize official medicine as inefficient and ineffective; on the other hand - as A. Ostrowska's studies show – they take more care of their own and their family's health as compared with members of the lower classes (Ostrowska, 1999, also Domański, 2005: 41). This category of people with such convictions as indicated by the survey data and by the results of the author's own research referred to in this book, most often use the services of 'other medicine' practitioners, not only when they are ill but also to increase their 'health capital' and improve their general feeling.

Another element of the transformation process that has an effect on the development of non-medical treatment systems in Poland is the migrations triggered by the 'autumn of the peoples' in 1989. This phenomenon is part of wider globalization processes that impact the character and form of the society under transformation. The Polish transformations have their own historical context and are driven by their own dynamics; they were, however, preceded by 'Soviet perestroika' initiated by Mikhail Gorbachev[6]. The 'offspring' of those changes was the object of the author's own studies: the unconventional therapist A. M. Kashpirovsky. This subject has been dealt with in Part III of the present book. The system transformation not only increased the subjectivity of individuals and released their initiative and business activity but also opened the frontiers to millions of citizens from the former socialist countries. As a result of radical political, economic and social changes, the stage of 'mass journeying' began. In the early 1990s different factors 'pushed out' people from their native countries (on account of the subject matter of the book we are mainly interested in the situation in the former Soviet Union countries). When the Soviet empire was breaking up, the masses of inhabitants in that country realized how backward, poor and lacking in prospects their region was; they were attracted by the vision of neighboring Poland as a better organized and richer country that was comparatively easy to enter, had no language barrier, and offered better earnings than their own country. The early 1990s was the period of mass migrations of Russians, Belarusians,

6 See entry 'transformacja ustrojowa'[political system transformation], (W. Gumuła, 2002:265).

and Ukrainians. These were external, temporary migrations.[7]. Apart from farm laborers, construction workers and domestic maids, the symbol of the migration were healers and folk doctors from the East who offered their services on the re-emerging healthcare market. For example, according to the Border Guard figures, in 1992 there were half a million foreigners staying in Poland on a lawful temporary residence basis (Rutkiewicz, 1994). The then special report on the trends in the labor market noted: 'The most popular are bioenergy therapists – employed both by private firms and the Polish Red Cross […].' (Gajdziński, 1992:22) Due to a huge demand for 'unconventional' medical service, numerous commercial and service companies sprang up, inviting healers from the East and employing them in specialist alternative medicine offices[8]. Visa relaxations introduced in 1994 for former Soviet Union countries increased immigration to an even greater level. In the Lublin province alone, the Provincial Labor Office issued 213 permits, 22 of which were for persons employed as bioenergy therapists or acupuncturists. In the mid-1990s, even 'door-to-door dentists' were reported in the Podlasie region villages; they used methods of treatment found in the nineteenth-century ethnographic records. (Odonus, 1993). 'Certified healers – specialists in unconventional medicine' worked in private practice in many convalescent homes and vacation centers, offering paid treatment of all illnesses including, for example, infantile cerebral palsy, and assuring that they guaranteed fundamental improvement in a patient's health condition. This radical increase in healing services offered by unconventional therapists from the East triggered protests by the Regional Medical Chambers, which objected to the violation of the Act on the Profession of Physician and the Code of Medical Ethics, and to the unpunished practice of what was termed 'pseudomedicine' (Dziadul, 1993).

In my studies I decided to use the extensive set of personal documents – letters sent to the Public Television broadcaster-by viewers who watched the program of the unconventional therapist A. M. Kashpirovsky. It is a paradox that the world-renowned 'Polish method', i.e. analysis of personal documents or, as Jan Szczepański writes, 'human documents', which was also developed by Florian Znaniecki, is not particularly popular in present-day Polish sociology (J. Szczepański, 1973: 615; see also Thomas and Znaniecki, 1976). At the same time the use of this method (or qualitative methods in general) in Polish medical

7 See entry 'migracje [migrations] H. Kubiak, K. Slany, (1999, 2: 243-249) and Bradby (2009: 81-82).

8 In one province, out of 27 applications for business activity permits 25 were about the legalization of paramedical treatment services provided by Ukrainians, Russians, and Belarusians (Grun et al., 1993:74-75).

sociology is extremely rare.[9] Commenting on the classical study by W. I. Thomas and F. Znaniecki, J. Szczepański points out that the analysis of letters enabled presentation of patients' **'own experiences'** and **'social conditions which gave rise to these experiences'**. [*my emphasis*, W.P.] (Szczepański, op. cit.:617). We should stress at once that the intention to reconstruct the patients' subjective experiences relating to health, illness and unconventional therapy methods, and to get to know the people who used them was a major reason for our own research presented in the book. The application of the method of personal documents analysis results in people's own accounts of their participation in the processes and events, which are the object of investigation. From the collected set of description the sociologist selects the data needed to solve the problem under investigation. The collected information can provide material to illustrate the adopted hypotheses. (Ibid: 620-621). Typical kinds of personal documents used in classical sociological research are letters, autobiographies, diaries and memoirs. In this interpretation we have an insight into the syndrome of subjective experiences, attitudes, aspirations or evaluation of people participating in the life of society in the area chosen. These elements may and do have a special value. Szczepański believes that the content analysis applied for interpreting personal documents can be an element that will systematize and structure the collected material. (Szczepański 1973: 640). In this study I describe the limitations and disadvantages of the method, but the idea of its application arose from its advantages as a way of leading to the description, interpretation and understanding of the attitudes of 'ordinary people' towards health, illness, being ill and recovering, as well as towards the process of treatment using unconventional methods, and their attitude towards the practitioners of the methods. The goal was also to learn the attitude of the letter writers towards medical professions and institutions. (Dulczewski, 1975:75 et seq.) The collected, edited and selected letters allow a certain insight 'from within' into the ways of thinking of lay people. They also allowed me to reconstruct their aspirations, underlying motivations, convictions and views. In the present book the method in question was the only way of gathering the necessary data. I personally watched the 'Kashpirovsky phenomenon', taking part as a commentator for over a year and a half on television programs, so-called 'teletherapy', and was able to have di-

9 Worth noting in his context is the book co-authored by M. Sokołowska (Sokołowska et al., 1965; see also (Piątkowski et al., 1993). At the Master's degree seminar in medical sociology conducted by the author of this study five Master's degree dissertations were written and defended, based on different qualitative methods, e.g. content analysis. One of those, by W. Kaliszuk, was published in an abridged version in the national journal "Promocja Zdrowia. Nauki Społeczne i Medycyna".

rect conversations with Anatoly Kashpirovsky himself; I met some of his patients in Kiev and the Ukrainian scholars interested in the 'Kashpirovsky method'. In June 2008 I was invited, as one of two commentators, to take part in the Polish TV production of a documentary on the 'Kashpirovsky phenomenon'. I met and talked with A. M. Kashpirovsky (now living in the USA), who handed me a DVD featuring the latest account of his healing shows. This Polish TV film is to be shown on Channel Two of the Polish Television service on the twentieth anniversary of the first 'teletherapy' performances. Furthermore, when I started to describe this subject I used specialist studies published in Poland and in Ukraine, and the results of surveys carried out by the OBOP. Zygmunt Dulczewski , cited above, accepts that the key directive in Znaniecki's methodological assumptions was the use of the humanistic coefficient, which enables interpretation and explanation of people's attitudes towards events and the motivations for their social behavior. It also makes it possible to understand the significance that people attach to situations that they encounter in social life. 'It is this characteristic of human behaviors that Znaniecki calls a humanistic coefficient. Without reference to the language of meanings of various things, which is present in people's experiences, we cannot speak of understanding and explaining their conduct. The application of the humanistic coefficient is therefore a necessary methodological directive in explorative inquiries of social sciences, especially sociology.' (Dulczewski 1075: 79) Florian Znaniecki characterized the concept of the humanistic coefficient in the following way: 'This feature of cultural phenomena, of objects of humanistic inquiry, this essential property of theirs that as objects of theoretical reflection they are already objects given to someone in experience or someone's conscious actions, can be called the humanistic coefficient of these phenomena. A myth, a work of art, a language word, a tool, a legal pattern, a social system are what they are only as conscious human phenomena […].' (Sitek 2002: 365)

At present we are witnessing a revival of qualitative methods although this phenomenon has a broader historical context. The social crisis in the 1980s and then the experience of 1980-1981 '[…] made', A. Sułek writes, 'our **everyday** [*my emphasis*, W. P.] life interesting: it became not only a practical problem for an ordinary man but also a cognitive problem for the sociologist. **New** [*my emphasis*, W. P.] phenomena emerged or those previously underestimated gained in significance, having become interesting by their **novel or unusual character** [*my emphasis*, W. P.] […] at the time.' (Sułek, 1989:22). If we took A. Sułek's words absolutely literally, we might say that they directly refer to the 'sociology of non-medical treatment systems'. In the early 1990s, on the eve of 'great social change', I found the studies on the phenomenon of social popularity of healing methods entirely new (because of the social context) and unusual. The implementation of two projects which I then initiated enabled me, in two stages, to collect and then analyze a total of 3218 letters. This material is an example of so-called everyday sociology, a recording of the knowledge that 'ordinary people' possess (Podemski 1989:77). A characteristic of this type of qualitative investigation (including analysis of personal documents) is the researcher's direct contact with reality at certain stages of the research process and reference to, as A. Wyka stresses, '[…] the competence of research subjects, expressed in different ways, with a different degree of the researcher's trust in that competence […] they try to open room for the activities of the subjects themselves during the research process, admitting a broad presentation of own views of research subjects […].' (Wyka, 1993:12). A situation like the one described by A. Wyka took place during my own investigations in 1990-1992; I was then invited by the Polish TV Channel Two to comment on programs by the unconventional therapist A. M. Kashpirovsky. When we realized (after OBOP surveys) that the programs were regularly watched by several million people, I asked the presenters to appeal to the audiences to send letters with their own impressions, opinions and assessments of this series of programs. The announcement emphasized that the healer would not answer the requests and questions in the letters but stated that all the material would be used for research purposes. As a result, Channel Two received several thousand letters, of which 1907 were used in the first stage and 1311 in the second stage of investigations. The area of accounts by those participating in the 'teletherapy' was defined by the following important, observation-structuring points of reference: participants in the sessions (Kashpirovsky's patients), the healer (using unconventional methods of treatment), physicians (medical professions), and the system of formalized medicine ('government' medical administration). Thus, the sociologist was, in these circumstances, not only a witness but also, to some extent, a participant in the presented social phenomenon. This, somewhat unconsciously, fulfilled A. Wyka's proposition that social sciences should come closer to life and the cognition of social reality, taking into consideration the viewpoint of subjects creating this reality. (Wyka, Ibid:34). When describing and characterizing general features of particular qualitative methods, K. Konecki points out that they enable respondents to tell the histories of their life experiences. In the case of letters to Kashpirovsky, the authors were the initial editors and censors of their own statements, and it was only afterwards that the sociologist selected the excerpts from them and made cuts in their narratives, trying to preserve their logic and meaning (Konecki, 2000:144). The collected qualitative data, the result of studies of the letters, have the form of words rather than figures. Their attractiveness seems to stem from the individual wealth of descriptions, interpretations and characterizations of personal experience caused mainly by illness development and by fulfillment of the 'social role of a sick person (patient)', and from the search (usually parallel to treatment in national health service institutions) for effective methods of fighting the disease, pain, and suffering. The researcher thus gains access to a world of individual emotions, stereotypes and subjective views on the causes of an illness, its course of treatment and prognosis for the future – for a medical sociologist this is a highly interesting area of exploration. Herein lies the attractiveness of qualitative data lies (Miles, Huberman 2000). The letters provided an insight into how their authors explained the phenomena of health and illness in everyday language, and how they arrived at their own ways at individual judgments and prognoses concerning treatment with unconventional and conventional methods, they also depicted their individual worlds of experience. The generalized knowledge derived from the ideas of 'television therapy' participants, expressed in letters, enabled us to reconstruct 'real life'. This kind of narrative expressed the individual, specific features of a letter writer's way of thinking and his/her attitude to the events experienced (here most often connected with health and illness). Despite the individual character of events and their 'subjective nature', it should be remembered that they all pertained to a specific series of TV programs with a similar scenario and to the real, highly popular idol-therapist, 'the inhabitant of mass imagination', and finally, to the method of 'television therapy (teletherapy)' well-known to the viewers. These elements were constant points of reference for the letter writers. It should be emphasized once again that a researcher cannot uncritically approach the collected material: that is why known deficiencies and limitations that mark these kinds of personal documents have been discussed throughout the present study.[10] In my studies, apart from sporadic encounters with Kashpirovsky's patients at the symposium in Kiev devoted to his methods, I had not contacts with the authors of the letters. The distance between the researcher and the subject grew larger because the 'intermediary agent' was the text of each letter. When speaking of social reality, we analyze it in this case 'via the text' (Palska 1999: 156-157). The study of a letter as a kind of personal documents requires, H. Palska emphasizes, 'that we study words'; we first perform here the role of the reader and then the interpreter of the text, and it is only on this basis that we interpret social reality. At the same time we, in a way, 'fish for meanings' that people attribute to facts and social phenomena. The point of reference can be F. Znaniecki's humanistic coefficient discussed above. Correct research procedures result in recognition of the letters as a legitimate sociological source. (Palska, Ibid: 164). We thus have to try to correctly read the intentions of the letter writ-

10 Janusz Sztumski describes in detail the defects and limitations o the material based on analysis of personal documents, (Sztumski, 1999:156-157).

ers and take into account the context and circumstances in which they were written (Domański, 1999:193-194). The content analysis consists therefore in recording and investigating human communications, letters being one of their forms (Babbie, 2003: 342). Here, we answer the questions: who writes, what does s/he write, to whom, why, and to what effect?

Letters are thus a special kind of message; it might seem that in the age of SMS texts and e-mails their significance will decline. This is not happening, however. An opinion-forming daily writes, 'Previously, a month before Christmas or Easter, we would start hunting for season's postcards [...] With the widespread popularity of mobile phones the custom of sending greetings in writing has almost disappeared. E-mails and SMS texts are in. Recently, another facilitation appeared. Rather than sweat blood over a text, we can choose from the mobile's server. Many addressees receive the same standard clichés – seemingly funny but in fact lamentably flat [...] someone remembers about us but with negligible, if any, respect.' (Małkowska 2005) It appears that after years of fascination with the technical transmission of information, there has been a gradual but noticeable revival of interest in the epistolary art. Many museums hold exhibitions of letters while their curators emphasize that they teach us proper language standards, the ability to exchange ideas, views, impressions, and consolidate our feelings and desires (Skrzypek, 2006). Respectable publishing houses publish large editions of letter collections, written by priests, cultural activists, writers and politicians.[11] Specialists in literary studies stress that, 'Epistolography is growing more and more popular in Poland, although we are still far behind Western Europe, where large editions of collected letters not only by writers [...] but also by popular actors, architects, musicians and pop-culture stars, have appeared for years. Will it be the same in Poland?' (Marzec, Sawuła, www.rzeczpospolita.pl, 2005). Readers want to learn more about the lives of famous people; the Poles are mainly interested in the letters written by eminent figures or in the correspondence that increases their knowledge about a period. Important historic events also arouse great interest (e.g. October 1957, December 1970, August 1980 etc.). [12]

To recapitulate this part of the discussion on the advisability of taking up studies in 1989 on the sociology of non-medical treatment systems, we

11 See for example (Dyczewski 1983, and Nowak, 2005).

12 Cf. the examples of letter collections, which were a commercial success: *Listy do Bobera. Nie tylko o gospodarce*, 1992; *Lata, Listy, ludzie. Adresat M. F. Rakowski*, 1993; *Listy do Rzecznika Praw Obywatelskich Tadeusza Zielińskiego*, 1994; *Listy do Papieża, o książce "przekroczyć próg nadziei"*, 1995; K. Mądel, *Wartości ogólnoludzkie i chrześcijańskie w ...* 1995.

can conclude that, if we accept the uncontroversial proposition that one of the main research goals pursued by Polish sociology after the groundbreaking events of twenty years ago has been the description and interpretation of successive stages of social transformation, then we should emphasize that health- and illness-related problems have been in the center of these changes. An important element of these transformations, in turn, was and still is the growing popularity of non-professional therapists, who managed to create a network of various commercial institutions providing health services outside the area of official medicine. This problem inspired me to design and implement a project aimed at complementing sociological knowledge in this field. Reports by opinion-polling institutions show that the area defined by the terms health – illness –medicine (medical system) has raised strong feelings, public criticism and interest from the very beginning of transformations. Health issues are for the Poles the main elements of plans for the future – people assess the quality of their lives from the health perspective. Health is invariably one of the most frequently declared values. The pro-ecological and prohealth lifestyle is becoming synonymous with modernity, especially among the growing group of young urban professionals. In the context of these changes, there has also been a growing interest in treatment methods not accepted by conventional medicine. The Poles are not only interested in such techniques of treatment and in improving general feelings of wellbeing, however, as demonstrated by the results of sociological studies presented in subsequent parts of this book, and by observations as part of the author's own study of the Kashpirovsky phenomenon, more and more often, from time to time or regularly, they also practice self-treatment or use the services of unconventional practitioners of folk medicine or modern healing. My own studies and the results obtained by other (also Western) authors indicate that non-medical treatment most often only complements the therapy that patients have already started, and that most of the clients of healers do not stop the parallel treatment at national health service centers. Unconventional methods, therefore, do not represent alternatives to the services of physicians but complement them. The practice of using the services of lay practitioners (non-physicians) is obviously nothing new in our culture (we are talking of course of the period when professional medicine was available), as I will seek to prove in the subsequent chapters, but it was only in the latter half of the twentieth century, at the time of the triumph of biomedicine and its increasingly high technical and scientific efficiency, that it lost a large portion of its patients. This book shows that the success of unconventional medicine does not come from the notion that 'alternative' therapists have solved some actual scientific or technical problem concerning health and illness. The popularity of unconventional medicine practitioners stems rather from the fact that they feel intuitively that modern medical sciences have largely lost their humanistic character, leaving sociopsychological problems on the periphery of training at medical schools. Meanwhile, the objective changes in the picture of health and illness (described in this study) – i.e. prevalence of chronic diseases, psychosociosomatic conditions, diseases of elderly people, those determined by stress syndrome and associated with terminal conditions – contribute to the rising importance of the issues having sociological or psychological contexts. Under such circumstances, lay people who attribute healing powers to themselves and offer, as a rule, only an 'amateur socio-and psychotherapy or try to use the placebo effect, become attractive to some patients. We should also remember that the people living at the turn of the twentieth and twenty-first centuries are not only interested in their own bodies when they are already ill, but more and more frequently tend to take care of themselves when they are well, wishing to consciously build their health reserve, capital and potential, and enhance their wellness. The 'other' (alternative) medicine has also increased its attraction by providing not only illness-related but also health-related services. These problems will be also dealt with in this study (Nettleton 1996:12; Giddens 2004:180).

Non-medical treatment systems would not have developed in Poland so rapidly without the syndrome, described here, of changes in the law, economy, culture and consciousness as well as in faith and religion, etc. A comparison of the range and quality of services offered by the non-medical treatment systems in the days of real socialism and now, at the beginning of the twenty-first century, shows that the growing public interest in and acceptance of complementary medicine was able to occur here and now in the conditions of liberal capitalist society. The transformation triggered off and accelerated new mechanisms of communal life; some citizens regained a sense of competence, initiative and subjectivity, including in the matters of health and illness. People now want to be more and more independent (including of doctors and medicine), they feel the need for self-actualization, and want to discuss which options concerning their own health interests are optimal in their subjective view.

Despite the objective weight and significance of health issues for the majority of people, the description of the Polish transformation mechanisms by general sociology often omits or marginalizes topics related to health and illness in the analyses of the general picture of society. An exploration of the reasons for this state of affairs is probably an essential research problem in 'the sociology of sociology'. On the other hand, we should add at this point that it was the encouragement by general sociologists that confirmed my determination to finish the research project in question.[13]

On the basis of results of my own research and of the studies by other authors the book has tried to answer the following questions: what is the range of the social phenomenon described, who uses the services offered by non-professional practitioners, and to what purpose, what is the non-medical treatment system, and what is its structure? Finally, it asks whether and in what way we can, using sociological tools (theoretical foundations, methods, taxonomy) investigate the problem, which is regarded as important not only for the sociology of health, illness and medicine, but also for general sociology. The sense of belonging to a subdiscipline with which we identify (here sociology of health and illness), and the awareness of still being an 'in-general' sociologist allows us to apply this discussion both to general sociology and medical sociology. Anthony Giddens's remarks, especially his extensive chapter on sociomedical issues, in which the author begins with a comment on complementary and alternative medicine and recognizes this topic as a research area significant for the sociologist, are a good example of the model of description of 'the whole society', without disregarding health- and illness-related issues, taking into account the problems related to studying unconventional methods of treatment, which are mass-practiced in present-day Western societies. (Giddens 2004: 164-191).

The present book consists of the *Introduction*, three complementary parts, *Conclusion*, *Index of Names*, and *Bibliography*. Part One *Non-Medical Healing Systems as A Sociological Phenomenon* contains two chapters. The first, *Non-Medical Healing Systems – An Attempt to Identify and Interpret the Social Phenomenon*, demonstrates that that the fundamental change, which took place within the system of academic medicine during the 150 years of medicine as a science, was the emergence of dissident healing doctrines attempting to present alternatives to the then medical sciences (chiefly homeopathy and mesmerism). Later, other 'heretical views' formed, most often developed outside medicine, or sometimes in its area. The creation of this kind of competition for medicine always had its more or less clear social context. It was brought about by

13 We are talking here about the decisions of the Editorial Board preparing the volume of Sociological Convention Proceedings, which would contain the most important reports delivered during the X National Sociological Convention held in Katowice. My report delivered at the Convention was accepted for publication. Consequently, I talked to the then President of the Polish Sociological Society's Executive Board Professor Antoni Sułek, who showed his kind interest in the results of the studies. As a result, the text on 'the sociology of non-medical treatment systems' appeared in the Convention Proceedings: *Śląsk – Polska – Europa. Zmieniające sie społeczeństwo w perpektywie lokanej i globalnej.* The revised and extended version of the text is contained in Part Three of the present book.

specific causes that changed in individual periods and it had measurable effects on the communal life of the people. Any scientific inquiry should be based on the nomenclature appropriate for a research problem and should define key terms as precisely as possible. For the issues discussed in this study, the central problems are definitions of two crucial and mutually determined concepts: evidence based medicine and non-medical treatment (or healing) systems (the term unconventional medicine is alternatively used). The first term was described in subchapter 1.1.1., the second – in subchapter 1.1.2. We tried to show the principal differences between the two concepts, pointing out their distinct scientific statuses (1.1.2.1), dissimilar legal positions (1.1.2.2) and ethical-deontological differences (1.1.2.3). The internal structure of non-medical healing systems is illustrated by the appended Table.

As I mentioned earlier, one of the major reasons for writing this book was the observation that no comprehensive study on the problems in question has appeared in Polish sociomedical literature since 1990. In my discussion of the problem I was also able to refer to a rather scant number of strictly sociological works; hence the same names and sources have repeatedly appeared in my book. Strangely enough, the paradox of the situation lies, among others, in that according to various representative sociological figures (GUS [Main Statistical Office], OPOB, CBOS) the interest in and use of unconventional medicine have been widely experienced by the Poles since the early 1990s. Certainly, sociologists of health and illness, when conducting studies in the last two decades, touched upon these problems, and in the 1980s Magdalena Sokołowska wrote several important articles on 'alternative medicine'. The presentation, assessment and recapitulation of Polish sociomedical investigations are the subject of the entire subchapter 2.1, one of the three parts of Chapter 2 (*Methods of Treatment Not Accepted by Medicine –State of Research*). The subchapter presents, analyzes and interprets several dozen different sociomedical studies which have been published chiefly in the last twenty years. Although the subject matter of the book is a sociological analysis of unconventional medicine developing in **Poland** [*my emphasis*, W.P.], I concluded that a research project with ambitions to generalize cannot omit a point of reference, which is the analysis of Western literature, mainly in English. The whole subchapter 2.2.. *Complementary and Alternative Medicine (CAM) As Interpreted by American and European Sociology of Health and Illness*[14] is entirely devoted

14 I am trying to prove here that the term complementary and alternative medicine is not the right one. We must recognize, though, that this term is most often used in Western literature. I eventually decided to use this concept; cf. Baer 2010: 373-390.

to this issue. It should be added that, in this part of my work, I also presented the main studies on CAM, which were published by the international socio-medical journal "Social Science and Medicine." Studies on non-medical healing systems point to the multidimensional and multidisciplinary character of the phenomena in question. Work on the methods and techniques of treatment not accepted by medicine is conducted as part of medical anthropology, history of medicine, and by clinical disciplines. The state of this research is presented in the last subchapter (2.3): *Other Research Perspectives (Medical Anthropology, History of Medicine, Clinical Medicine*).

Part II is titled *Polish Folk Medical Systems and Self-Treatment – Continuity and Change*, and discusses two of the three elements that make up the non-medical treatment system. The two systems of help with illness named in the title were the main ways of coping with the trouble of being ill before widely available medicine developed. It seemed that self-treatment and folk medicine, so important in the 'premedical era', would be marginalized or perhaps even eliminated during the triumphs and successes of biomedicine. Such forecasts were wrong, however. The first chapter of Part Two deals chiefly with the methodological problems that the researcher encountered in this field (difficulties in defining terms and concepts, reliability of the sources, and discussions on the irrationality of folk medicine form the content of Chapter One's subchapters). A separate problem pointed out here is the manner of conducting sociological-historical investigations by medical sociologists. The next chapter of Part Two is entirely devoted to the broadly understood social context in which traditional folk medicine and self-treatment functioned from the early twentieth century. In order to show the full picture of the phenomenon, I chose to present the health condition of the rural population from the early twentieth century until today (2.1). Chapter 2.2 presents a description of behaviors in illness in peasant families, with emphasis on the principal role of women as home therapists (2.3), pointing out their activity in self-treatment and in performing the role of folk practitioners (2.3.1 and 2.3.2). Another block of problems (2.4) covers the determinants of behaviors in illness: macrosocial (including political, economic, cultural), meso-social(including attitudes to medical institutions and professions), and, finally, micro-social (dietary patterns, hygienic habits, etc.). Part III is titled *Therapies of Modern Healers. Specificity. Contexts. Interpretations* and consists of three subchapters. The first two are: *Sociological Description of Non-Professional Ways of Meeting Health Needs in A Pluralistic Society* and *Lay Healing Practices – A Theoretical Approach. Symbolic Interactionism, Phenomenology and Ethnomethodology as the Sources of Research Conceptions Used in the Sociology of Non-Medical Healing Systems.* Subchapter 1.1 again returns to the methodological themes already touched upon in various contexts The next subchapters discuss the social factors which prompt and determine the use of healing services offered by non-professional practitioners (1.2), indicating the range of utilization of such practices, and finally, the cultural context of the phenomenon (1.4). The entire subchapter 2 is an attempt to define the theoretical framework enabling effective investigation of our field of inquiry. The goal is to show the perspective from which to investigate views on health and illness with subjective, emotional, and irrational features. The investigation of the area of attitudes, needs and behaviors associated with non-medical treatment appears possible when we are guided by the directives of phenomenology, symbolic interactionism and ethnomethodology. This part, devoted to the elements of sociological theories, which can be helpful in solving the research problem in question, also refers to the classical standpoint of a founder of medical sociology, Eliot Freidson (2.1. The *Analysis of Everyday Knowledge about Health and Illness - Eliot Freidson's Approach*; the next subchapter (2.1.1) discusses one of the main themes explored by this sociologist, the concept of the lay referral system. Subchapter 2.2 presents the results of the author's own pilot studies conducted on the basis of Freidson's conception, and the next (2.3) reconstructs 'treatment theories' that healers themselves tried to create, e.g. S. Nardelli and A. M. Kashpirovsky.

The latter unconventional therapist has been discussed in the last (third) chapter in Part Three of the book, where the results of my own studies on the so-called Kashpirovsky phenomenon are presented. This portion of the book consists of three subchapters, which set the Kashpirovsky phenomenon in the context of the changing society: Subchapter (1) describing the scale of public interest in the method employed by the healer and in himself, subchapter (3.1) discussing in detail the features of the so-called 'Kashpirovsky method' and seeking to answer the question of how it can be classified (3.2). The last, third, subchapter returns to methodological issues running through the present book, showing the author's observations and reflections on sociological inquiries based on the analysis of personal documents [letters] (3.3). In the broader context the subchapter also presents the arguments for the need to start, within medical sociology, investigations based on qualitative techniques, which allow us, I believe, to describe better and in-depth the social context of every person's vitally important spheres of life such as health and illness.

When trying to build the foundations of the sociology of non-medical healing systems I set myself a difficult task; it stemmed *inter alia* from the lack of points of reference - similar sociological studies - which would make my work easier. However, a sufficient inspiration for work can, after all, be the uncontroversial conclusion that we should study important, universal phenomena, the more so if they have not yet been fully investigated.

PART ONE

NON-MEDICAL HEALING SYSTEMS AS A SOCIOLOGICAL PHENOMENON

1. Non-Medical Healing Systems. An Attempt to Identify and Interpret the Social Phenomenon

Health and illness are basic categories that define the course and character of social life. The concepts of health and illness determine behavioral patterns in human communities, influence ways of thinking, hierarchies, values, aspirations and human needs, define hopes and fears as well as life quality and the feeling of social satisfaction (Cockerham 2004:3 et seq.) Health and illness also influence and shape lifestyles in postmodern societies, determine the course of legislation processes and the form of social policies, describe integration and exclusion mechanisms, place an individual in social space, thus being one of the elements dividing human populations into winners (the healthy) and losers (the sick, old, and disabled) (Cockerham 2000: 159-170). Public discourse on health and illness issues also changed the face of consumer movements over the last three decades of the twentieth century, stirred up discussions within contemporary feminism, provoked antiglobalization disputes, set ecological priorities, influenced the definition of human rights, etc. (Gabe et al. 2006: xii et seq.). How then do the concepts of health, illness and medicine influence the form and character of macrosocial processes and the functioning of public institutions, and how do they determine phenomena at the microstructural level revolving around 'ordinary people'? When analyzing and interpreting the social processes occurring over the last three decades, we clearly perceive that the phenomena in question are *per se* a product of specific societies, definite historical time, and of a special cultural context. The result of the weight of phenomena associated with health and illness is the status of a subdiscipline describing this area of social life: the sociology of health and illness. It is regarded as one of the fastest growing branches of general sociology. Additionally, we should emphasize that fore casts on the development directions of postmodern societies indicate that the role of broadly understood health factors for individual citizens, local communities and finally for globalized society will systematically increase. One of the latest editions of a popular handbook on the sociology of health, illness and healing asserts that the vitality of medical sociology can be accounted for not only by the energy and commitment of its founders but also by the fact that '[...] today's health sector constitutes an extraordinarily broad and vibrant arena of the society.' (Weiss, Lonnquist 2006: 2). Health and illness, as biomedical and sociopsychological studies show, constitute a shaky and yet fundamental foundation for the social functioning of individuals, groups, and communities. Health disorders not only bring about dysfunctionality, discomfort, deprivation, feeling of pain, or experience of exclusion at the level of the everyday life of an ordinary person (individual dimension), but are also important for the condition of the whole society (the public dimension of illness) (Parsons 1951; see also Freidson 1970; Giddens 2004: 181). Ever since the scientific revolution caused by the discovery of the actual etiology of most diseases, medicine conceived of as knowledge and the system of institutional activities has dominated and even appropriated the area defined by the concepts: birth – health – illness – being ill – dying – death. For the last hundred years the canon of natural science has determined what science is and what it is not, based on the dominative biomedical paradigm. However, by the mid-twentieth century it had already turned out to be impossible, exclusively on the grounds of the set of propositions that are the foundation of allopathic medicine, to fully understand or explain either the term 'health' or the concept of 'illness'. As a result of long-lasting changes and transformations medical knowledge has been partially enriched by the achievements of behavioral sciences: sociology, psychology, pedagogy, anthropology, political science, etc. (Brown 2000: xiii-xviii). We might also add that the present dominative biomedical model of health and illness tends to be criticized not only by many behavioral scientists but also by the growing category of lay people who usually do not have medical training (or indeed any training at all) but are convinced that nature (Providence, God) has endowed them with supernatural powers to diagnose and cure all diseases, and with the ability to prevent many ailments, and that they have also mastered the art of enhancing health (Nettleton 1966: 209-214).

1. 1. The Sociology of Non-Medical Healing Systems – Taxonomy

1.1.1. Evidence-Based Medicine (EBM)

If we understand the scientific term taxonomy as an attempt to systematize the object of research, and to give it an optimum structure, clarity and coherence (the Greek *taxis* is 'order') (Kopaliński 1968: 743; Bradby 2009: 177-179)[15] then to able to understand the phenomenon of non-medical healing systems it is crucial to distinguish (insofar as it is necessary for lucid argumentation) between that which is science, where we shall refer mainly to the definition of medicine, and that which is not: here the point of reference will be methods of treatment not accepted by medical sciences and not recognized as tested, reli-

15 Cf. also Connecting to Medicine: The Profession and Its Organization in: Pescosolido et al. 2011: 173-201.

able or effective. We approach here the complex interrelations (changing in time and space) between qualitatively different ways of helping in illness, offered on the one hand by evidence-based medicine, and on the other by lay practitioners employing diverse treatment methods and techniques that fail (now or in the past) to meet the criteria of 'being science'. Differences between the two different strategies of helping in illness appear to be best described by the features of contemporary medicine as one of the natural science disciplines (the lack of most characteristics of science being the *differentia specifica* of the non-medical healing systems). Another criterion enabling the distinction between academic medicine and its 'alternative imitation' is the legal status of both systems of treatment. Finally, the last kind of dissimilarity can be seen in reference to deontological standards. We shall therefore look at the three main categories of differences. [16]

Obviously, it is difficult to decide precisely what is and is not science, especially when we are dealing with such complex and interpenetrating areas (particularly by the end of the nineteenth century) which were defined, on the one hand, by academic medicine, and on the other by complementary and alternative medicine (CAM). Handbooks of history of medicine provide many examples of criteria for 'being or not being medicine' that have changed over time (Weiss, Lonnquist, op. cit.: 12-33; Bradby 2009: 177-170; Busby, Williams, Rogers, 1997: 81-83.).

American medical sociologists Lonnquist and Weiss point out that what used to be medicine is no longer within its scope. An array of therapies once tolerated on the fringe of medicine are now regarded as scientific fraud and usurpation. This process of gradual exclusion has recently affected homeopathy, for example. It is generally assumed that the differences between a knowledge of the characteristics of being scientific on the one hand and everyday lay views on health, illness and treatment on the other concern theoretical assumptions, heuristic capacity and values, ontological and epistemological foundations, and the goals of scientific cognition. 'True science' has to have a transcultural and universal character based on repeatable, verifiable standard techniques of data collection; it has to have methods enabling exact assessment of experimentally obtained research results; and it has to use objective criteria for distinguishing between the genuine and the false. The classic conception of science also emphasizes the autonomy, independence and objective character of the cognitive subject (Amsterdamski 1999: 296-301). In the age of Enlightenment, medical sci-

16 I am aware of difficulties and certain inconsistencies and imprecision in the use of terms, e.g. CAM and 'non-medical healing system'. I hope that these problems will be solved at the next stages of my own research.

ences gradually broke free of mystical-magical and thaumaturgical elements, becoming empirical disciplines with time. Beata Tobiasz-Adamczyk writes: 'medicine was initially an "art of healing" based on accidental empirical observations and faith in the supernatural. It was only after the mid-eighteenth century that there was a breakthrough in its history, chiefly as a consequence of the development of natural sciences [...] As it developed, medicine became a knowledge based on scientific foundations, utilizing achievements in other disciplines, at first biology, physics, and chemistry [...] The basis of clinical disciplines emerged in the latter half of the nineteenth century' (Tobiasz-Adamczyk 1999: 395). We should stress that the same author, when discussing the subject matter of medical sociology, observes: 'One of the controversial problems of the present day is that official medicine competes with non-conventional medicine, which often derives from folk medical systems. To explain the phenomenon of non-conventional medicine in the age of rapid development of scientific medicine requires sociological analysis and reference to insufficient satisfaction with practices used in the official health care system.' (Ibid: 308). We should add that the World Health Organization (WHO), when determining the quality of binding medical standards, requests that clinical and epidemiological research into CAM be conducted as soon as possible (Chodhury 82; Ernst 2000, 78 (2)). A characteristic of holistic medicine encompassing the whole body of knowledge of health and illness is that it also draws on the achievements of behavioral sciences (Barczyński, Bogusz 1993: 216). Consequently, as a discipline of science medicine should meet basic, standard quality criteria, which most often include a requirement that it be based on structured and strictly defined methodological norms and patterns. This type of knowledge also needs to have a scientific character in contentual, functional and institutional terms. Medicine thus interpreted is based on universal criteria governing natural sciences as a whole and on its own, and on specific measures of scientificity that stem from the special area of theoretical research and practical activities. Generally accepted criteria of scientificity usually include critical scientific rationalism (grounded on experience and correct reasoning) and the creative and revealing results of scientific cognition. In the context of these criteria, the results should contribute as much innovation as possible to the development of medicine, seek to construct new theories explaining the reality investigated, put forward new hypotheses and systematize previous achievements in sciences of health and illness, follow research procedures in accordance with scientific methods governing natural sciences, use terminology that makes it possible to formulate research results in an exact and unambiguous way, recognize as scientific only sufficiently justified propositions, ensure the internal non-contradiction of a set of propositions relating to the object of research, admit criticism of scientific theses that enable verification of the propositions, and assess and publish the obtained results to submit them for a discussion of their substance, etc. This long list of requirements appears to remind us that adherence to the canon of research procedures increases the chances of achieving results in the form of tested and reliable scientific knowledge characterized by a high degree of truth, objectivity and epistemological certainty as well as by a considerable level of exactitude and intersubjective verifiability, and by a high accuracy of the predicted course of the investigated facts and scientific phenomena (Kraszewski 2003: 381 et seq.). Medicine as a system of knowledge is based on the foundations that have been generally accepted and uniformly applied as permanent standards and procedures governing routine medical management (Youngson 1997). Additionally, the framework of scientific medical management is formed by such standardized and repeatable procedures as universal use of standardized statistical methods and techniques allowing the exact recording of scientific acts, randomized controlled clinical trials, and reference to the placebo effect (an apparent treatment) as a way of enabling one to assess the actual value of the analyzed method of proceeding (Linde and Jonas, 2000: 60 et seq.). The conduct of long-term randomized clinical trials on animals and then with patients, and the use of the 'double-blind trial' rule thus define the basic qualitative criteria that permit us to separate medicine from that which is not medicine, which also includes many highly diversified techniques, methods and treatment attempts to which the healers themselves and some of their patients attribute some degree of effectiveness, although their efficacy cannot be proved based on the generally adopted and accepted scientific criteria.

1.1.2. Non-Medical Healing Systems

The following remarks and comments refer to the Euro-American cultural circle and to Judeo-Christian civilization. When considering the question about the common traits of these types of alternative and complementary healing attempts, we can answer somewhat perversely that what distinguishes them is, on the one hand, their dubious scientific foundations which allegedly legitimate their effectiveness, and the lack of medical qualifications of the overwhelming majority of therapists, and on the other, the widespread use of CAM in Euro-American countries. These methods with their lack of scientific legitimation, and 'alternative therapists' who practice them, do not use, for example, a single taxonomic system to describe their procedures; they do not refer to universally accepted theoretical foundations and do not observe the universally recognized code of ethics, which determines the fundamental standards of management in the treatment process and defines the precise scope of the healer's rights, obligations, and responsibilities for the patient's health (*Wielka Encyklopedia Medycyny* 2003: 204; cf. Thomas 2003: 78-81). Apparently, the only mechanism most often produced by healers, which might explain miraculous recoveries is the placebo effect and the ability in some patients utilizing such methods to spontaneously recover, with some help, as the author's own studies show, derived from the parallel use of evidence-based medicine (Piątkowski 1990: 104). It should be stressed that the results of the author's own studies, referred to in subsequent chapters, on the effects obtained by the non-conventional therapist A. M. Kashpirovsky show that health deteriorations declared by his patients, which are attributed to the use of non-conventional treatment systems, stand at two or three percent (Piątkowski et al. 1993: 49). The use of 'nothing' as a therapeutic means cannot therefore pose real danger to the health of patients utilizing healers' services.

When conducting studies on the sociology of non-medical healing systems under conditions of social transformation, I propose using permanent criteria for the most precise distinction between scientific methods of treatment employed within the academic medical system, and diverse, often mutually contradictory, subjective, emotional views of lay people deeply convinced of their ability to provide fast, effective, painless, long-lasting and risk-free treatment of almost all diseases. Consequently, the above-mentioned description of medicine as knowledge and a system of procedures defines a set of health-oriented activities, which are not medicine but which derive from different socio-cultural traditions and draw upon diverse healing experiences of old medicine, traditional folk medicine practiced by peasants (folk healing methods) and self-treatment methods. As the first part of this text explains, between professional, scientifically substantiated treatment methods and the therapies offered by lay practitioners (non-physicians) there are significant qualitative differences, enabling us to separate medicine from 'non-medicine' (non-medical healing systems). We should bear in mind, nevertheless, that sometimes the dividing line is blurred and difficult to mark since there will always be zones of contention and borderline areas. We should also remember that dynamic changes are occurring at the two levels examined because both medicine and non-medical healing systems are undergoing changes. For example, the emergence of holistic medicine, socio-ecological health models and acceptance by the medical system of many self-treatment methods have brought the two fields closer to each another. In turn, we are witnessing growing criticism of various homeopathic theories and new definitions of medicinal products are being formulated by the European Court of Justice which recently ruled on 15 November 2007 that the fundamental criterion for recognizing a marketed product (in the case in question it was a therapeutic agent used in traditional folk medicine) as medicinal is that it should have the proven function of 'preventing or treating disease' (The Wall Street Journal –Poland, 2007:16) As has been stated earlier, there are three basic qualitative criteria that distinguish non-medical healing systems from academic medicine: **scientific status, authorization by law**, and having (or not having) a consistent **deontological-ethical code** which defines standards of conduct in the treatment process.

Non-Medical Healing Systems – Internal Structure

Character of information related to health and illness	**Types of healing systems**		
	Self-treatment	**Folk medicine**	**Practices of healers**
	1	2	3
Information on causes of disease	Limited scope of information on the causes of typical, most frequent diseases, generalized by patient's own life experience in this area, and by his/her closest friends and relatives as well as by stereotyped knowledge of causes of diseases obtained from official scientific medicine (present and past), from folk medicine and healers' practices.	1. Material causes of disease: a) *internal* etiological factors, 'turned uterus' and the like, b) *external* etiological factors: injuries, worm infestation etc. 2. Mystical-magical and psychological causes of disease: charms, spells, witchcraft, demons, a committed sin, loss of 'vital force', excessive worries (distress), etc.	1. Material causes of disease: errors and iatrogenic causes by MDs, use of medicines inconsistent with homeopathic doctrines, disease as a consequence of disturbing 'magnetic forces of the organism', illness as a result of water vein radiation etc. 2. Mystical-magical and psychological causes of disease: loss of 'divine grace', loss of 'life energy', disease as a result of emotional imbalance, etc.
Information on disease prevention	Widely used and recognized effective preventive procedures and means, first tried on the patient him/herself and his/her close family and friends, stereotyped knowledge of disease prevention obtained form official scientific medicine (present and past), from folk medi-	1. Material preventive measures: disease-protecting diet, house building on 'healthy sites', leeching, etc. 2. Mystical-magical and psychological preventive measures: use of holy relics, amulets, talismans, avoidance of excessive worries, etc.	1. Material preventive means: natural-immunity-enhancing substances prepared according to healer's own prescriptions, use of special relaxation techniques (rebirthing, bio-energy regulation, etc). 2. Mystical-magical and psychological preventive

	cine and healers' practices, e.g. diet regarded as disease prevention, taking vitamin supplements for prevention, reasonable rest etc.		measures: contact with spiritual healer to strengthen the organism's immunological forces, prayers for divine grace, psychophysical relaxation while experiencing 'Universal State of Consciousness', etc.
Information on disease diagnosis	Widely used and recognized effective, simple and easy diagnostic ways, first tried on the patient him/herself and on his/her close family and friends, stereotyped, popular diagnostic knowledge borrowed from official, scientific medicine (past and present), from folk medicine and healers' practices., e.g. examination of feces color or urine color, taking body temperature etc.	1. Material diagnostic ways: examination of feces, and blood color, examination of patient's hand, examination of objects belonging to patient, etc. 2. Mystical-magical and psychological diagnostic ways: diagnosis via revelation, inspiration, clairvoyance, diagnosis based on omens, signs etc.	1. Material diagnostic ways: diagnosis using radiesthetic methods, iridoscopic methods, Kirlian photography, or PROM diagnostic test, etc. 2. Mystical-magical and psychological diagnostic ways: diagnostic occult methods, magical diagnostic methods, diagnosis based on analysis of the superconscious, etc.
Information on disease treatment	Widely used and recognized effective, simple and easy treatment methods and techniques first tried by patient him/self and his close family and friends: methods of treating the most frequent, usually trivial illnesses, borrowed from official medicine (past and present), from folk medicine and healers' practices: kinds of treatment: compress, embrocation, fasting, etc. kinds of therapeutic agents: honey, fruit juices, animal fat, basic, easily available medicines, etc.	I. Material therapeutic means 1) Folk surgery: a) kinds of treatment – trepanation, reduction of fractures and dislocations by means of splints, removal of bladder stones, etc. b) kinds of therapeutic means/tools: pliers, knives, awls, splints, etc. 2) Folk pharmacy: a) kinds of treatment – therapeutic agents administered orally, e.g. tinctures, infusions, herbal mixes; therapeutic agents for external use, e.g. compress, poultices, ointment rubbing, etc. b) kinds of therapeutic	1. Material therapeutic means: a) kinds of treatment: osteopathy, chiropractic, etc. b) kinds of therapeutic means: innate or acquired characteristics of the therapist (healer), natural therapeutic agents – amber, minerals, products with microelements, etc. 2. Mystical-magical and psychological therapeutic means: a) kinds of therapy: hypnosis, suggestion, mesmeric methods, b) kinds of therapeutic means: individual potential of the healer's psychic powers, simple

		agents – plant agents (herbs, flowers, bracket fungus), animal agents (urine, blood, internal organs), human agents (urine, placenta), mineral agents (therapeutic peat, kerosene). II. Mystical-magical and psychological therapeutic means: a) kinds of treatment: casting charms or spells to banish illness, heading off illness, burying illness, etc. b) kinds of therapeutic means/tools: objects (requisites) used during treatment – crosses, pictures with images of saints, blessed candles, holy water, holy chalk.	devices intended, as healers maintain, to enhance and stimulate their healing capacity, etc.

1.1.2.1. Scientific Status

We shall begin by discussing the first distinguishing criterion, which is the scientific status of so-called alternative medicine. Regardless of the heterogeneous character of various treatment methods and techniques employed as part of the three traditions delineated within non-medical healing systems (self-treatment, traditional folk medicine, practices of present-day healers), to which 'alternative' therapists attribute healing powers and efficacy, four permanent structural elements relating to the concepts of health, illness, and treatment process can be distinguished in each of the currents. These are: specific etiological views, lay methods of disease prevention, common-sense diagnostics, and most developed treatment methods recognized as effective. These highly diversified treatment methods and techniques practiced in our culture **are not** [*my emphasis*, W. P.] based on some codified, comparatively consistent system of knowledge of health, illness and treatment processes. We might add that even scientists favorably disposed towards those methods estimate that special benefits to patients are attributed to many CAM systems, which are not confirmed either by conventional medicine or by other CAM approaches. There are few levels that these systems share except for the opinion that they can provide patients with benefits that are not found outside of conventional medicine (Jonas and Levin 2000; and Ibid: 59-75). In the context of differences between academic medicine and non-medical healing systems the expression 'advantages [...] **are attributed** [*my emphasis*, W. P.] to many CAM systems' used in the *Introduction* to this book, which is extremely tolerant towards 'alternative medicine', appears to be highly telling. The first systematic and genuine attempts to verify the actual value of CAM methods were not made until the 1990s. We should add that most of the evaluation tests conducted at the time, , did not produce conclusive and convincing evidence of the effectiveness of various methods used by healers and folk practitioners (Jonas, Levin 2000:2-7; and Pescosolido 2011: 3-20). An additional, characteristic trait of therapies offered by some CAM practitioners is frequent fraud for gain. A separate problem and at the same time a characteristic of these healing systems is the practice of deliberately misleading the patient and unnecessarily prolonging therapy which increases the costs of these methods. Comparatively few scholars have tried to assess as accurately as possible the quality of treatment methods and techniques applied by healers and folk practitioners, but the results are similar. For example, studies by the British authors, J. Trevelyan and B. Booth suggest that there is no hard evidence for the effectiveness of fourteen of the most popular treatment methods in Europe practiced by 'alternative medicine', not counting the placebo effect and results of sometimes spontaneous processes of self-healing. They emphasize that the overwhelming majority of tests conducted by the healers themselves to verify the results of their own investigations lack objective features (Trevelyan and Booth 1998: 237-239). Unconventional therapists use arguments based on their subjective conviction about the value of therapies applied, make patients write letters allegedly documenting the effects of treatment, and use all manner of direct or indirect self-advertising in popular high-circulation media, emphasizing that the effect on the patient is achieved by means of 'cosmic energy', 'spiritual forces', 'astral bodies', and 'different kinds of energy', which is why these methods cannot be assessed by standard criteria used in natural sciences, and it is very difficult to conduct studies on the phenomenon of non-medical healing systems. At the same time, healers insist that, because it is based on the 'false paradigm' of empiricism, scientism and rationalism, academic medicine is itself to blame for its failure to understand and assess 'complementary and alternative therapies'. Dissemination of this way of thinking only increases distrust and skepticism among the many scholars trying to investigate the character and effectiveness of CAM methods without prejudice. The aforementioned classic modes of investigation used in studies enabling assessment of the effects of treatment process - randomization, use of a control group, utilization of the placebo effect, blinding, application of the cross over method, prospective and retrospective methods, as well as employment of standard statistical methods - are applied extremely rarely in the area of complementary and alternative medicine (Ibid: 241-142). It is not possible, as some healers would have it, to exempt a large group of mass-provided health services from the responsibility of being subject to factual (scientific), legal and social supervision. The analyses to date assessing the quality of results of such treatments show that the overwhelming majority of these do not meet most of the criteria for effectiveness and efficiency adopted in the science of health and illness. (*Wielka encyklopedia medycyny*, 2003: 204). The foregoing remarks may lead us to a conclusion that the term 'medicine', often used by healers to name their own treatment methods and techniques, is not justified and legitimate. (Youngson 1997: 267). We might make one more general remark: the sociologist of healing understands that when it is promoted by the power of the popular media and the internet and supported by more and more professionalized marketing methods and public relations techniques increasingly utilized by healers (see the case of businessman, bioenergy therapist and spiritual healer Zbyszek Nowak), complementary and alternative medicine is essentially not interested in the use of objective criteria to assess the effectiveness assessment of its own methods. It appears that recognition by clients, high incomes and a lasting tendency for people to utilize the services of 'other medicine' is enough for most healers.

The legitimacy of this thesis seems to be supported by an examination of the content of the "Uzdrawiacz [Healer]" periodical published by the CAM-promoting community in Poland between 1995 and 2007. In most of the editorial material declarations and announcements that scientific studies will be conducted on the efficacy of the treatments used are never put into practice, while the occasionally published efforts in this field do not meet the criteria of scientific accuracy and correctness. See for example, the criteria for selecting 300 'best and most credible' therapists of all Poland ("Uzdrawiacz" 2006, 3(183): 1). In the February 2006 issue, the regular column *Uzdrowiciele rekomendowani* [Recommended healers] recommends 'phantom surgery' using spiritual healing for bloodless no-touch 'energy operations' employed to eliminate tumor, myomas, and cysts ("Uzdrawiacz" 2006, 2(183): 6). Again, the column *Porady wybitnych terapeutów* [Advice by distinguished therapists] recommends distance healing after prior sending of the 'photo of the patient' ("Uzdrawiacz" 2006, 1 (182): 3). The no. 7 (176) July 2005 "Uzdrawiacz" publishes interpretations by the miraculous healer H. S. of the curing of the pituitary gland tumor, tumor in the lung and cirrhosis, hearing recovery, regaining eyesight, altering of the immune system, etc. The healer tells patients that he underwent specialist examinations in the 'Laboratory of Subtle Energies' in W., which demonstrated *inter alia* that, '[…] if a normal man emits an energy of four to eight watts, a prospective therapist should emanate an energy of minimum 15 watts. An average bioenergy procedure releases a momentary power of 20-40 watts. On the basis of several years of experiments and studies […] he found that the upper limit of power emitted by the bioenergy therapist is the result achieved by H. S. During one of his transmissions the electrocomparator showed 70 watts. Visualization of the aura around the hand was also carried out. During a therapeutic procedure the streaks of light grow considerably longer. The closer the hands are to the person being healed, the more the therapist's aura comes into contact with the patient. In the case of a touch procedure this impact is direct' (Uzdrawiacz 2005, 7 (176): 8-9). These selected examples of 'scientific research' in the field of bioenergy therapy show the patterns of 'procedures in the experiments conducted' with the participation of well-known healers, as well as how the results of such procedures are interpreted and to what conclusions this reasoning leads.

1.1.2.2. Legal Status

Another qualitative difference that distinguishes medicine from its 'bioenergy-therapy imitations' is the legal regulations defining the status of both modalities of treatment in the territory of Poland. Adopting a chronological order, which best shows the dynamics of changes, we should refer to the first documents, legal acts and administrative decisions concerning healing practices provided by non-physicians (lay practitioners) by the 1970s/early 1980s, when the popularity of 'alternative treatment methods' started to grow rapidly. On 29 March 1983, the Health and Social Welfare Minister's Scientific Council issued a communiqué on 'the ways of therapeutic management formerly outside the activities of medicine as a science of human health and illness, to which significance in diagnosis and treating illnesses is attributed' (*Komunikat…*, 29 March 1983:1). The document stated that the effectiveness of each method of treatment had to be verified according to the principles of scientific reasoning in an authorized research center prior to its introduction into practice. It emphasized that there could be no exceptions to this rule. At the same time the Scientific Council declared that research would commence on non-conventional methods of treatment, including bioenergy therapy. The communiqué also warned against 'the effects dangerous to health and life that may ensue as a consequence of replacing scientifically verified medical procedures by other methods, to which popular opinion attributes significance in diagnosing and treating illnesses' (Ibid1). The document clearly stressed the lack of proven scientific value of healing methods and warned against possible adverse effects of their utilization. One more formal opinion on the status of 'other medicine' was the then Public Prosecutor General's letter on 'healing methods falling outside the scope of conventional medicine' defined as 'illegal treatment practices'. Violation of the law consisted in healers failing to comply with Article 26 of the 28 October 1950 Act on the Profession of Physician: consequently, 'the public prosecutor has the duty to start preparatory proceedings regarding this offense if s/he has obtained information indicating reasonable suspicion of its commission' (*Leczyć mogą tylko…* 31 March 1985). The Public Prosecutor General stressed that public and state institutions which became aware of the commission of a criminal offense prosecuted *ex officio* were obligated to immediately notify the competent public prosecutor about 'illegal practice of the profession of physician' (Ibid: 8). In reference to the growing popularity of the contemporary healers it was also restated that the operation of companies offering healing services was a contravention of the provisions regulating the practice of the physician's profession, while the right to provide medical services could be granted only to 'a Polish citizen upon completion of medical studies in a Polish medical university' or 'in another country […] if this education is recognized in Poland as equivalent' (Ibid) The letter also emphasized that under Polish law the physician was not allowed to sell medicines. When commenting upon the documents issued by the Ministry of Health and by the Public Prosecutor General, a proponent of studies on alternative medicine, Professor Julian Aleksandrowicz wrote: 'If an African shaman came to me - the doctor - and experimentally proved, which I believed impossible, that he was able to stop the progression of a leukemic disease by means of spells and incantations, I would not hesitate to employ him in my clinic, heedless of the fact that it might substantially undermine my scientific reputation' (*Poszukać prawdy o…*, 1989, 2). We might add that Professor Aleksandrowicz , although keenly interested in non-medical healing systems, personally never encountered convincing evidence of the efficacy of such methods (Piątkowski, "Kamena" 1987). The systemic transformation in Poland brought changes in the law and new legislative solutions concerning the status of therapeutic methods not accepted by scientific medicine. More and more often opinions were published by representatives of the newly established medical self-government and of Regional Medical Chambers. Doctors saw the origin of expansion of non-conventional medicine in the liberal provisions of business law which permitted *inter alia* registration of the practice of non-conventional treatment without the required qualifications as a business activity in crafts. Dr Graba, Vice-President of the Regional Medical Chamber in Gdansk, emphasized at that time that '[…] any applicant can start a business activity, for example in health care' (Klemens 1993, 19: 7). Representatives of the medical community stressed that many healers 'after completing three-day courses in Kiev provided healing services in contravention of the binding Act on the Profession of Physician'. The medical community was indignant at the fact that the commercial media promoted the fashion for 'alternative methods of treatment', often accepting advertisements and commercials for 'painless and fast treatment of all diseases'. It was demanded that Regional Medical Chambers verify the value of every registered healing activity. Official spokespersons for the Medical Chambers spoke of the 'legal impotence' and widespread practices of public prosecutors who, as a rule, decided to discontinue inquiries 'on account of lack of features of a criminal offence' (Ibid: 7). In their statements, the Chambers pointed out that healers used a special kind of marketing technique by ordering enthusiastic articles on 'miraculous health restorations' in the yellow press (Popielski 1993, 3: 6). These practices violated not only the Act on the Profession of Physician but also the 1991 Code of Medical Ethics. When commenting upon this situation, B. Popielski pointed out that, even if it did not have adverse effects on health, treatment by means of methods not accepted by medicine was in contravention of the Misdemeanor Code. In his analysis of the systems of paramedical services in Poland he insisted that the rise of interest in these types of pseudotreatment systems was '[...] a surprising sociological phenomenon' (Ibid: 7). The opinions of doctors and lawyers in the early 1990s stressed that the only formally accepted non-conventional method in Poland was acupuncture. However, it had to be practiced by trained and certified MDs. During the period in question, the Minister of Health's Scientific Council stated, however, that the character of the method 'is still not fully explained'. Representatives of Medical Chambers dealing with the formal aspects of the functioning of 'other medicine' also signaled delays in starting proper oncological treatment among patients utilizing healing therapies without any effect and who often postponed visits to health care service centers (Ibid: 40). In this context we might well refer to the 'case of Julek Czarodziej [Julius the Wizard]' who for many years placed adverts in the popular press, proclaiming that he 'eliminates hunchbacks, scoliosis [...] limb paresis, and restores innervation [...]' ("Gazeta Kielecka" 10 February 1993). In his adverts the healer promised fast, non-operative, painless and inexpensive treatment. His healing practices triggered a response from the Medical Chambers of the Świętokrzyskie and Lublin provinces, resulting in his indictment brought by the District Prosecutor in Przysucha. During the trial the defendant argued his case by emphasizing that he had never prescribed any medication or injured the 'bodily tissues', treating his patients exclusively with his own mental powers (Krasnowska 1994). The case of Julek Czarodziej ultimately ended up before the Supreme Court because after acquittal judgments in the lower courts the subsidiary attorney for the Regional Medical Chamber in

Lublin petitioned for annulment of the judgment acquitting the healer. The lawyers representing the Chamber argued that 'the healer in fact provided services reserved for the medical profession' (Wąsik 1997). They also pointed out that first- and second-instance courts made errors in the establishment of facts and violated procedural law provisions by ignoring evidence detrimental to the healer. A dissenting opinion on the groundlessness of the annulment petition was submitted by the Public Prosecutor in Radom, emphasizing that the 'non-conventional therapist' did not pose as a doctor and informed his patients of the need to contact medical practitioners. The activities of these kinds of healers have evoked increasingly intense emotions in the medical community since the mid-1990s, and culminated *inter alia* in a parliamentary question asked by Zbigniew Kułak in Poland's Senate. The senator indicated the powerlessness of Medical Chambers in combating 'alternative medicine' and stressed that public prosecutors routinely discontinued proceedings in such cases 'on the grounds of low degree of harm'. The interpellant demanded that the Minister of Justice and the National Public Prosecutor take firm action in order to eliminate completely worthless methods of pseudotreatment. ("Gazeta Lekarska" 1994, 5: 7). Another element that contributed to the legal status of 'alternative methods of treatment' was the opinion by the Supreme Administrative Court on the practices offered by immigrants who came in large numbers from the former Soviet Union countries. The problem was that such therapists used all manner of diplomas and certificates issued by the Russian Federation or Ukrainian authorities while these documents were not recognized in Poland. Competent employment agencies refused applicants permission to start healing activities of this type. The situation was especially dramatic in the provinces where unemployment among medical university graduates was signaled in the mid-1990s. When justifying their decisions at that time, the administrative authorities emphasized that refusals to employ healers from the East were chiefly motivated by protection of Poland's labor market against the occupational activities of foreign citizens because the law imposed on state institutions the duty to take into account the current employment situation. An additional formal circumstance was that the person providing health and illness services had to have his/her diploma certified by Poland's Minister of Health and have it recognized as equivalent to completed medical training in Poland ("Gazeta o Pracy", 3 March 1995: 1). It should be recalled that in the mid-1990s, before the new law on the medical profession was enacted, the binding legal status was regulated by the abovementioned Act of 28 October 1950 (Dziennik Ustaw [Journal of Laws] no. 50, item 458), which provided for the penalty of jail up to six months and/or a fine for illegal practice of the medical profession ("Gazeta Lekarska" 1994, 9: 11). This Act explicitly stipulated that a form of illegal practice could also be both treatment and diagnosis or prevention of illness. At the same time the 1994 Code of Medical Ethics stated that '[…] the physician **cannot** [*all emphases are mine*, W. P.] use methods regarded by science as **harmful or worthless**. Nor **should he cooperate** with persons treating illnesses without certified qualifications' (Ibid: 11). The then legal opinions pointed out that there were legal grounds to prosecute persons treating illnesses without appropriate qualifications; in practice, however, these persons most often went unpunished despite advertising their activities in daily newspapers, magazines, and commercial TV programs (and then on the Internet). Sometimes it was reported that the inefficiency of the prosecuting agencies was the result of public pressure: the public demanded that 'other medicine' be tolerated. Furthermore, the Ministry of Health lawyers found that in light of the current law healers who perform such procedures as 'iridoscopy, touch treatment, manipulations on the spine, palpation of the patient, and recommendations concerning therapeutic management satisfy the conditions of Article 1 of the Profession of Physician Act and are thereby liable to prosecution under Article 26 of the said Act' (Ibid.). The next stage of legal actions against non-physicians providing health services was the legislative initiative by the Republic of Poland Senate's Committee for Health and Social Policy concerning the supervision of the occupational activities of persons offering health services **without an MD diploma** [*my emphasis*, W. P.]. The main reason for the initiative was the awareness of a legal loophole making it possible for medical advice and health- and illness-related procedures to be offered by persons who lacked the right to practice the profession of physician but who were operating only on the basis of an entry in the records of business activities. The intent of the initiative was to restrict non-conventional healing practices often provided by incompetent persons who committed errors and gave incorrect therapeutic recommendations. ("Gazeta Prawna" 25 January 1995). The legislators thereby sought to eliminate poor-quality practices and to strictly supervise paramedical professions. Fundamental changes in the legal status of folk doctors and healers appeared with the new 5 December 1996 Act on the Profession of Physician. In Chapter 2, Article 5 it explicitly defines a number of criteria for the award of the right to practice the profession of physician (stomatologist). These include *inter alia*: Polish citizenship, possession of a medical diploma obtained in Poland or another country but recognized in the Republic of Poland as equivalent pursuant to separate regulations; completion of a postgraduate internship, earning a final State qualification closing the postgraduate internship; and demonstration of impeccable ethical conduct ("Gazeta Lekarska" 1997, 3: 1). At the same time Article 58 (Chapter 6) reads, '[…] whoever, without due certified qualifications, provides health services consisting in diagnosing and treating illness is liable to the penalty of a fine (paragraph 1) […] if the perpetrator of the act defined in paragraph 1 acts in order to obtain financial gains or intentionally misrepresents possession of such qualifications, is liable to the penalty of imprisonment up to one year [..] or a fine' (Ibid: 4). For their part the community of healers, responding to legal actions by doctors, asserted that, by the decision of the District Court in Katowice on 26 September 1996, legal personality was given to the National Guild of Bioenergy Therapists and Radiesthetic Practitioners, which was entered in the guilds registry by the Court's Commercial Division. The healers' guild also planned to join the central, national crafts organization – the Polish Craft Association. Healers' organizations claimed that that decision provided an opportunity to dissociate themselves from, '[…] charlatans and swindlers of all descriptions, from those who disregarded principles and values in pursuit of fame and money' ("Uzdrawiacz" 1966, 11(90)). Bioenergy therapists also declared they would observe the 'never instead of a doctor' rule. They also announced that by decree of the Minister of Labor and Social Policy dated 20 April 1995, radiesthetic and bioenergy-therapy services were included in the list of occupations. (Dziennik Ustaw 1995). The editors of the healing business periodical "Uzdrawiacz [Healer]" representing the interests of 'other medicine' believe that bioenergy therapy and radiesthesia have become service professions classified as crafts. It was also restated that, prior to registration the healers' corporation submitted to the court the principles of training bioenergy therapists as 'non-medical specialists' and the manner of verifying their skills as well as the rules of apprentice's and master craftsman's examinations. The healers' community believes that a physician differs from a healer in that the former uses 'material instruments of impacting on the patient while the latter operates with energy instruments' (*sic*!). The healer operates without encroaching in any way on the sphere reserved for the physician, especially the domain of diagnosis in the medical sense or inadmissible prescription of medications. The declared objective of healers was to make it easier for clients to choose, and to serve 'their interest through harmony of their energy structures.' Another procedural element which regulated the status of non-medical healing systems was the Charter of Patients' Rights. During a discussion on detailed provisions in this document Tadeusz Brzeziński, a medical historian, held the view that the provision stipulating that, 'the patient has the right to be treated by physicians and healers practicing branches of medicine other than those taught at medical universities' gives the patient the right to utilize services offered by lay healers on the hospital premises, in which case the costs of treatment would have to be covered by the public health service. T. Brzeziński strongly criticized such solutions, maintaining that these were incompatible with 'both the law in force and the provisions of the Code of Medical Ethics, which prohibited cooperation of doctors with all manner of healers' (T. Brzeziński 1996: 11).

Another legal fact pertaining to non-medical healing systems and emphasizing qualitative differences between scientific knowledge about health/illness, and lay views was the Supreme Court judgment of 4 February 1998, which deprived H. Słodkowski, an actively practicing bioenergy therapist, of the right to practice the profession of physician. In adjudicating the case, the Supreme Court invoked the content of the abovementioned Act on the Profession of Physician and the binding Code of Medical Ethics. The judges found biotherapy (bioenergy therapy) a harmful and worthless method. Endeavors to finally determine the legal status of treatment methods and techniques regarded by the law in force as harmful and worthless were made at the same time in Poland's Senate. The immediate reason was the parliamentary question addressed to the then Minister of Health and Social Welfare, Wojciech Maksymowicz. The issue of regulating this problem by law had been discussed earlier in the Senate Committee for Health and Social Policy in consultation with the Supreme Medical Council. The new initiative by Senator Z. Kułak concerned the 'restriction of the scope of and freedom in providing health services by non-physicians' (Diariusz Senatu Rzczypospolitej Polskiej 1998). This initiative was backed up in the voting (58 votes 'for' and three 'against'). The grounds for the motion emphasized the growing phenomenon of advertising and self-advertising of non-conventional methods of treatment, which was observable in the daily and weekly press, and in the electronic media, both public and private. The motion reads *inter alia*, '[…] all these methods do not serve the patient, these are exclusively profit-seeking activities' (Ibid: 1).The motioning Senator also pointed out the legal and administrative loopholes that permitted treatment of patients by persons without qualifications on the pretext of business activity. The interpellant proposed that the problem be solved by '[…] licensing, under the supervision of physicians or the Ministry of Health, of business activity in the field of health services provision' (Ibid: 1). Senator Kułak emphasized that this might be a means of minimizing the risk to patients posed by non-conventional therapeutic methods. Further contributions to the reconstruction of stages of the battle fought by the medical community seeking to uphold respect for the Act on the Profession of Physician could be found in the opinions of lawyers representing Regional Medical Chambers as well as decisions of the statutory authorities of the medical self-government. Such moves were most often inspired by the grassroots pressure from the medical community, condemning the conduct of those medical university graduates who, by practicing and '[…] advertising pseudomedical practices debased the dignity of the medical profession.' (Kamiński, 2000, 5: 2). For example, the President of the Regional Medical Chamber in Lublin S. Kamiński, pointed out that promotion of healing practices was an obvious infringement of the rules of professional responsibility because the use of such methods of treatment violates the rules of the Code of Medical Ethics, especially Articles 57, 63 and 65, and contravenes Article 56, Act on the Profession of Physician, and Article 18b, Health Care Institutions Act: consequently, it is in obvious contravention of the legal order in force in the territory of Poland. The practicing by doctors of methods not accepted by present-day medicine also conflicts with regulations passed by medical self-governments (The Supreme Medical Council resolution No. 18/98/111). In view of the expansion of non-medical healing systems and the growing dishonest (as many doctors believe) competition on the part of 'botchers', determined actions were taken by the Supreme Medical Council, the main objective being 'legal protection of the title of physician'. In 2000 the Council submitted a motion to the Justice Minister that persons practicing alternative medicine be prohibited from using the terms 'doctor', **'medicine'** [*my emphasis*, W. P.], and clinic (*Pytanie o uzdrowicieli*, 2000). Giving the reasons for his motion the Council's President K. Madej stressed that in Poland there was no actual protection for the physician's profession because this title was unlawfully used by healers. In advertising leaflets and brochures they often use typical medical terms such as 'outpatient clinic', 'hospital', 'therapy'; moreover, they describe their activity unlawfully as 'non-conventional medicine'. The Supreme Medical Council President requested an answer to the question whether 'medical shamans' would be allowed to register with the National Court Register and on what principles. K. Madej also added that the main motive for his action was clinical reports about more and more cancer patients who were utilizing 'alternative medicine' services instead of immediately taking up treatment in authorized national health care facilities; this delay in starting conventional treatment was also resulting in more frequent mortality. After 2000, the Supreme Medical Council also took parallel action in the Ministry of Foreign Affairs in order to restrict the application of the so-called 1972 Prague Convention, which granted equal status to the medical university diplomas issued in the COMECON countries. If the law passed under entirely different political circumstances were changed, the foreigner holding an MD diploma obtained outside Poland would not automatically have the right to practice medicine because in such cases the final decision would be made by a competent Regional Medical Chamber only when a person seeking employment in Poland fulfilled all the strictly defined criteria (Guttman 2000). In their letter to the Health and Justice Minister dated 5 November, 2000 the medical self-government also requested that appropriate rules of registration or refusal to register be laid down for economic entities offering health services '[…] that involve paranormal phenomena and magical procedures' (*Dokument* 2000). In a special letter the Supreme Medical Council President emphasized that he hoped that '[…] Health and Justice Ministers would take firm actions protecting the social interest, which is the qualified treatment of patients, and also safeguarding the authority of medicine and health care as well as the authority of the law' (Ibid.). The central authorities of the medical self-government also encouraged local Regional Medical Chambers to request competent District Public Prosecutors to prosecute healers providing illegal medical services; however, it turned out that the prosecutors hardly ever instituted legal proceedings, most often discontinuing prosecution on the grounds of 'low degree of damage to society' caused by healers' activities (*List prezesa* 2000). For the author of the present study it is obvious that the medical community did not always seek (as they asserted they did) to protect the patients' interests and their rights to effective treatment or to eliminate non-scientific methods. A significant element of 'activities against healers' was the physicians' battle to preserve domination, or better still, exclusive control of the health services market, and thereby their wish to maximize profits. This phenomenon has been dealt with in another book (Piątkowski 1990, 5-11). It appears that the next step on the way to defining procedural differences between medicine and methods of treatment provided most often by lay practitioners but not accepted in modern medical science was the establishment by the Health Minister of a special Council for Non-Conventional Methods of Treatment. This body was eventually composed of eleven members and had the task, under paragraph 3 of its Rules, of '[...] laying down the relevant guidelines of how to regulate in legal provisions the issues of non-conventional methods of treatment, taking into special consideration the criteria for activity in this area, rules of granting permits for such practices, cooperation of such therapists with doctors, and the starting of scientific research on non-conventional treatments and the use of its results' (*Zarządzenie Ministra Zdrowia*, 2002). For the first time in Poland a Ministry of Health agency took a stance on the assessment of non-conventional treatment methods. The document pointed out that tens of thousands of people were currently involved in this activity, while permits to practice such treatments were obtained under the 1988 law on business activities. The Council stressed that under the binding procedure for issuing licenses no institution checked any qualifications whatsoever of practitioners of methods that are outside the realm of academic medicine, nor is the quality of such therapeutic services verified in any way. In a special statement the Council also said that many [alternative] therapists 'prey on other people's misfortunes', being motivated solely by financial gains. Under such circumstances it recommended regulations and solutions by law, the more so that the existing legal state (penal sanctions for provision of health services without certified qualifications) was no genuine obstacle to the practice of the methods in question. (*Stanowisko Rady* www.gazeta.ani.wroc.pl). It was emphasized that such practices could be performed **exclusively** [*my emphasis*, W. P.] under the supervision of doctors.

Moreover, the Council stated that on account of its interdisciplinary nature the problem required studies and expert opinions also in **sociology** [*my emphasis*, W. P.]. It pointed out that the task of this Ministry-appointed body was to initiate, advise and express opinions on activities concerning non-conventional treatments (including biotherapy, aromatherapy, chromotherapy, homeopathy, etc). The document underlines the fact that the methods in question **do not fall** [*my emphasis* W .P.] in the scope of conventional medicine and that is why they have to be verified by scientific methods. The Council members also indicated that it was impossible to eliminate non-conventional treatments in Poland by legal sanctions; at the same time the experts expressed the view that the main problem was to determine whether it was possible to develop any methods of cooperation between academic medicine and the healing systems falling outside its realm. What they regarded as a significant objective was to **eliminate** the term **medicine** [*my emphasis*, W. P.] from the names of various disciplines, which healers describe as effective (Ibid: 2). It should be observed that in general, despite many efforts by medical self-governments to oppose violation of the 1966 Act on the Profession of Physician, a characteristic of the actions taken in specific cases by local Public Prosecutor's Offices and police was an almost entire lack of effectiveness in combating medical services offered by persons without appropriate certified qualifications. Most often, after starting and conducting an inquiry at the behest of the local Medical Chamber the police 'did not find any features of a prohibited act'[17]. Healers from the former Soviet Union countries usually tried to excuse themselves by saying they had valid temporary residence cards for Poland and practiced 'biotherapy and manual medicine', having registered their activity in competent offices[18]. After an examination of selected cases of ineffective enforcement of the law by prosecuting supervisory agencies it should be said that the legal element enabling the definition and codification of the formal status of treatment methods and techniques not accepted by and outside the scope of academic medicine but offered by persons without required formal qualifications is also the current medical law in Poland (Nestorowicz 2004). Describing the 'abandoned' or 'unreliable' methods, M. Ne-

17 See for example the District Public Prosecutor's decision dated 2 September 2003 to discontinue an inquiry (the document is stored in the author's files).

18 See also other decisions to discontinue an inquiry by the District Public Prosecutor in Lublin of 18 November 2002 concerning illegal medical practice. A similar decision was taken by the Lublin-Północ Public Prosecutor's office in the case against a healer from the East on the motion of the Regional Medical Chamber concerning 'provision of health services without qualifications', the enquiry was discontinued 'on the grounds of a lack of data sufficiently substantiating the commission of an offense'. See the decision dated 30 June, 2003.

storowicz writes that procedures performed by the physician have to conform to '[…] the state of medical knowledge and have to be carried out according to the rules generally adopted in science and in medical practice' (Ibid: 148). In the meaning of the law 'procedures unable to achieve a therapeutic goal are not therapeutic procedures'. This rule is consistent with the 1 December 1998 judgment of the Supreme Court (III CKN 741/98, 3 SN 6/1999, item 112). Therefore, in light of the binding law in Poland, the doctor cannot use methods 'condemned and abandoned' (Ibid: 149). The doctor should employ only 'generally recognized methods' and '[…] cannot [..] use methods regarded by science as harmful or worthless. Nor should he cooperate with persons offering treatment without certified qualifications' (Ibid 150). At the same time Nestorowicz emphasized that 'it is risky for the patient to use a placebo except in cases of a lawfully admissible medical experiment. A placebo can cause the patient's negligence in starting treatment, the consequence of which may be deterioration of health or death. A placebo cannot **replace** [*my emphasis*, W. P.] treatment' (Ibid 150).

We have examined here selected regulations and official documents legally binding in Poland, issued by the Ministry of Health and the Supreme Medical Chamber and by Regional Medical Chambers. The subject of interest also extended the provisions of the Polish medical law in force and related comments. The purpose of this discussion was to show one more area where we can observe qualitative differences between medicine and non-medicine.

In conclusion, we can say that:

1) Various methods and techniques of treatment, the value of which has not been scientifically confirmed by standard evaluation methods accepted in medical sciences and which are most often practiced by persons without the required formal qualifications, are regarded as unlawful in light of the binding law.
2) The previous measures taken by the Ministry of Health in order to enforce the binding legal order in the territory of Poland have so far been ineffective.
3) Actions taken by individual Public Prosecutor's Offices, usually on the motion of Regional Medical Councils, almost always ended in discontinuance of legal proceedings because of a lack of features constituting an offense.
4) Opinions of clinical doctors, especially oncologists, indicating that in light of the conducted research and case-studies there is an actual danger of delaying cancer treatment because of long-lasting utilization of 'pseudomedical services', did not become the topic of public debate or did not contribute to eliminating cases of law violations by healers.

5) Quick legal solutions are needed both for verification of all 'certificates', 'diplomas', or 'qualifications', which healers exchange among themselves or buy in foreign countries to legitimate their practices, and for inspection of mass advertising of unlawful treatment methods and techniques prohibited by Polish law on the Internet, in the electronic media, and in the press.
6) It is also necessary to check whether the registration procedure of the guild of bioenergy therapists and radiesthetic experts in the National Chamber of Crafts (1996) was performed in compliance with the law, e.g. whether this procedure took into account the stance of the Ministry of Health.

1.1.2.3 Ethical Aspects

The third qualitative criterion which distinguishes between evidence-based medicine and methods whose effectiveness has not been proven using standard evaluation criteria applied in medical sciences and which are most often employed by lay people without appropriate qualifications (CAM) is ethical aspects. In this context an obvious question is in order to what extent these ethical and deontological standards in biomedicine are respected and observed in medical practice. Modern-day sociological studies show that these are violated as social assessments indicate. We should begin by stressing that these issues are diametrically differently assessed by the medical and healing communities. As has been observed earlier, from the mid-1990s onwards, professional medical corporations repeatedly voiced their stance on the widespread provision of 'paramedical services' by lay practitioners who lacked appropriate qualifications. The abovementioned medical historian, Professor T. Brzeziński had already pointed out, in 1996, the danger arising from the new Charter of Patients' Rights, which guaranteed that the patient could be treated by means of methods neither recognized by medicine nor taught at medical universities (Brzeziński 1996: 11). In his article T. Brzeziński indicated that the patient's right to be treated had to be a genuine one and **must not be in conflict** [*my emphasis*, W. P.]with other rights (Ibid.). In particular, this was about the free choice of a therapist and at the same time the patient's utilization of consultations and therapies offered by healers in out-patient and in-patient health care centers. The historian maintained that the situation was in contradiction of both the provisions of the Medical Ethics Code, which prohibited a doctor from cooperating with a healer, and the Act on the Profession of Physician. Brzeziński referred to Article 57 of the Medical Ethics Code, which stipulates that the physician '[...] cannot use methods regarded by science as harmful or worthless. Nor should he cooperate with persons treating illness without certified qualifications' (*Kodeks*

Etyki Lekarskiej 1994:18). We might add that the last (2004) edition of the Medical Ethics Code stipulates in Chapter IV that the rules of conduct in medical practice are contained in Article 56-68, while the wording of Article 57 remains unchanged as compared with the 1994 version (Medical Ethics Code 2004: 18). Regional Medical Chambers also repeatedly voiced their opinions on unlawful 'paramedical practices', presenting frequent cases of law violations by healers. In this context the Chamber spokespersons also spoke of infringement by non-conventional therapists of deontological and ethical norms and imperatives which should apply to all persons offering and practicing treatment. For example, one of the Regional Medical Chambers received a petition to consent to provision of rehabilitation of children with cerebral palsy using '[…] stimulation of the central nervous system (CNS), Bernard's currents, and galvanic currents' (*Działanošć paramedyczna…*, 2001: 21). In answer to the request, the president of the Regional Medical Chamber stated that no doctor could give an opinion on this method, and even less cooperate with persons engaged in paramedical activity because it was in contravention of the Medical Ethics Code (Chapter IV, Art 570 (Ibid 21). The Regional Medical Chamber also based its stance on a special clinical expert opinion, which read *inter alia* that, '[…] The methods of CNS electrostimulation as methods of treating children with infantile paralysis […] are not listed in any of the present-day handbooks of child neurology. The clinical syndrome in question, on account of its incurability, has long been the area of activities by the authors of "miraculous" healing methods. The professionals who have taken care of these children for years know about it very well' (Ibid.). According to the report commissioned by the "Wprost" weekly, one out of four medical practitioners in Poland violates the 5 December, 1996 Act on the Profession of Physician and the Code of Medical Ethics by working with healers or opening so-called natural medicine offices (Konarska 2006: 76 et seq.). The Silesian Medical Chamber estimates that 'some money-minded doctors deliberately use the authority of their medical university diploma to legitimate harmful non-conventional methods' and try to encourage patients to use them in the treatment process. In the area under the authority of the Gdansk Medical Chamber, some doctors are involved in publishing a periodical for the patients "Vilcacora – Żyj Długo [Live Longer]", which presents information about the alleged curing of advanced tumor using this Indian therapy. I. Konarska's report shows that medical university graduates, motivated chiefly by profit, even open whole complexes of 'alternative medical services' and 'non-conventional medicine centers', for example the so-called Health Institute in Gliwice. At the same time the "Wprost" report authors point out that in the last two years there has been a declining interest in 'alternative methods of treatment' in many EU countries, *inter alia* as a result of figures presented in the

British Medical Association's Report, which warns against more and more frequent frauds, spiritual healers and after a series of media-publicized lawsuits by patients in Germany against the local non-academic medical community [*Ausserschulische Medizin*]. In Poland, some parts of the medical community appear to have a lax and permissive attitude towards the current rules of ethics. Interviews with doctors who break the regulations in this field show a picture of typical excuses: persons summoned to the competent Medical Chambers justify their conduct by 'difficult financial situation and the need to seek additional income'; there are also arguments that healing methods are less harmful when practiced by 'graduates of medical universities'. The problem is not marginal, though, because many year-long studies (since 1983) carried out by the oncologist Professor M. Pawlicki show that over five thousand patients 'unnecessarily' die of cancer every year in Poland, mainly as a result of delayed contact with conventional medicine, especially oncological health care, due to persistent use of healing services. The Krakow Medical Chamber believes that from the ethical and legal standpoint, the participation of doctors in 'medical fraud' is a 'hideous practice' (Ibid: 80). I. Konarska also points out that the widespread application by doctors of methods, which are increasingly questioned, and the effectiveness of which remains unproven, may cause not only a further decline of ethical standards but also growing skepticism among patients about medical institutions and professions. As a side note to this discussion, we should observe that the aforementioned comprehensive studies on CAM conducted by W. B. Jonas and J. S. Levin repeatedly stressed the significance of ethical aspects in light of the current US standards. That discussion applied to specifically American realities but we might well emphasize that in the chapter devoted to ethics H. Brody and J. M. Rygwelski write that in each procedure, whether medical or healer-administered, one expects results such as an improvement in the patient's health and the avoidance of harm (H. Brody et al. 2000: 48). The main thesis of these authors is the belief that medical ethics apply **equally** [*my emphasis*, W. P.] to both non-conventional and conventional medicine. Brody, Rygwelski and Fetters name four main universal ethical principles, which, they believe, apply both to evidence-based medicine (EBM) and CAM: the principles of autonomy, beneficence (do the best good), nonmaleficence (do no harm), and justice (Ibid: 51). In their interpretation they also assume that the most important decisive criterion of harm or benefit in the process of treatment is the patient's autonomous assessment, and only then the doctor's. In this context we might refer to the bioethical dispute which recently divided the US medical community. A cancer-suffering teenage boy from Virginia decided to choose treatment methods by himself, preferring the non-conventional ones ('herbal tonic') instead of standard chemotherapy, his parents having backed up his decisions. In that situation, there was a growing ethical and legal dispute about the limits of patient autonomy. The local Federal Court ruled that Abraham Cherrix had no right to refuse chemotherapy, which, the patient's attending doctors insisted, was the only way to stop the disease. The boy had been diagnosed with Hodgkin's lymphoma. The cancer attacked the lymph nodes and lymphatic tissue; in hospital he underwent intensive treatment with cytostatic drugs. Due to strong side effects the patient was convinced several times that he was dying. After several months of remission the symptoms intensified again and then the patient refused to consent to a resumption of chemotherapy. The boy said, '[...] chemotherapy has almost killed me, I am not going to return to it' (Gillert 2006: 6). With his parents' complete approval, the patient tried non-conventional medicine, using the Hoxsey method offered by an 'alternative clinic' registered in Mexico. The therapy consists in following a diet and in regularly drinking 'special herbal mixtures', this manner of treatment was borrowed from American traditional folk medicine, and was used in the early twentieth century by farmer Harry Hoxsey to treat domestic animals suffering from neoplastic diseases. It should be added that, in the early 1960s, Hoxsey fell ill with prostatic adenoma and treated himself with his own method, which proved entirely ineffective. By the judgment of the local court his clinic was closed down although it then moved to Mexico. Despite the known fact of the ineffectiveness of 'Hoxsey mixture' in treating cancers, supporters of the method claim that it is 80 percent successful when properly used. In a special statement the American Cancer Society says that systematic research on this 'miracle drug' has never yielded positive results. The oncological report emphasizes at the same time that conventional chemotherapy has good results in the treatment of Hodgkin's lymphoma. The patient's and his parents' decision was challenged by the attending doctors in the local court in Virginia, which ruled that decisions concerning treatment would henceforward be taken by a specially appointed guardian. As a result of these decisions sixteen-year old A. Cherrix was formally forced to resume therapy in the local cancer hospital. The boy's attorneys presented the situation as an extreme case of legal institutions and medicine violating the liberty and rights of the patient and his family to freely decide about their lives and health, including the free choice of methods of treatment, even those not proven effective by academic medicine but trusted by patients. This case once again turned the debate into a dispute about whether we can decide on the value of a treatment method on the basis of its being formally part of academic or alternative medicine. Jonas and Levin believe that this is wrong and unjust because there are **no** fundamental differences between the general and main principles of conventional medicine and complementary medicine, both of which are identical in their aspirations to achieve a high professional level and accuracy of actions (Brody et al. 2000: 52)[19]. Brody, Rygwelski and Fetters also criticize medicine's dubious strivings for power and economic domination. In their argument the underlying principle is to emphasize patients' and their families' freedom to choose a treatment option. Patients can be guided by their own views on health and illness and their own vision of 'holistic treatment'.

We can conclude that it is possible to prove the thesis that one of the essential differences between academic medicine and 'its alternative imitations' is *inter alia* the lack of a single clear-cut and consistent code of ethical principles universally used by healers (e.g. on a domestic scale). It seems particularly important that such a system be established because 'complementary therapists' without formal qualifications to practice treatment, using methods of unproven effectiveness, advertise their ability to treat almost all diseases (even cancer cases) in a fast, effective, inexpensive and painless manner. Despite the fact that the social scale of the phenomenon has been growing for over thirty years, the healer community have so far failed (in spite of v arious endeavors) to develop their own consistent code of ethical principles – a kind of equivalent of the Code of Medical Ethics. Under these circumstances the questions I asked in my studies on creating the foundations for the 'sociology of non-medical healing systems' still remain relevant. Some of them are as follows:

Should lay practitioners be held responsible for the effects of the treatments, diagnosis, rehabilitation and prevention they provide in the same way that doctors are?

Do healers have the right to perform acts on their own, which they call 'treatment', or should they perform such procedures only under a doctor's supervision?

Should healers be allowed to treat all diseases or should their activities be confined to sociopsychosomatic conditions where the placebo effect can be achieved?

Should formal-legal and ethical guarantees protect the patient undergoing an alternative-medicine treatment and, if so, what are these guarantees?

Does the healer, before performing procedures that he believes constitute treatment, have the obligation to inform the client about the scope of risk involved and the chances of genuinely curing the disease using the methods not accepted by allopathic medicine?

Who and in what mode (and based on what criteria) would settle possible disputes between healers and their patients?

Can the healer demand that his patient cease treatment in health service institutions?

---

19 In the earlier discussion the authors stress that both kinds of medicine are almost the same: it appears that it is 'almost' that makes the essential difference.

Is it admissible to publicly claim (in the media, Internet, advertising) that a folk doctor can treat all diseases?

Is it is admissible to publish surreptitious advertising materials including letters of thanks from allegedly cured patients?

Should the established legal regulations (e.g. The Act on the Profession of Physician, Medical Ethics Code) binding in the territory of Poland be actually enforced, for example by penalizing both healers and the doctors who cooperate with them?

Should the National Health Fund reimburse expenses (partially or in full) incurred by patients who decide to use 'alternative' therapies?

The foregoing questions, which exemplify both formal-legal and deontological-ethical problems, require scientific investigations and the start of a wide public debate (Piątkowski 1999: 99-106).

2. Methods of Treatment Not Accepted by Medicine. The State of Research

2.1 Non-Medical Healing Systems in Light of Polish Studies on the Sociology of Health and Illness[20]

If we accept the chronological order as the criterion for this presentation, the first Polish research project in the field of sociology of health, illness and medicine, concerned with description and interpretation of treatment methods offered by village practitioners as part of traditional folk medical systems, was a study on the system of medical knowledge of the Podhale [Polish Highlands] rural population. (Bejnarowicz 1969: 251-268). The goal of field investigations was to show, in the context of the 1960s cultural and social transformations, the changing character and function of traditional folk medical systems (folk medicine). The study described the health awareness, attitudes towards health and illness, health needs and behaviors of the rural (farming) population at that time. The project also involved free-form interviews with local folk healers ('internists', 'surgeons', 'herbalists', etc.). In the early 1960s, in the poorly urbanized Podhale region the status and prestige of folk medicine were high; the then healing methods covered both 'folk surgery and folk internal medicine', and practices involving mystical-magical and religious elements (Ibid.). When reconstructing folk knowledge of health and illness, it was found that the basic criterion for the division and classification of diseases was most often the dominant symptom and its location. The term 'illness', largely conventional, was widely applied. An interesting feature of popular 'medical thinking' was that some diseases including their actual symptoms were quite well-known; however, parts of this medical knowledge had been reinterpreted, distorted and mingled with traditional folk beliefs and convictions. Popular disease etiology comprised natural and supernatural (thaumaturgical) elements. The former were most often caused by material factors. Popular thinking on diseases caused by material factors was usually inconsistent with medical knowledge, e.g. folk healers commonly believed that the material cause of women's diseases was a twisted uterus. Tangible, noticeable and identifiable factors were regarded as those that could be defied. Supernatural causes of diseases in turn stemmed from charms, spells and the work of demons. Interpretations of the system of everyday knowledge of health showed that this type of knowledge was a heritage of centuries-old tradi-

20 The author's own studies have been presented in other parts of this book. Polish medical sociologists only touched upon the problem in question in their own investigations.

tions and local folk culture, overlapping and interwoven with selected, often distorted hearsay elements of both old and present-day medicine. The result was a syncretic store of popular information on diseases, expressed for example as a statement: '… […] female cancer has reproduced and metastases are flowing in the veins.' (Ibid: 256). It turned out that diagnostic information was far closer to medical knowledge than views on the etiology and pathogenesis of individual diseases. The contemporary cultural (modernization) and civilization changes influenced everyday lay knowledge of many diseases. More and more widespread, for example, was the view that some infectious diseases, e.g. tetanus, could not be treated at home and had to be dealt with exclusively in hospital. Terms like bacteria, vaccinations, serum and stomach ulcers were known especially to the younger members of the studied community. On the other hand, opinions on cancers were based on the belief that one could become infected with cancer, that the disease developed when someone was bitten by a fly that had first fed on a crayfish [=cancer] carcass, that there were two forms of cancer: male and female, that malignant cancer was red, etc.

The social status of rural folk healers (men or women) who specialized in preventing very serious diseases such as rheumatoid disease or erysipelas was high: they enjoyed respect and prestige among the local community, and it was generally believed that the therapeutic knowledge of such people and their magical powers were considerable. In the 1960s, faith in spells was also very widespread – almost all folk healers interviewed admitted that they were able to undo charms. Symptoms characteristic of spells could apply to any disease, both in animals and in people, and their cause was the conscious or unconscious action of another person, old women being most often likely to have cast them. A remedy was to undo the spell; the rite involved taking both material measures (lighting a blessed candle, throwing burning coals into water) and religious ones (saying the right prayers at a specific time and in an exactly specified manner). The Podhale population was also convinced that an especially effective way of overcoming the effects of spells was to burn incense. It was reported that, although some of those surveyed believed in charms, they would not reveal or describe such incensing practices, in contrast to the eagerly volunteered information on spells. When it proved necessary to use spells, a sorcerer or gypsy specializing in fighting them was brought in: they, some informers insisted, had some relations with the devil. A special variant of charm application was the domain of so-called *boginki* (nymphs) responsible *inter alia* for the death of children. The most extensive part of healing knowledge among the Podhale rural population was information on treatment methods and techniques, these covering natural and mystical-magical measures, or mixed ones combining both strategies. As part of natural methods, traditional medicines of mineral, animal and human origin were administered while, at the same time, medicines and other medicinal products were used, these were prescription-free and available in drugstores (peroxide solution, iodine, antiseptics, aspirin, etc.). The J. Bejnarowicz project was an attempt to conduct sociological field research on everyday views on health and illness among the farmer population in one of the typical Podhale villages. Its author used various parallel research methods (interview questionnaire, free-form interview, participant observation). The respondents were both local farmers and representatives of the local intelligentsia (gmina officials, the priest, doctor in the village health center, teachers) and selected folk healers. Great importance was also attached to interviewing people regarded as especially well-informed (old women). The results obtained permitted a reconstruction of the character and internal structure of folk medicine and self-treatment in the early 1960s, taking into account the social context. Groups of etiological, diagnostic and treatment elements were distinguished, with natural and mystical-magical measures being identified in each group. The sociological analysis demonstrated that, despite intensive, large-scale propaganda and information campaigns in the late 1940s and 1950s launched by the political and administrative authorities and directed against rural folk healers, it proved impossible to eliminate and marginalize self-treatment and traditional folk medicine until as late as the 1960s. The study showed that, under the influence of cultural modernization changes (the role of education, access to the press and radio) and more frequent contact with medical professions and institutions, folk healing gradually but slowly changed and was transformed. Magical practices were almost entirely eliminated (although interestingly enough, there was still widespread belief in the influence of spells at the same time), the services of unqualified village midwives were marginalized, prescription-free pharmaceuticals available in drugstores were used more and more frequently for self-treatment, and all village inhabitants accepted the situation that acute and infectious diseases were treated in medical institutions. Nevertheless, vestiges of old beliefs, practices and superstitions, especially those relating to the alleged causes of many diseases, were still present in the minds of the population of Podhale villages.

In the 1960s practically no other sociomedical research projects related to non-medical healing systems were carried out (apart from a Master's dissertation written in Warsaw University's Institute of Sociology, which was marginally contributory) (Uramowska-Żyto 1976). As in Western countries, medical sociology at that time focused on describing the system of institutional, professional medicine rather than on lay health practices. In this context an exceptional position is occupied by Jadwiga Szaro's early 1970s study, in which the goal of field investigations was to describe the system of folk medicine and self-treatment as in the J. Bejnarowicz project. Field studies were carried out in one of the districts (*powiat*) of the Beskid Niski region. Discussion of the results obtained pointed out that the lack of medical infrastructure (10 practicing doctors and a ten-bed hospital for the whole district) was the reason why, in the 1940s and 1950s, **the majority** [*my emphasis*, W. P.] of the rural population in the area utilized various forms of self-treatment and folk medicine: '[…] during that difficult time special opportunities opened to folk healers, from whom the people sought help in different diseases.' (Szaro 1976: 465). Despite subsequent development of the infrastructure of institutional medicine (14 health centers in the early 1970s) and radical improvement in available health provision (74 medical doctors, 22 dentists, 398 nurses employed in the district), the report said: '[…] there are still practices of unofficial medicine derived mainly from folk medicine (Ibid: 466). Like the J. Bejnarowicz studies, the report emphasized the continuing high prestige of folk healer in the local village communities, and the solidarity and discretion of patients utilizing these practices. Repressive administrative measures and restrictions of the 1970s did not so much eliminate folk healers' practice as create a kind of underground practice, where health services were provided by persons without formal qualifications. Consequently, those persons who, the study author knew, were folk healers denied engaging in such practices. The studies distinguished between folk healers who earned their living in this way exclusively ('professional folk healers') and those who occasionally performed the social roles of 'backstreet health advisors'. The former enjoyed especially high prestige: therefore patients sometimes waited weeks for an appointment. These 'professionals' normally used so-called natural methods, e.g. herbal medicine. In the past they had had longer or shorter contact with medicine (as former army nurses or ward attendants, etc.). An entirely different kind of therapists was the folk healer who used mystical-magical methods with religious elements. These methods were employed mainly by old women, who practiced, among other things, casting spells or charms to cause or prevent certain diseases. By using the dominant therapeutic technique criterion, which was the result of professing special views on the etiology of the most frequent conditions, 'folk pharmacy specialists' were also distinguished. Like the Bejnarowicz project, studies by J. Szaro conducted a decade and a half later demonstrated that despite the pressure from modernization factors in education, cultural communication, and in access to medical professions and institutions, there was still a kind of 'folk healing infrastructure' in the district investigated, with the elements of the social role of folk healers being somewhat modified. Some of them started to administer injections and apply antibiotics acquired on their own, etc. Interestingly enough, in the 1970s illegal health services provided by folk healers were utilized by people of higher social status – the well-off and educated.

The patients were divided into three principal groups: those treated only by folk healers, those utilizing parallel treatment (by folk healers and medical doctors at the same time) and those who sought treatment by non-medical practitioners only when their disease was declared incurable. The J. Szaro project showed folk medicine in the process of transformations, in the one hand the stability of its principal elements (traditional etiological and diagnostic views) and, on the other hand, in the high vitality of the system and its capacity for adaptive changes (new elements in therapeutic methods and techniques, use of drugstore medicines, etc.). Another significant reason for the popularity of the then illegal practices was psychological factors: provision of fast acting, painless and effective treatment, as folk healers assured, and the comparatively inexpensive methods of treatment of all diseases. It turned out that traditional folk medical systems, under severe pressure from administrative law from the mid-1940s onward, not only avoided atrophy or decomposition as an element of the old world of superstitions and prejudices but also began to win new clients; this apparently, foreshadowed the expansion of 'other' medicine in the 1980s, when non-medical healing systems became a noticeable, real and mass social phenomenon. Like those of J. Bejnarowicz or J. Szaro, a project of sociological investigations into the folk medical system's changes over time was designed and carried out by I. Jaguś. This research approach could be termed as sociological-historical (Jaguś 2002). In the chapter *Theoretical Sociological Conceptions versus Health and Illness*, she writes *inter alia*: 'To sum up, we can say that the growing number of studies on 'non-medical' healing systems, a result of transformation of medical sociology into the sociology of health, allows us to learn everyday knowledge in this field. It should be emphasized that more and more often the professional and non-professional ways of perceiving reality function side by side. They interpenetrate and sometimes complement one another. The […] selected elements of sociological conceptions discussed here may be used for studies in health sociology, including folk medicine.' (Ibid: 23). Following W. Piątkowski's research pattern, I. Jaguś investigated folk views on disease etiology, treatment and prevention; she also analyzed relations between the folk healing system and medical institutions and profession at the turn of the nineteenth century. She showed the changing attitude of folk practitioners and their patients to transformations brought about by the progressive process of institutionalization and professionalization of the contemporary medicine. In the section on the present-day folk healing system she took into consideration the role of such factors as the spread of the health insurance system in the countryside, the impact of the first postwar 1950 Act on the Profession of Physician (which provided legal grounds for the total elimination of so-called 'medical bungling'), etc. At the conclusion of her research I. Jaguś emphasized the strong position of folk medicine, or more broadly, non-medical healing systems in Poland in the 1980s, stressing that mystical-magical elements had been entirely eliminated from folk medicine. At the same time the popularity of traditional herbal medicine grew considerably. The author pointed out that folk medicine was an integral part of folk knowledge, which in turn is a constituent of rich and complex folk culture. The research project in question also had some diagnostic value, permitting identification of important health needs that are satisfied outside the system of institutional medicine. This, Jaguś believed, might have improved the functioning of medical institutions so that they could fulfill the patients' expressive needs more fully (Ibid: 124).

The circumstance, which could be described as the specific characteristics of Polish sociomedical studies in the late 1970s and 1980s on treatment methods not accepted by medical doctors, was a paradox consisting in that this kind of medical help in illness was utilized on a mass scale by the sick and healthy alike. The context of this mass social phenomenon was not, however, the subject of systematic sociological investigations [I omit here the results of my own continuing studies since 1990 because they have been presented elsewhere in this book]. At the end of the 1970s, the founder of Polish medical sociology, Magdalena Sokołowska, suggested that such projects be carried out in the sociology of health and illness on the grounds that only one spiritual healer, Clive Harris, during '[…] his two-day stay in Poland saw about 240 thousand people out of 600 thousand registered […] As we can see it was a **mass** [*my emphasis*, W. P.] phenomenon and at least for this reason it could not be ignored by sociologists.' (Sokołowska 1980:99) In her paper, M. Sokołowska outlined the sociological perspective for investigation of the phenomenon of spiritual healers, accentuating the scope of public interest in such practices and the description of the individual 'Harris Institution' – a certain formal structure which arose as a response to the immense popularity of these types of practices, to which many people attributed healing powers in the late 1970s. She pointed out that it was the first time that a new, previously unknown type of healing and that kind of therapist had appeared in Poland. This was not a traditional folk healer practicing folk medicine, an integral, larger whole, which was traditional rural culture. This time treatment was provided by a 'Western man', a professional healer, a multilingual Canadian who offered his services all over the world, with his own office in London, etc. (Ibid:102). The first reactions of the Polish academic community (including sociologists) to this previously unknown phenomenon seemed to display some confusion and surprise. During a special panel session organized by the Polish Sociological Association's Medical Sociology Section at the Polish Academy of Science Institute of Philosophy and Sociology, experts emphasized that they were surprised that the healer's patients (unlike those of village folk practitioners) were largely persons of high social status, well-off and well educated. The survey results presented at the session showed that one out of five persons polled had had earlier contact with 'non-professional medicine' (as M. Sokołowska put it), while more than half of those surveyed accentuated their faith in the treatment effects during this kind of therapy. Pilot studies headed by J. Dziatłowicki enabled a description of three basic patients' groups that utilized the services of the 'Harris Institution'. The largest group were chronically ill patients, while another comprised those who did not want to undergo long and expensive hospital treatment without a guarantee of recovery; the last category were those who suffered from no ailments but wanted to undergo 'touch treatment' hoping to gain greater health capital. The first sociological analysis of the Clive Harris phenomenon also emphasized that the healer's arrival and the mass participation of the sick and healthy in his sessions initiated a spontaneous rise of a new individual 'civic structure'. Organization committees emerged that piloted and created conditions for so-called 'big meetings' in 14 Polish cities, and prepared the healer's sessions with huge masses of patients (in some cities the crowd was 10-12 thousand strong); the contribution of church institutions to coordination of such events, and the friendly attitude of many rank and file priests and even bishops in particular dioceses toward these activities were also emphasized. Interestingly enough, these mass phenomena (it was the period before John Paul II's first visit to Poland) were favorably received by the then administrative and political authorities, which even employed the Civic Militia (police) to control traffic and ensure safety at these large-scale events. At that time Magdalena Sokołowska's standpoint was characteristic: she opposed many opinions voiced by prominent clinicians, who believed that Harris was an ephemeral phenomenon to be explained by a collective delusion, hysteria and faith in superstition fuelled by the sensation-seeking media. In her analysis Sokołowska stressed the rational character of the presented phenomena and processes, emphasizing the fact that sick persons behaved logically, seeking any assistance when their life and health was threatened, while 'biological' medicine did not notice, or ignored or disregarded specific, important emotional needs of the patients, these being at least partly satisfied by contact with, as she put it, **non-medical** [*my emphasis*, W. P.] healers (Sokołowska 1980: 103). It should be pointed out that this was the first time an analysis was undertaken of the response of institutional medicine, treated as part of the social supersystem, to a new entity entering the health service market. In this context Sokołowska also suggested re-interpreting institutional and ideological transformations occurring in the area of contemporary medical sciences. She maintained that it was necessary to revise the binding dogmas of official medical epistemology and recognize that he practice of healing was not confined to medical doctors and specialized institutional medicine centers; the period when science was centers; the period when science was arbitrarily contrasted with non-science or correct methods with incorrect methods was drawing to a close. In order to actually know the social context of health and illness, one also had to oppose the medicocentric attitude of Western civilization. Sokołowska's approach distinguished four basic physician attitudes towards the emerging phenomenon of 'other medicine'. These were attitudes oriented towards investigating the phenomenon (interest in and distance from), active participation and acceptance, rejection and criticism, and ambivalence. At the same time the prevalent view among sociologists was that we were witnessing the collapse of the empirical-scientific medical paradigm and revision of the category of rationality/irrationality in relation to the concepts of health and illness. But '[…] the waning of faith in "pure reason" does not mean an increase in irrational behaviors, it is rather a harbinger of new reason […]' (Ibid: 112-113).

In the early 1980s Polish sociomedical studies on so-called traditional medicine entered a new stage: it was the description of the emerging forms of cooperation (especially in Asian and African countries) between 'local medicine' systems and the structures of institutional healthcare. These solutions were promoted in the 1970s and 1980s by the WHO. The opening of the WHO to local, indigenous treatment methods was believed to be the most characteristic manifestation of medical evolution. At present we cannot yet estimate the great significance of this phenomenon and its results (Sokołowska 1980b: 252-269). M. Sokołowska was convinced that the end of the twentieth century brought both spectacular success and many failures to institutional medicine. Expensive treatment systems failed to solve core health problems in the third-world countries, and their dysfunction was also noticeable in affluent Western societies. In the underdeveloped countries the influence of medicine on a radical drop in mortality and morbidity rates was highly problematic, availability of institutional medicine to ordinary people being incomplete. For Sokołowska the axis of the contemporary discourse in medical sociology was the following question: why do most doctors practicing in the Euro-American cultural sphere not notice and not recognize the fact that in by no means all communities that is treatment provided solely by practitioners of 'technochemical medicine'? And why does this have to be a symptom of backwardness? Following this reasoning, present-day medical doctors have to face the fact that they have lost their exclusive monopoly on treating people, and should accept the patient's right to freely choose a therapist s/he trusts. From this discussion stemmed a practical conclusion that while recognizing '[…] plurality of human experiences in suffering […] we do not want to acknowledge the plurality of forms of seeking help in suffering' (Ibid: 255). At that time a demand was explicitly expressed that traditional medicine be further investigated, '[…] because of the medicocentric attitude we know next to nothing about other healing systems. There is no large contemporary Polish publication on the subject, if only to systematize the terminology and practice types of a great number of non-scientific healers; nor do we have Polish equivalents of the names of their professions' (Ibid). The sociological canon of studies on the subject would consist *inter alia* in the assessment of their efficacy from the perspective of behavioral science. The model and point of reference would be the contemporary WHO reports on this issue, the more so that it was recognized that '[...] traditional medicine became one of the fundamental fields of WHO operation.' (Ibid: 256). The project of combining the pro-health activities of this institution with local, folk treatment methods was to be a remedy for solving many problems related to the inadequacy and unavailability of various institutional forms of assistance in illness. In addition, it was stressed that model cooperation could gradually bring the two systems together, for example on the basis of the adopted ecological-holistic conception of health. The principal reason, M. Sokołowska claimed, why healers are popular both in developing countries and in Europe and the US is that they are highly open to different human needs and well integrated with the communities in which they practice, also putting emphasis on partnership relations with clients; moreover, they see illness in sociopsychological rather than biomedical terms. The summation of M. Sokołowska's views on alternative medicine at that time was the opinion that the entry into and popularity of healing in the health service market could help the systems of institutional medicine to revise their conceptions of health and illness. Doctors should draw conclusions from such a situation and carry out 'a scientific-humanistic revolution', the ultimate result of which would be to create 'a holistic, biopsychosociomedical system of care of the entire man'. Therefore, further development of medicine can take place by overcoming its crisis (Sokołowska 1980b: 272-276)

A new stage of analysis in the sociology of health and illness of methods not accepted by academic medicine was defined by Sokołowska-inspired field studies on the phenomenon of the popularity of Harris in the late 1970s and into the 1980s. This was the first attempt in Poland to describe the phenomenon in question using sociological research methods and was an effort to devise the theoretical foundations for analysis of the phenomenon of healing. The project authors also wanted to inquire into the real reasons for the growing popularity of non-medical healing systems in Poland (at the end of 1978 and beginning of 1979 the number of those wishing to consult with Harris exceeded 1,200,000 people) (Kański and Wasilewski 1981, 3(82):103).

The authors decided to employ a rare research strategy – participant observation, which they carried out in 13 cities between the autumn of 1978 and the spring of 1979. Sociologists participated directly in a series of healers' meetings with many-thousand-strong crowds of patients, working as ushers or stretcher-bearers helping to transport the sick. To interpret the phenomenon, the research pattern developed by American sociologists A. C. Twaddle and R. M. Hessler was used (Twaddle and Hessler 1977: 139-159). They distinguished the following categories of sociological description of healing: The Symbolic, The Technical, Theories of Disease, and The Social Organization of the Healing Role (Ibid: 140-143). This original research concept, the first in Western sociology, will be discussed in the next subchapter. The Hessler and Twaddle analysis framework was thus adjusted to entirely different social and cultural realities. Having undertaken to investigate the first group of elements – the symbolic – the study found out *inter alia* the reasons why many sessions with the healer took place in churches, monasteries, convents and similar church buildings. It was pointed out that Harris, as a spiritual healer, intentionally preferred such venues as traditional places of concentration and prayer. These elements allow the healer to achieve desirable therapeutic effects. The technical elements investigated consisted in turn in the reconstruction of the 'Clive Harris Institution'. The study was able to establish that there was a formal but discreetly operating national staff, which coordinated the whole organization of the healer's visits to Poland (invitations, technical organization of big meetings, verification and collection of applications, printing of invitation cards and their distribution, etc.). Apart from the central management staff, all over Poland there were about 1500 local organizers of mass healing events. While conducting observations, researchers noticed that further growth in Harris's popularity was the effect of a series of enthusiastic articles in the press and the premiere of Marcel Łoziński's documentary *Dotknięcie* (The Touch), which was shown together with the then popular movie by Zanussi *Spirala* (The Spiral). The researchers also managed to ascertain the criteria that qualified patients for meetings with the healer (patients diagnosed by doctors, patients with certified cancers, or those with other severe somatic diseases were preferred). It was also possible to reconstruct the big meeting as a typical form of the healer's operation, and to describe the manner of using the healing technique, the touch for health and the emotional context of healing sessions. The study also sought to reconstruct the 'disease theory', to which the healer referred; it turned out he was not interested in knowing the etiology of diseases that he tried to cure. At the same time he stressed his complementary role in relation to medicine, recommending that all his patients continue hospital treatment. Harris recognized that his mission consisted in fulfilling emotional (interactive) needs disregarded by allopathic medicine. The healer also emphasized the supernatural nature of his abilities, which he believed were a God-given gift. At the same time he stressed that he had innate healing powers and that is why he could not pass his skills on to anyone else. In his opinion, healing consisted mainly in eliminating the causes of illnesses. Moreover, good effects of his therapy did not require any special faith in his therapeutic capacities. In accordance with the research pattern described earlier the social role of healing was also identified. Its most important element proved to be the healer-patient interaction patterns and detailed elements of the relationship (motives for choosing a healer, mutual expectations of healer and patient towards each other, the healer's social status, etc.). Harris emphasized that the principal motive for his actions was his selfless desire to help others; he did not own or wished to own any personal property or tangible assets. This declaration, he insisted, was necessary because it determined his own capacities for therapeutic influence. The studies in question marked a significant stage in the sociological exploration of the phenomenon. Sociologists no longer described only traditional, rural folk healing systems; now the object of their interest was a new 'urban', 'international' model of mass treatment using methods not accepted by present-day institutional medicine. In order to describe and interpret this phenomenon, an innovative (and effective) research method was used – participant observation and the theoretical pattern developed in American sociology of health and illness, which was applied to Polish sociocultural realities. Clive Harris himself and the mass phenomena that he created became the symbol of breaking the monopoly of institutional biomedicine and, as we said earlier, provoked discussion in medical science. For the first time patients had the option to choose a therapist and the manner of treatment, doctor-patient relation patterns changed, and an opportunity appeared to interact with healers. From then on all these issues were sporadically the subject of sociomedical inquiries. At that time the research area in question again became the subject of further analyses, comments and evaluations by sociologists of health and illness. Studies were initiated on the role of social factors in medical practice, with discussions on the role played by 'unofficial/informal medicine' or 'medicine of traditional ethnic groups' in this field (Sokołowska 1986: 81-90). M. Sokołowska insisted that biomedicine never had a monopoly on offering health- and illness-related services. The core reason why healers were successful was that they fulfilled emotional, social and physical needs **outside of** [*my emphasis*. W. P.] the medical system. As the author of the first Polish handbook of medical sociology, she regarded the contemporary studies as fragmentary and chaotic. She sought the origin of contemporary healing in traditional folk medicine, '[...] quackery [or folk healing systems] has many meanings and suggests many associations. There isn't [...] any single generally accepted meaning of the terms, the more so that folk doctors are discussed in fictional literature and the media rather than in scientific disciplines (Ibid.). As a side note to the demands repeated since the late 1970s that the taxonomy be standardized and systematic sociological research be undertaken, we should observe that such projects began after undertaken, we should observe that such projects began after Magdalena Sokołowska's death, after 1989. Their most important results are set out in the present book. In her handbook *Sociologia medycyny* [Medical Sociology] the author also tried to identify which factors accounted for the fact that healing did not prove a transient passion but became a permanent part of modern Western medical systems. Sokołowska maintained that non-medical healing systems in the developed Western European countries are becoming institutional and professionalized, thereby becoming an imitation of medicine to some extent (the cases of homeopathy and chiropractic), because there is professional qualifying training, formalized educational modes, handbooks, etc. However, even these techniques and methods of treatment seemingly closest to medicine itself are very far apart; consequently, the former are not recognized by medical doctors (Ibid: 84). The process of convergence between academic medicine and alternative methods, even the least controversial (homeopathy, chiropractic) was very slow in Western Europe because the obstacle were qualitative differences: '[…] If acupuncture alongside homeopathy and chiropractic were to be the official subjects taught at medical schools this would be tantamount to recognizing models of illness that **fundamentally differ** [*my emphasis*, W. P.] from the accepted model based on natural and exact sciences' (Ibid: 86). To sum up, we may say that the overall contribution of Magdalena Sokołowska to the presented sociological research on treatment methods and techniques not accepted by medicine was fundamental. From 1978 to 1989 she was constantly interested (although with varying intensity) in the development of 'other medicine', and tried to explain the social causes of complementary and alternative medicine (CAM); she described the reaction mechanisms of the medical system to mass activities of healers in Poland and in Europe, devoting much room to the role of WHO. Finally, and of most importance to me as the author of the present book, she recognized many years ago this set of issues as one of the most important research problems both for medical science and medical sociology as a subdiscipline of general sociology (Ibid: 89-90).

One the main themes investigated by medical sociology is the problem of behaviors and attitudes towards health and illness (see Cockerham and Glasser 2001: 89-169; Weiss and Lonnquist 2006:109-129). Until the late 1970s, Polish sociologists investigating health and illness did not have to ponder on the boundaries and content of the term 'medical behavior' because our subdiscipline described the reality entirely monopolized by institutional medicine. When conceptualizing the contemporary Polish studies on the subject it was observed that 'medicine not only moulds and makes the content of medical culture in society but is a generally accepted source of models and norms for all behaviors related to health and illness' (Titkow 1983: 4). In the 1980s it was commonly pointed out that in Polish society almost all activities associated with health and illness are realized in medical institutions in contact with a physician. The first Polish research project devoted to health behaviors examined *inter alia* the social mechanisms of choosing the method of treatment. It turned out that, in the early 1980s, apart from the prevalent offer of the formal medical system, a patient could already utilize the complementary modes: self-treatment and the services of practitioners of magic and folk doctors. It should be stressed that the use of a 'non-medical (or non-biomedical)' option was treated at that time as a kind of **deviation** [*my emphasis*, W. P.] Anna Titkow wrote, 'In modern societies characterized by a highly developed medical centers network, the most frequent are forms of partial deviation of behaviors in illness. A deviation is to avoid official medicine as long as one can or to utilize it inconsistently. Sometimes this is oriented towards healthcare provided by the lay system (non-medical or paramedical circles). An example from Poland would be in order at this point: the use by the Poles of help offered by healer Harris.'(Ibid: 67). When systematizing variables distinguished in the study of health behaviors, the set of dependent variables describing the 'way of assuming the social role of patient' contains *inter alia* 'alternative choices of help when illness appears', including unofficial medicine utilization labeled as 'deviation.' (Ibid: 210). The summing up of sociological studies on health behaviors concluded that 'At the same time those surveyed declare having reservations or qualms about using medicine; in addition those who utilize alternative forms of healthcare to a greater extent, have a better financial standing or are more involved in communal life, and have a greater perception of inequities of access to effective treatment regardless of frequency of their contact with medicine.' (Ibid) The results obtained in the now classic research project confirmed *inter alia* the 'growing emotional autonomy of lay people towards medicine and its representatives'. Ordinary patients were becoming increasingly emancipated and independent, and most of those surveyed (80%) felt negative emotions when contacting physicians. Although the greater majority of Warsaw residents used the assistance provided by institutional medicine in illness, regardless of their social position, for the first time sociological analyses recorded the emerging opportunities of, most often complementary, parallel treatment of the patient's illness outside the formalized medical system. The gradual breaking of the monopoly of medical services provision, noticeable in light of A. Titkow's results, initiated a discussion on the legitimacy of use of the term 'medical behaviors' when some patients sought help in illness from- self-treatment or from therapists who, not being physicians, offered treatment by means of methods not used or accepted in medicine.

Research projects on behaviors in health and in illness were continued by the Łódź team of medical sociologists in the 1990s (Gniazdowski 1990:2). The purpose of their investigations was to characterize prevalent health behaviors in Polish society in the 1990s. The studies were carried out as part of the all-Polish project ‘Health attitudes and behaviors of Polish society’. An especially interesting theme for our discussion was the description and sociological interpretation of ‘everyday behaviors’, which we will now present. A further goal of the analyses was to develop theoretical foundations for such discussions with reference to sociomedical and socioecological paradigms. When presenting the term ‘alternative society’, Krzysztof Puchalski wrote, ‘A distinctive feature of health-related activities analyzed in the conceptions of alternative society is to realize these activities outside official healthcare institutions [...] Especially noteworthy are individual or group ways of fulfilling health needs not satisfied by the institutional system of official medicine or fulfilled in a not accepted way’ (Puchalski 1990: 39-40). Another theme that students of non-medical healing systems may find interesting is discussions on the character and features of everyday consciousness. The analysis of the term ‘everyday consciousness’ and related special needs, attitudes and behaviors appears very interesting. Without examining the terms ‘rationality’ and ‘irrationality’ (which will be dealt with in the section devoted to traditional folk medicine), we should remember that the features of everyday thinking include the following: heterogeneous ways of reasoning, incomplete validity of judgments expressed, ambiguity and overgeneralization of opinions voiced, lack of logical continuity in reasoning, failure to see a cause-effect relationship between classes of phenomena, internal inconsistency of actions undertaken. These and other features of everyday thinking appear especially useful for characterizing, describing, interpreting and conducting research both on self-treatment and folk medicine, and on the practices of present-day healers, which is the aim of this study.

Highly interesting sociological studies on health behaviors in the context of transformations in the healthcare system were carried out by Marek Latoszek in Gdansk. This project, in a sense, complemented the analyses of the Łódź team. As in all studies presented in this chapter, it deals with the issue of non-medical healing systems. The objective set by the Gdansk team was to describe and interpret the dynamic changes taking place in the sphere of health aspirations and attitudes towards the rapidly changing healthcare system during the transformation period (Latoszek 2000). As a result of the field survey (questionnaire by mail) 504 questionnaire forms were obtained by return mail (Ibid: 12). The Gdansk study showed that 12% of respondents utilized healer services, as many as 86% of those surveyed having rated them favorably. ‘[...] in the 1990s new forms of medical services appeared i.e. [...] non-conventional medicine, mainly bioenergy therapy – however, the use of these services appears to be less frequent than everyday knowledge would indicate.’ (Ibid: 33). Another traditional issue that is part of the canon of classic sociology of health, illness and medicine is the description of the character and determinants of the patient-physician relationship, presented against the broad background of social and cultural conditions (Waitzkin 2000:271-283). Antonina Ostrowska, when discussing these relationships in light of the earlier survey conducted on an adult population sample in Poland, pointed out factors that in some way anticipated the later expansion of non-medical healing systems in the 1990s. The analysis of the results obtained showed that only one out of five of those surveyed (21%) felt a fully satisfying interaction with his/her physician, while distance and mutual distrust of the parties to this social relationship was becoming wider and wider (Ostrowska 1981, 3 (82): 69 et seq.) New phenomena and processes modifying this old scenario were then observed: the growing health consciousness of patients and a gradual sense of their own interest, a growing knowledge of the side effects of medical interventions, and risks of iatrogenic errors, etc. At the same time, in Western societies for example, there was an increasingly widespread conviction that the whole medical system had only an actual 10% effect on the phenomena of health and illness (Ibid: 78). These analyses also demonstrated that, while characterizing the 'sociology of medical professions', we should understand that from the perspective of both the patient and of the physician new options (complementary and alternative) appeared, which the patient could utilize when dissatisfied or not fully satisfied with his/her relationships with medical practitioners. It should be borne in mind, though, that many such opportunities were provided in the developed Western countries; it was there that phenomena described as the (partial) demedicalization of social life began to occur. Those dynamic processes were also a social reaction to the criticism of commercialized, capitalist, corporationist and profit-oriented medicine. Many citizens sought to define 'the alternative style of living' and while seeking, they encountered offers of different versions of self-treatment or numerous variants of alternative and complementary medicine. It was then that some citizens started to try out and then practice these forms of help in illness. (Ibid: 86). At that time the patient-healer interaction also appeared, to be subsequently described and interpreted. This is how A. Ostrowska characterized that situation, 'An alternative are healers **from outside of** [*my emphasis*, W. P.] the domain of official medicine. Over the last years their growing popularity has been reported, which makes the medical world ponder. Is this popularity a response to the technicized point of view represented by many physicians? […] the feature that characterized the patient-healer relationship is close emotional contact (Ibid: 87). The analyses presented at the time showed that institutional medicine was unable to respond adaptively to the emerging competition, in terms of knowledge and practice based on foundations other than the natural science paradigm applied in biomedicine. It is also worth noting another perspective observable, for example, in Chinese medicine, where the perspective observable, for example, in Chinese medicine, where the mutually non-antagonistic systems of traditional healing practices and modern biomedicine have coexisted for many years. The analysis of the contemporary social reality also demonstrated that the absolute biomedical monopoly of exclusivity in defining criteria for the rational and the scientific was untenable in the long run. In summing up the description of changes in the patient-physician interaction, Ostrowska remarked: 'What does it mean, though, that physicians and healers have nothing to learn from one other? The example of the coexisting systems in China can certainly be followed in other countries. The solutions existing in Poland as alternative should rather be complementary.'(Ibid: 88).

Trying to outline the stages defined by diverse research themes 'touching upon' the issues of non-medical healing systems, we cannot ignore the situation created in the early 1990s by certain institutional measures advanced by the Ministry of Health. As we remember from the observations in earlier subchapters, the first sociomedical studies of folk medicine appeared in the early 1960s; this subject became an element of interest to some Polish sociologists investigating the issues of health and illness in the 1980s (although systematic, large-scale investigations were not conducted); it was only in the 1990s, including transformations in the domain of medical systems, that opportunities for and prospects of qualitatively implementing new research projects were provided. It was then that the proposal to conduct extensive sociomedical research on 'non-conventional methods of treatment' appeared, inspired by a decision of the Ministry of Health and Social Welfare Scientific Council of September 1993 (Official letter of 28 September 1993). One of the measurable effects of this proposal (although formally they were not caused by the said institution) was a series of publications on non-medical healing systems, which appeared as separate volumes edited by Professor Kazimierz Imieliński. One of the first volumes contained a text by medical sociologist Anna Firkowska-Mankiewicz of the Polish Academy of Science Institute of Philosophy and Sociology, which analyzed research then underway on non-medical healing systems in Poland and Europe, and stressed the social determinants of the phenomenon (Firkowska-Mankiewicz 1994: 174-181). At the macro-level the article described the cultural and civilization mechanisms triggered and accelerated by the system transformation in Poland and their indirect or direct influence on the rapidly growing market for alternative healing services. We should agree with the major point of the article that free market mechanisms, the growing ideological and cultural pluralism, the development of the commercial media independent of the State, easier contact with the world, and the opening of frontiers, which *inter alia* made possible mass immigration of all manner of healers from the former Soviet Union countries, were some of the social factors with an accelerating effect on the fast-growing market for services of 'other medicine' (Ibid: 176). There also seems to have been slow parallel demedicalization of social life in Poland, which was associated not only with the breakup of the monopoly of the national healthcare system on the provision of health- and illness-related services but also with the growing role of self-treatment, greater availability of prescription-free medicines, greater level of medical self-knowledge, more frequent preventive measures and health promotion undertaken on one's own initiative. A great role in promoting natural therapy methods was played by the pluralist, commercial media, the so-called women's press, tabloids and then the Internet. Attitudes towards health and illness gradually became more self-creative and less and less demanding, while the Poles treated their health in an increasingly active and subjective way. Under such circumstances a physician or a healer were often merely health advisors or consultants, the emancipated patient taking decisions on his/her own. The sick and healthy became not only independent but also increasingly certain of their choices and behaviors. An important role was also played by all kinds of fashions and trends in culture (ecologism, feminism, popularity of the esoteric, subculture and pop-culture trends, fascination with the Orient, etc.). On the one hand, Firkowska-Mankiewicz maintains that there was a slow but steady tendency towards demedicalization of social life, on the other hand, we witnessed rapid institutionalization, professionalization and commercialization of the whole 'alternative medicine industry'. Health consortia emerged that provided comprehensive complementary medicine services, healer diplomas were certified, dynamic associations and trade unions of healers were organized, specialist thematic channels that promoted 'holistic medicine' (e.g. EZO TV) proliferated on commercial TV, and mass-circulation periodicals (usually monthlies) sponsored by the wealthiest healers began to be published, chiefly as hobby or how-to magazines ("Szaman [Shaman]", "Uzdrawiacz [Healer]"), which in fact covertly advertised natural medicine companies. Firms and consortia in this business began to use increasingly effective marketing, psychotechnical and PR techniques in order to win new masses of clients.

One more research theme in the Polish sociology of health and illness, in which there are references to non-medical healing systems, is the studies conducted on the borderline between family sociology and medical sociology. These investigations were initiated in the late 1980s by Magdalena Sokołowska and Zbigniew Tyszka. The conceptualization of the new, interdisciplinary research trend in Polish sociology was defined by the concepts of health – illness – family. Family was treated as one of the links in the system of lay care (E. Freidson's concept of lay referral system has been discussed elsewhere in this book). When planning these studies, it was pointed out that 60% of health- and illness-related actions are taken spontaneously at the family level: these are non-medical measures outside of official medicine, e.g. self-treatment (Firkowska-Mankiewicz 1990:17-21). The project in question (in which I participated) took into account three specific, non-professional forms of help in illness: the first was family, while the others also covered practitioners of non-professional medicine: folk doctors, herbalists, and all kinds of healers (Ibid: 21). We should add that projects carried out on the borderline between medical and family sociologies also included diverse field studies. For example, as part of the project "Sociomedical aspects of the functioning of families in different environments" one of the main themes was analysis of the influence of family on creating elements of medical culture (Woźniak 1991: 193-215). A section in the report "Illness and disability in relation to family" reads *inter alia* that in modern urban families 'Use of classic folk medical practices has almost vanished but folk doctors were replaced by all manner of healers.' (Ibid: 203). In farming families, in turn, health- and illness-related behaviors '[...] usually draw on the store of folk knowledge [...]' (Ibid). The section of sociomedical studies by W. Wozniak on families with cerebral palsy children shows that 42% of such families sought bioenergy therapy services, 27% used herbalism, and 25 used acupuncture (Ibid: 207).

We will now focus on another perspective in post-1990 research as part of a Polish sociology of health and illness: this was an approach aimed at enriching the theory of medical sociology. For example, Barbara Uramowska-Żyto writes: 'recently sociologists have borrowed other theoretical patterns that make it possible, unlike the functional concept of illness, to focus on some other informal areas related to maintenance of health and treatment of illness [...] On the basis of these patterns sociologists have analyzed common-sense knowledge and everyday life [...] These analyses are part of the trend of humanistic sociology, *inter alia* in phenomenology and symbolic interactionism.' (Uramowska-Żyto 1992: 9) When discussing the theoretical foundations of medical sociology (T. Parsons's structural-functional conception) the study reads, '[...] the functional definition of illness and its limitations have excluded from sociological investigation two **huge** [*my emphasis*, W. P.] areas of social reality: the subjective meaning of illness and **health activities of lay people** [*my emphasis*, W. P.]' (Ibid: 24). The research approach in question presents a comprehensive account of three main conceptions useful in describing phenomena associated with non-medical healing systems and their sociological interpretation: symbolic interactionism, ethnomethodology, and E. Freidson's classic conception of the lay referral system. All these theoretical themes will be discussed in the subsequent sections of the present book.

As I have emphasized above, of great significance for the development of studies on the sociology of non-medical healing systems were the research themes on the borderline of medical and family sociologies. In the mid-1990s one more kind of investigation was initiated, this time on the borderline between medical sociology and the sociology of religion (Libiszowska-Żółtkowska 1998: 39-61). We will start with general introductory remarks on the broader context of the presence of religious content and elements in the non-conventional methods of treatment and healing (this theme has been dealt with in the present book in a different context when describing folk medicine). The observations by religious (and medical) sociologist Maria Libiszowska-Żółtkowska refer predominantly to present-day healing. The Catholic Church Catechism in its section on divination and magic reads 'All practices of magic or sorcery, by which one attempts to tame occult powers, so as to place them at one's service and have a supernatural power over others - even if this were for the sake of restoring their health - are gravely contrary to the virtue of religion. [...] Recourse to so-called traditional cures does not justify either the invocation of evil powers or the exploitation of another's credulity (Catechism of Catholic Church, para 2117). A good example of the skepticism and caution of Catholic Church institutions towards so-called miraculous recoveries is the procedure that needs to be followed prior to declaring such facts to be miracles. The Lourdes Sanctuary Medical Bureau examines each case for six years and gives an appropriate opinion only afterwards. Recovery itself must meet a number of stringent parallel criteria: it should be quick and unexpected (without convalescence), immediate, complete and permanent; hence there is a prolonged and thorough-going examination of each case. At the same time the disease that precedes recovery should constitute a direct threat to life and be incurable and organic (not functional). Each case is subject to a long-term process of clinical analysis (it is emphasized that medical treatment must be ineffective or that no biomedical measures were applied earlier). In addition, in 1954 the International Medical Committee was established; this verifies the Medical Bureau's decisions. The Church makes a decision to recognize a recovery as miraculous through the bishop of the diocese, of which a patient is a member. The bishop expresses his opinion only after he has familiarized himself with medical expert opinions and examined all the circumstances in which the recovery took place. By the mid-1990s only 65 officially confirmed recoveries were recognized as miraculous (Cuda dzisiaj... 1994: 17). When commenting on miraculous recoveries, theologians wrote, 'The effort to confine man to himself is being made today by so-called natural medicine. It regards the discovery of the Earth's divine nature as the main thing [...] It disseminates the view that the condition of health is associated with the balance between life-giving forces and man's energy, illness being a disturbance of this inner energy' (Jedynak 1995). Priests point out that the popularity of various healers gives rise to the danger of deceit and dishonesty. People posing as healers want to make the patient emotionally dependent on them by promising speedy recovery; in addition, practices of this kind may be accompanied by a series of superstitious rites (signs, incantations and the like). The theologian cited maintains that human curiosity, credulity, lack of distance, and skepticism are the basis on which new sects and pseudo-religious groups develop, also offering 'pseudo-philosophy of miraculous treatment', and thereby posing a danger to the physical and mental health of the contemporary man. An example showing the significance that the Catholic Church attaches to the questions of healing is the document issued by the Congregation for the Doctrine of Faith, containing instructions on prayers for healing. The Congregation, headed by the then cardinal Joseph Ratzinger, warns against speaking hastily of 'healing charisma' in the case of people who organize, for example, prayer groups. It also reminds the faithful that all recoveries are the work of the Holy Spirit, who endows some people with special healing charisma. The Congregation seems to have a reserved approach to some types of miraculous recoveries; it recommends that prayers for this purpose be held in a church and be conducted by a priest, whereas combining them with liturgy is prohibited. Similarly, the syncretic set of pseudo-religious beliefs, which is a constituent of some orientations defined as New Age, was pronounced to be anti-Christian. The February 3, 2003 Vatican document "Jesus Christ the Bearer of the Water of Life" emphasizes that movements of this type containing views on alternative medicine may constitute a danger to believers by denying Christian revelation (*Nasz Dziennik* 2003). Sometimes, so-called biomagic was mentioned by the Bishops of the Polish church. For example Bishop Edward Frankowski, in his homily delivered in the Jasna Góra Sanctuary on 15 July 2000, stated *inter alia* that, 'It is a sin – our helplessness in the face of all manipulators, yielding to their most foolish, primitive and meanest suggestions and ideas [...] when we are feeling very ill we fall into the traps set by various charlatans and healers' (Nasz Dziennik 2000: 12). When summing up the results of studies, M. Gajewski, Director of the Center for Research on New Religions "Rafael", says, 'Non-conventional medicine is not entirely verifiable. Those who practice it do not have any reliable qualifications. They are very often quack doctors' (Żukowska 2001:4). Gajewski stresses: 'By contrast, a bioenergy therapist is someone who has become sensitized to energy, he can manipulate and control it [...] No one is able to measure this energy. We do not know if it exists [...] Criticism of non-conventional medicine should run at least two ways. On the one hand, we should evaluate such practices from the scientific and rational standpoint, whether they are well-founded in medicine or physics. The other way is theological and dogmatic criticism. We are asking to what extent they – bioenergy therapists, folk doctors, pseudo-medics – indeed offer help in treating the body, and how much they exceed their competence entering the area of the spirit [...]' (Ibid: 4). Another kind of argument against the manifestations of the 'powers of evil' at work was advanced by a Licheń sanctuary exorcist, 'One of the most harmful actions of the Satan, into which man lets himself be drawn, is occultism and divination, spiritualism, Satanism, sorcery, magic and superstitions. Utilization of services offered by fortune-tellers, astrologists, healers, and the practices of parapsychology and magic rituals [...] open man to the actions of demons' (Czaczkowska 2004: A4)

To sum up the foregoing remarks, we can treat them as a kind of introduction to and comment on the problems on the borderline between medical sociology and religious sociology. The Catholic Church appears skeptical about the problem of miraculous healings and the activities of various healers, especially spiritual ones, although it observes, analyzes and assesses the new phenomena in the area defined by the concepts: health – illness – faith. Utilization of services provided by charlatan-healers is sometimes regarded as idolatry because magical practices and invocation of 'secret gods and energies' tend to be used to dominate patients and to manipulate their behaviors (Baranowski 2005:10). We will now discuss the borderline area between medical sociology and religious sociology (Libiszowska-Żółtkowska 1998: 39 et seq.). Until the 1990s, research areas determined by the terms 'family' and 'health' were not regarded as complementary concepts; similarly, the terms 'religion' and 'health and illness' were treated as incompatible fields. In actual fact, as M. Libiszowska-Żółtkowska observes, these spheres complement and overlap with one another. It is commonly accepted that a natural characteristic of the development of each discipline (including sociology) is progressive specialization and a growing number of subdisciplines; on the other hand, a side effect of this phenomenon is the excessive partitioning of the reality presented and the rise of somewhat artificial barriers between individual areas of social life described by particular specialist disciplines.[21] Suffering, which accompanies illness, disability, or impairment is treated in Christianity as a way to salvation and reformation, while God's forgiveness gives one a chance to recover (Libiszowska-Żółtkowska 1998: 40). For their part, medical sciences try to reduce pain and suffering, and attempt to control such psychophysical conditions in order to eliminate them. Pain and suffering are something dysfunctional: 'the sacrifice of pain is not necessary'. Emphasis is placed on a special paradox of the development of knowledge-based civili-

21 It appears that we were dealing with a similar situation at the end of the 1980s and in the early 1990s when, on the initiative of Professors M. Sokołowska and Z. Tyszka we started interdisciplinary studies on the borderline between medical sociology and family sociology (see Firkowska-Mankiewicz 1990)

zation, whose element is contemporary medicine: the more rational the world is as a result of scientific development, the more a great number of people feel a growing need to seek thaumaturgical, esoteric, magical sensations. Changes in culture and in morals (*inter alia* the fashion for New Age philosophy) have also given rise to a growing interest in alternative medicine. A religious sociologist can discern health themes in '[...] confessions derived from Adventist, Pentecostal, or Bible student traditions, in the Christian Science association, and in some new religious movements (Ibid: 43). The concepts in question - health and illness, and religion can be analyzed (without blurring their differences) at the same cognitive levels: intellectual, emotional and institutional. In the Catholic Church's teachings, health is presented in the theological dimension (as God's gift) and in the practical dimension (Church-defined rules of conduct towards one's own body and health, and towards the health of other people) (see references to health in the Catechism of the Catholic Church, paras 1293, 1421, 1459, 2010, 2117, 2185, 2275, etc.). In relation to health, religion thus fulfils many functions: explicative and sense-making, normative, controlling, protective, charitable, therapeutic, and healing functions (Libiszowska-Żółtkowska 1998:45-460). References to the New Testament show Jesus as a physician and healer (Matthew 9, 35; Matthew 12, 15). Jesus passed his healing powers onto his disciples. The many Marian centers that have developed since the nineteenth century attract masses of the faithful, including thousands of sick persons, some of whom feel healed. Most often, the healings recorded by the Catholic Church occurred through the intercession of a deceased saint or in the recognized holy places of worship. In the case of the concept in question - healing - a clear transition from passive faith in the healing powers of chosen saints to one's own conscious religious activities (the Catholic Charismatic Renewal) was noticeable. The Pentecostals in turn stress the religious possibility of overcoming illness and the healing role of Jesus. In 1974 the Malines (Belgium) conference, attended *inter alia* by Cardinal Joseph Ratzinger, attempted to develop a model of (physical and spiritual) healing ministry treated as an act not incompatible with medical care. The Catholic Charismatic Renewal avoided public testimonies to healings without reliable evidence; it prohibited the use of special attire or specific characteristic prayers during such practices. The form of healing was praying (also at a distance or without the patient's knowledge) and the gesture of putting on hands. The patient has to meet a number of specified, detailed conditions so that a healing can take place and be effective (Libiszowska-Żółtkowska 1998:49). An interesting phenomenon, studied by both religious sociologists and medical sociologists, was the activities (discussed earlier) of a typical representative of American spiritual healers – Clive Harris, who 'opened Polish parishes to healing practices' (Ibid: 51). Political, cultural and moral changes and the initially permissive attitude of many priests to healing practices resulted in many visits in the early 1990s by priests and monks claiming to be healing practitioners (e.g. Fr. E. Tardif from Canada). Mass services were organized, combining long prayers and healing sessions. Fr. Tardif was able to conduct healing séances with the assistance of the Catholic Charismatic Renewal's All-Polish Coordinator Team and to the Łódź [Lodz] Jesuits. More and more such meetings took place, developing into a form of direct contact with the charismatic healer. Those favorably disposed towards such activities believed that it was an opportunity to overcome the phenomenon of crisis of faith, especially noticeable in urban environments. Healings were presented as the symbol of new, dynamic Christianity taking especially attractive forms for young people. Great achievements in the promotion of a pro-health lifestyle and natural therapies (natural medicine, water treatment, heliotherapy) can be boasted by the Protestant community's Seventh-Day Adventist Church.[22] The healing theme can also be found in the teachings of Christian Science: its principles are set forth in the book *Science and Health with Key to the Scriptures* by Mary Baker-Eddy, the founder of the First Church of Christ the Scientist. She was convinced that healing was possible through faith and the power of the Divine mind. A form of healing consisted of the patient or the healer reading a freely chosen excerpt from *Science and Health* (Piątkowski 1990). The Christian Science movement attaches great importance to revealing and propagating spiritual testimonies to healings through prayer; it also publishes names and addresses of the most effective spiritual healers.

The phenomenon of spiritual healers (especially when they are priests) is without doubt an interesting subject of inquiry shared by religious sociology and medical sociology. One of the recent editions of the well-known American sociomedical handbook contains a separate chapter devoted to faith healers. W. Cockerham (2004:171-75) writes that they are persons who use the power of suggestion and faith in God to treat others and promote health. The author believes that the efficacy of such treatment generally concerns sociopsychosomatic diseases. He describes five kinds of spiritual healing: self-healing through prayer; healing by a lay person able to communicate with God; treatment by an official religious leader, for whom healing is one of their activities; healing by individuals or groups unrelated to or not associated with religious congregations; and healing by a religious leader, for whom healing treatment is their main and only kind of activity (Christian Science healers). Sociological investigations

22 I invited Adventist physicians to conduct a three-month workshop on healthy diet for UMCS Institute of Sociology students majoring in health promotion. See also G. Kruczek et al. 2001.

show different forms of faith healing practiced in the United States: healing in churches, in houses of prayer, at big meetings with the faithful, or over the radio, by phone, on television, and recently via the Internet. Cockerham points out that some religious groups rely exclusively on diverse healing forms, prohibiting their members from using pharmacy medicines and contacting medical institutions, which may, in cases of severe diseases, lead to conscious refusals to consent to active biomedical treatment and consequently carries the danger of disease progression and the risk of death. In such cases the medical, legal and ethical problem is the discussion of the State's interference in the citizen's personal views and decisions and whether followers of different religions can be subjected to compulsory, treatments without their wish and consent. More recent research in the US on the role of religious factor impacting the course of treatment indicate a great significance of religious faith as an element strengthening for example the patient's immune system, motivating his/her pro-health behaviors, and reducing depression and neuroticism (Ibid).

The questions related to non-medical healing systems appeared in Polish literature on the sociology of health and illness in yet another context, showing the importance attached to it by those conducting key research in this field. For example, under the extensive headword 'medical sciences' in the *Encyklopedia Socjologii* [Encyclopedia of Sociology], Beata Tobiasz-Adamczyk writes *inter alia* 'One of the controversial problems of the present day is "competition" between official medicine and non-conventional medicine, which often derives from folk medicine. To explain the phenomenon of popularity of non-conventional medicine at the time of the rapid development of scientific medicine requires **sociological analysis** [*my emphasis*, W. P.] and reference to insufficient satisfaction with practices applied in official healthcare.' (Tobiasz-Adamczyk 1999, 2: 308). The same author gave a broader treatment to the foregoing research themes, pointing out the interdisciplinary character of the presented issues and the overlapping of different perspectives (sociology of religion, ethnology, history of medicine). Tobiasz-Adamczyk emphasizes, on the one hand, the significance of matters related to 'non-medical healing systems', and on the other, the methodological, terminological and theoretical difficulties that we encounter trying to account for this social phenomenon (Tobiasz-Adamczyk 1998, 4: 111-113). The key question, she contends, that the sociologist investigating the problems in question needs to ask should concern the limits of the term 'non-medical healing systems', making a distinction between methods that do not produce dispute or controversy in the medical community and others that do arouse criticism from biomedicine. Another problem is the criteria that differentiate medicine from non-medicine. [These questions have been dealt with in detail in this book]. One more key problem concerns the reasons why patients choose non-conventional therapies in a period of rapid development of medicine as science and the modern technologies that it employs. The demand that the causes of popularity of 'other medicine' in modern societies be explained was strongly emphasized. Tobiasz-Adamczyk (like A. Ostrowska) appears to attach special importance to changes in patient-physician interactions (2002: 128-130). In her opinion the reason why people shun institutional medicine may take the form of a syndrome made up of many constituents, including the following: dissatisfaction of some patients with the content and character of doctor-patient interaction; family tradition (associated with the practice of self-treatment); inefficacy of medicine in treating some (chronic) diseases, discomfort felt by some clients who feel that the physician is focusing mainly on controlling disease symptoms without trying to find out the causes of breakdown in health condition; anxiety about using medicines that the patient distrusts, fears of medicinal products whose action is assessed as too invasive or carrying the risk of undesirable side effects,; and finally, a sense of a deficit of social support by medical personnel (especially in chronic diseases). This discussion emphasizes that there are different variants of utilization of alternative or complementary methods of treatment: occasional experimenting with offers of this type, regular use of 'other medicine', selective attempts to try one or another treatment strategy for one specific disease, etc. The key role in this line of argument is attributed to the features of patient-healer interaction, in that the non-conventional therapist satisfies many emotional needs more effectively than a medical doctor can offer in this area (Ibid: 130).

A different, interesting way of presenting the issues of the sociology of non-medical healing systems is to include these questions in the context of the sociology of illness. Tobiasz-Adamczyk made a comprehensive description of this key research area in medical sociology, presenting a systematization of diverse studies conducted in this field. Investigations may cover the historical context of the rise the sociology of illness with the distinction of description and interpretation of social determinants of diseases, characteristics of illness as a social phenomenon, description of its consequences, and finally, the development of a sociological model of illness. When characterizing the evolution of sociological studies on illness, the following are listed: analyses of the social context of chronic diseases; investigation of the significance of life events; the spheres of lay actions taken in the face of illness; the impact of diseases on the course of everyday life; biographical approach in interpreting the effects of illness; individual perception of illness symptoms; and research into the quality of life of the sick (including the aged). Among the nine main research themes in the area of sociological studies on illness, two were deemed of most significance: the sociology of self-treatment, and seeking alternative forms of help (Tobiasz-

Adamczyk 2005: 36). We should emphasize that inclusion of the issues of non-medical healing systems (and self-treatment) in the context of the already classic sociomedical research area can be regarded as legitimation of this theme in the research mainstream of the subdiscipline.

The foregoing remarks present various themes related to the sociology of non-medical healing systems, which were not systematically analyzed in Polish studies in the sociology of health and illness starting from the 1960s. To sum up, the first studies were based on the results of field research carried out in one of the Podhale villages and showed constant elements in traditional folk medicine and changes taking place in it triggered by the growing modernization processes. It should be emphasized that the results obtained by J. Bejnarowicz showed the comparatively strong and stable position of folk medical systems in the local community investigated. A continuation of such research work was J. Szaro's project, also devoted to characterizing self-treatment and folk medical systems in the early 1970s. The project was implemented in the selected district of Beskid Niski. The author was interested in the position of folk doctors and in the characteristics of the social role that they performed. Traditional folk medical systems turned out to be undergoing further changes (elimination of mystical-magical elements, disappearance of practices of village midwives, etc.); however, the popularity of those non-conventional methods did not diminish but grew to increasingly high levels in some of the investigated regions. Another author, I. Jaguś adopted the sociological-historical perspective in her analyses of folk medical systems. On the basis of legacy materials (official documents, press articles, memoirs and diaries) from the Kielce and Lublin regions, she studied the evolution of folk medical systems over the last century. A turning point in the sociological studies on 'complementary and alternative medicine (CAM) came with the involvement of Magdalena Sokołowska in this work. She made an interpretation of the phenomenon of mass utilization by the healthy and the sick of the service provided by spiritual healer Clive Harris - a sociological analysis of the 'Harris institution'. She showed the changing attitude of the world's medical organizations (WHO) towards utilization of non-physician services by the societies in developed and developing countries; she outlined the main difficulties in studies on this type of problem and indicated the ways of overcoming them. Inspired by Magdalena Sokołowska, this work was continued by M. Kański and S. Wasilewski, who first used the Hessler and Twaddle model and implemented an interesting project of applying a qualitative method (participant observation) to investigate the phenomenon of spiritual healing. In the 1980s the theme of non-medical healing systems was present in large-scale studies by A. Titkow on behaviors and attitudes towards health and illness. The study found that at the end of the 1970s and beginning of the1980s, patients assuming the 'social role of the sick person' had a choice of other, emergent 'alternative sources of help in illnesses. A. Ostrowska, in turn, included the motif of 'complementary medicine' into the description of changes in patient-physician interactions in the early 1980s. An interesting stage in the investigation of the place occupied by 'other medicine' in Polish society was the studies on the borderline between medical sociology and family sociology, coordinated by A. Firkowska-Mankiewicz, which described forms of lay care created by family circles (self-treatment) and by all manner of folk practitioners and healers. Z. Woźniak's field research covered a similar subject. In the early 1990s long-term studies on health behaviors commenced under the supervision of A. Gniazdowski. That project also reported the growing phenomenon of selecting other treatment options than those provided by institutional medicine. It described changes in the sphere of behaviors and attitudes towards health and illness, stressing the features of 'popular awareness' characterized by K. Puchalski. This line of studies also included M. Latoszek's field research on health attitudes and behaviors under the conditions of rapid institutional changes occurring in the healthcare system. An entirely different perspective was opened in the studies by B. Uramowska-Żyto on the theoretical foundations of medical sociology, which described theoretical orientations especially useful in exploring non-medical healing systems: a symbolic interactionist approach, a phenomenological approach and ethnomethodology. Freidson's concept of the lay referral system, inspiring for the sociology of non-medical healing systems, was also characterized. While the subject of 'other medicine' had previously been integrated into the broader context of investigations on the borderline between medical sociology and family sociology, at the end of the 1990s studies on the sociology of religion related to health and illness began. Maria Libiszowska-Żółtkowska initiated an exploration of the problem of 'miraculous healings' and the description of practices by faith healers. Her examinations implied and determined the framework for broader discussion on the attitude of Church institutions and men of the Church towards various non-conventional methods and techniques of treatment. The sociology of non-medical healing systems also found new impetus in the studies by Beata Tobiasz-Adamczyk, from her entry 'medical sciences' in *Encyklopedia Socjologii* [Encyclopedia of Sociology]; here she emphasized the importance of and need for sociological analysis of wide acceptance of non-conventional methods of treatment offered by folk practitioners and then mainly by healers. She also stressed the need to take account of these issues in examining one of the classic sociomedical themes: -physician–patient interactions -and the demand that this area of social reality be investigated in the context of description of the present-day object of 'sociology of illness'.

To sum up, numerous themes associated with non-medical healing systems in various ways were discussed, usually on an ad hoc basis, by diverse authors. However, this key subject matter (as rated by Magdalena Sokołowska) was never the object of systematic and comprehensive socio-medical research. It is that element of diagnosis of the state of art of Polish present-day medical sociology that was the main reason for writing this book, which is an attempt to include the problems in which I have been interested into the canon of the subdiscipline.

2.2. Complementary and Alternative Medicine (CAM) as Interpreted by American and European Sociology of Health and Illness[23]

The goal of this study is to present a monograph of the sociology of non-medical healing systems. That is why the preceding subchapter described in detail the state of research on the subject, referring mainly to literature in Polish. However, we must not forget that from the moment it emerged, the Polish version of the sociology of health, illness and medicine had strong institutional, ideological, and personal ties with its European and American currents. Antonina Ostrowska pointed out these relations, stating that 'this often provoked a question whether we were closer to Europe or the United States. These questions seem to be very far away from the problems of medical sociology yet they show in a more general aspect that Poland's striving to be Westernized always had its separate American and Western European contexts. [...] for many years Western Europe from one side, and the United States from the other, fulfilled model-making functions in Poland in many aspects of life, including science. As for Polish medical sociology, we may ask: where did it derive its main inspirations, theoretical base, or research conceptions from? Do the social forces, which created demand for its studies, diagnoses and expert evaluations, more resemble the American or West European context?' (Ostrowska 2004: 31). The assessment by A. Ostrowska, co-founder of Polish medical sociology, is not only a scientific diagnosis but also an opinion of a 'witness to events' because while working on Magdalena Sokołowska's team, she was involved in many joint editorial, teaching and expertise projects realized by Polish and Western medical sociologists. Another argument for the need to take into account the achievements of European and American medical sociologies in this study is the fact that the first pub-

23 See remarks on the term 'complementary and alternative medicine' on page 19

lications on healing appeared in the US in the 1970s (1977), these conceptions being the reference point for the first Polish sociological studies devoted to non-professional methods of treatment.[24] It is not without significance that M. Sokołowska's publications on 'alternative medicine' referred mainly to Western literature (Sokołowska 1986:83-90). These texts are a major point of reference for me as the author of this book. The subsequent sections of this chapter present the main stages and results of studies on CAM, from the aforementioned innovative conception of Hessler and Twaddle to the textbook treatment of these themes in the 2006 book by Gregory L. Weiss and Lynne E. Lonnquist, *The Sociology of Health, Healing and Illness*. The two publications on the sociology of healing, the former from the 1970s, and the latter from the first decade of the twenty-first century determine the framework and chronology of presentation. We might also add that it is symbolic that the Weiss and Lonnquist 2006 handbook on health and illness (chapter entitled *Complementary and Alternative Medicine*) already indicates in its title that the classic term 'sociology of health, illness and medicine' should be complemented with a new constituent – healing - which shows the growing importance of the sociology of non-medical healing systems within the subdiscipline (Weiss and Lonnquist 2006: 219-243). It is not possible to give a complete presentation of the abundant achievement of Western sociological studies on CAM; consequently, we will only refer to a dozen or so basic concepts and research patterns comprehensively treated in the classic literature on the subject. A complement and supplement to the description of the state of research will be an outline of CAM issues discussed in an important sociomedical journal "Social Science and Medicine" between 2000 and 2007.

The first comprehensive description and interpretation of the healing phenomenon was the extensive chapter *Types of Healers* in the Twaddle and Hessler handbook (1977: 139-159).

The authors begin by emphasizing that the dynamic development of biomedicine in the latter half of the twentieth century created medicocentrism (medicocentric ideology), gaining control over diverse areas of social life and

24 One of the first texts on CAM was the chapter *Types of Healers* in an American handbook of medical sociology. Cf. Twaddle and Hessler (1977: 139-159). Earlier Polish studies on healers referred to the ideas of Twaddle and Hessler (Kański and Wasilewski 1981, 3 (82): 103-118). In 2010 (as has been said earlier) an interesting text by the medical anthropologist Hans A. Baer appeared, which discussed the CAM taxonomy, relations between medical professionals and healer; the text also contained a sociological characterization of patients who chose complementary methods and it analyzed relationships between the medical system and institutions of non-conventional medicine. See H. A. Baer, Complementary and Alternative Medicine… in: Cokerham: 2010: 373-399.

imposing its professional point of view on people in many matters (Ibid: 137). Gradually, the term ‘treatment’ became synonymous with intervention by physicians and, more broadly, by institutional biomedicine. Institutional biomedicine failed to see the fact that in the multiethnic American society there are other traditions of folk medicine practiced by native Americans (Native-American medicine), by Americans of Latin descent (Mexican-American curanderismo) or immigrants from Continental China (Chinese-American medicine). There was also a tendency to ignore faith healing, popular among some ethnic groups, in which therapists often utilized religious and mystical-magical elements. Twaddle and Hessler stress that their conception, which de facto expressed the striving for equal rights for and enhancement of various treatment methods and techniques, may be difficult to accept as it undermines certain stereotypes, habits and patters commonly adopted in developed Western societies. The authors believe it is time to break the information monopoly of medicine and to describe other healing traditions that are not based on the canon of natural science and are not practiced by traditionally trained doctors. Western medicine and its representatives (i.e. representatives of medical professions) must accept the fact that the processes of pluralization, demonopolization, and democratization take place on the health services market, where different entities can provide various treatment offers. Consequently, the rules of competition, rivalry and free choice begin to function, to the apparent advantage of patients (Twaddle and Hessler 1977: 139). In many societies, the process of healing, and practitioners who assume the role of healers, enjoy respect and prestige due to the significance of the actions performed; for that reason healing is one of the most important roles practiced in those communities. Processes of healing have a long history and take many forms (healing systems of the Mayas, the ancient Greeks, etc) but in order to describe diverse versions of healing we need only four basic elements: the symbolic, the technical, theories of disease and/or illness, and social organization of the healing role. The symbolic refers to the healing systems’ past, when the symbols of good and evil were contrasted. The healer’s special attire (e.g. white robes symbolizing good and innocence), his/her characteristic language and the tools (instruments) s/he applies, and communication with the community in which he practices, resemble the elements that Western biomedicine employs in the physician-patient interaction (white coats and stethoscopes as symbols of professional membership and competence, Latin as a hermetic way of communication between doctors, etc.). Symbols in the patient-healer relationship are also important since they communicate to healing service recipients that they are dealing with a highly qualified, honest person of great prestige, who is, therefore, thus trustworthy (Ibid: 140). Another descriptive category is technical factors. This is a combination of diverse therapeutic methods and medicinal substances used by the healer. Elements of this type are for example special herbal cures or the therapist's healing power. Healing techniques are modified depending on whether the therapist diagnoses an ailment as internal or, conversely, external. Therefore, different therapeutic procedures will be used in curanderismo, chiropractic, and faith healing. In healing practices, it is diagnosis that largely determines the manner and strategies for treatment. Another element connected with the ways of treatment by the healer is the theories of diseases that he accepts. Etiological conceptions are especially significant because it is they that imply the use of specific symbolic and technical elements. All these are subordinated to a belief that some assumed factor/factors is/are the main cause of the disease treated by a particular healer. Theories of diseases (causes of health disorders, or conditions of ill-being) explain two classes of phenomena: they say what the cause of the poor state of health is and make it possible to precisely classify diseases that a therapist is treating. The causes of typical diseases in the healing practice may be based on taking into account the following factors: natural, human (disease as evil done by another man) and supernatural. Other healing traditions name five basic disease categories: magical (witchcraft, disease is deliberately caused by a person using sorcery); breaking of taboo - illness is the result of divine punishment for violation of religious or social norms; illness is caused by penetration of the organism by foreign substance detrimental to health; illness is the effect of the presence of an evil spirit (demon) in the patient's body; finally, illness may be the result of soul loss, the soul leaving the patient's body. Theories of causes of disease are meant to explain to the patient in a simple and clear way why people fall ill (and sometimes die) and how they can be treated effectively and healed permanently. One more element of healers' practice is the social organization of healing. Apart from symbols, treatment techniques, and theories of the causes of disease causes, there has to be a socially acceptable behavior pattern enabling the healer to start treatment in a particular community. A classic example is the patient-healer relationship, both in its expressive and instrumental dimensions. The essential element of this interaction is that the healer has to understand the causes that make a patient come to a specific healer, the diagnosis of the healer's expectations from a patient also being important. If there is a close relationship between the two sides, the efficacy of therapy may be higher. The expectations of both sides sometimes remain divergent (for various reasons) and are sometimes contradictory, which practically prevents the spiritual healer from starting treatment (Twaddle and Hessler 1977:142-143). Another determinant of healing efficacy is the healer's prestige in a society; high prestige which usually raises the patient's level of faith, trust and expectations in regard to the treatment process. When the patient has similar experience and represents a similar system of values and preferences to those of the healer, therapy can be certainly more successful. At the same time Twaddle and Hessler emphasize differences between the healer's and the physician's social role, showing a separate character of educational training and different understanding of the terms 'science' and 'magic' by both parties. The conclusion of the foregoing argumentation is the opinion that present-day patients will have more frequent opportunities to choose (and change) preferred forms of treatment, deciding to utilize 'Western orthodox medicine' or diverse 'alternative or complementary forms of healing', or most often choosing the two parallel forms of help in illness. For the goals of the book, the most interesting remarks are those of the above-cited medical sociologists on the method termed 'spiritual healing'. This method of treatment or its main elements resemble the previously presented procedures used by healers who were the subject of my studies – C. Harris and A. M. Kashpirovsky; it is also very close to bioenergy therapy, which is very popular in Poland. Hessler and Twaddle believe that this oldest method of treating the soul and body is universal (many cases of faith healing combined with the technique of laying on of hands were described in the Old and New Testaments) and at present, paradoxically, it is enjoying increasing popularity in the secular Western societies. Healers who invoke the therapeutic power of prayer or religious faith are usually associated with some concrete religious community or church, but there are also therapists without such affiliations. Most often such persons (which is the case with Harris) do not attribute to themselves any special healing powers; they rather emphasize that they are a kind of transmitter of God's will, who has given them the ability to treat people effectively. Many such healers felt a sudden vocation for healing; they then gave up their professional careers and family lives in order to devote themselves to the sick. Twaddle and Hessler refer to many testimonies of individual spiritual healers, who described the beginnings of their vocation to serve the sick (Ibid 143-144). In the previous chapter, while discussing Polish studies on non-medical healing systems, we characterized the Hessler and Twaddle conception in its version adjusted to Polish sociocultural realities by M. Kański and S. Wasilewski. At this point we are showing the whole of the original idea. Most religious symbols used in spiritual healing are of a religious or para-religious character (prayers, sweeping robes resembling liturgical vestments, crosses, etc.). The most important aspect of contact is prayers, which constitute a special kind of bridge between God with His healing power and the therapist who sees his person as 'an instrument in the hands of God'. Some healers of this type are so convinced of the efficacy of their skills that they do not even expect their clients to believe in the success of treatment (Ibid: 145). Many of the best-known healers formalize and institutionalize their activities, setting up special foundations, creating their own programs in the media and on websites, in order to legitimate and strengthen their position in a community. The fundamental technical element is the therapeutic touch and numerous variants of the laying on of hands. The moment of touching is not only the moment of establishing physical contact with the patient but also the symbol of focusing and concentration. Touch can have different forms including touching the temples, forehead and the back of the head; it may also be combined with other gestures, such as crossing oneself with the sign of the cross, anointing with oils, etc. Technical elements are modified depending on whether interaction is a face-to-face relationship or in the form of contact with large groups of patients at big meetings; such relationships can be also indirect (e.g. via the media as was the case with Z. Nowak or A. Kashpirovsky) (Ibid: 146). The Hessler and Twaddle model devotes most room to theories of disease causes. The authors point out that there are four basic etiological conceptions (or combinations thereof) in healing: spiritual, psychological, biomedical and parapsychological. Explanations that invoke spiritual elements emphasize the role of sin as the cause of loss of divine grace, and the occurrence of illness as a result. Psychological theories are more frequent and more widespread; they emphasize the importance of the stress factor as the main cause of sociopsychosomatic diseases and mental health disorders. Stressors may have diverse causes, e.g. conflicts of roles, or awareness of needs without fulfilling them. Biomedical theories emphasize that diseases may be caused by material factors (viruses, bacteria, traumas). Healers attaching importance to these causes seem to appreciate biomedical achievements and are inclined to advise their patients to continue contact with institutional medicine. Spiritual healers who profess these etiological views often cooperate with psychiatrists in particular. Healers often express an opinion that the future of medicine belongs to holistic conceptions, which they find particularly close to their position. When they are dealing with, for example, motor organ injuries, these therapists suggest that their clients first contact an orthopedic surgeon or traumatologist in order to start effective treatment; in this variant a spiritual healer can only support the process of treatment or convalescence. A similar kind of doctor-healer cooperation is especially desirable in the treatment of psychogenic diseases, where cooperation between healers and psychiatrists is possible or sometimes even necessary. Of parapsychological theories, the most influential among spiritual healers are the conceptions of Gross and Rolle, which draw upon the elements of Jung's psychology (Ibid: 149). In this approach, emphasis is placed on energy that arises and accumulates between the healer and the patient during big meetings, it is then that some participants in therapeutic meetings may experience revelations or fall into a trance. Healers believe that, at this moment, an exchange of energy occurs between spirit and body, between mind and psyche. Healers emphasize that it is God who acts through them, and they are only His instrument. The Creator also ultimately decides whether He will bestow His grace on someone and heal them. When asked about the mechanism of spiritual healing, healers answer that it is God who is exclusively responsible for the therapy and its success. Another element is the organization of the healing process. The overwhelming majority of spiritual healers are solo practitioners, some of them working with individual patients, others healing large patient groups at the same time; others such as C. Harris use both techniques alternately. During individual sessions, therapists usually want to learn as much as they can about a patient's personal problems that may be related to his/her health. With mass audiences the therapist's knowledge about individual diseases of participants is next to nothing. Healing can be effected for example on several patients randomly selected from the audience or the therapists might touch for several seconds the sick organ of each person in the queue of session participants. The financial aspect of the organization of a healing session is also important. Those participating are informed beforehand that they have to make offerings (most often without the sum of money being specified). Experienced healers also use conscious or unconscious psychotechnical or sociotechnical manipulations in order to control the crowd and try to make use of the influence of a mass audience to initiate healing (self-healing) processes. When organizing various kinds of sessions, technical means (radio, television, telephone) are employed more and more frequently, which enables contact between one therapists and the mass audiences expecting his/her help (Ibid: 150).

The Twaddle and Hessler conception was the first comprehensive attempt to interpret healing practices, which were becoming increasingly accepted in the US in the mid-1970s. Despite the growing secularization tendencies in this liberal society, many patients increasingly sought help from spiritual healers. Their services are utilized not only by people of poor financial standing, or belonging to ethnic minorities (Native Americans, Chinese-American and Mexican-American families) but also by many Anglo-Saxon upper- and middle-class Protestants. Since the 1970s, modern Western institutional medicine has paid more and more attention to other healthcare and healing systems developing outside its paradigms and its tradition of helping in illness. According to Hessler and Twaddle, an important objective of natural and behavioral sciences should be to thoroughly investigate these kinds of activities. Highly specialized medicine, based on advanced technologies, could be reformed by adopting a holistic perspective, useful both in building new theories of treatment and making medical practice more effective. Such changes would make it possible to better learn the patient's emotional and spiritual needs, and thereby provide him/her with better care and help during treatment and convalescence.

Another example of comprehensive research on and interpretation of CAM in American medical sociology are Michael Goldstein's analyses. His text reports on and sums up his studies in the 1980s and 1990s (Goldstein 2000: 363-372). In the 1990s the popularity of 'other' medicine in the US grew systematically, having been triggered by a wave of enthusiastic publications in the opinion-forming high-circulation media, which announced the advent of the healing revolution. For example, a panel of expert organized by "Time Magazine" and "Newsweek" forecasted that the canon of helping in illness would radically change because non-conventional healing systems would assist in treating the majority of diseases, from trivial and frequent to life-threatening conditions. The analysis of the social phenomenon, which was the growing wave of interest in and acceptance of 'unorthodox medical practices' emphasized the immense role of the commercial media, which publicized, promoted and encouraged utilization of alternative medicine services. The press and the Internet published tens of thousands of usually favorable items providing information on CAM. The book by one author alone - D. Chopra's *Ageless Body, Timeless Mind, The Quantum Alternative to Growing Old* has sold seven million copies since 1993 (Ibid: 364). A very important factor that enhanced interest in and even fascination with CAM were testimonies of well-known public figures (actors, film directors, pop culture stars, journalists) who abandoned conventional medicine for alternative methods: 'some of the media attention and popular concern comes form the vivid personal testimony offered on behalf of various alternative treatments. Celebrity accounts have received a good deal of attention' (Ibid). Public debate on the equal legitimacy of both treatment systems and the rights due to CAM was also provoked by well-known literary critic Norman Cousins and became the symbol of fashion for utilization of what Cousins termed 'better medicine'. In the "New England Journal of Medicine" he contended that the hospital as a symbol of biomedicine was not a good place for the sick (Cousins 1976, 295: 1458-1463; and Colt 1996: 35-50). Apart from journalistic articles, in the 1990s reports were first published on surveys carried out on representative samples of the US adult population, showing the scope and reasons for the growing popularity of non-conventional medicine. It turned out that, in the 1990 surveys, one third of Americans declared that they had personal experience of CAM utilization (Goldstein 2000: 365). The predominant users of treatment strategies of this kind (1997) proved to be wealthy, well-educated middle-class whites, who accounted for 42% of users of 'other medicine'; two thirds of them did not inform their family doctor about this, and those who used the services of non-conventional practitioners visited their offices 19 times a year on average. According to the 1997 survey this amounted to a total of 629 million appointments, which cost US$ 27 billion (Ibid: 366). For example, one third of patients suffering from chronic back pain chose the help provided by non-conventional medicine as part of chiropractic. Goldstein points out that it is difficult to carry out sociological studies on CAM because of unsolved taxonomic problems, which prevent *inter alia* a precise answer to the question of where alternative (complementary) medicine ends and biomedicine begins. Such specific questions arise when classifying medicinal herbal treatments. Is this a method of non-medical healing systems or of biomedicine? It should be observed that CAM has so far defended itself successfully against strict supervision and control by evidence-based medicine, e.g. by trying to use unclear, blurred and imprecise terms to describe its methods, and by claiming that the efficacy and safety of CAM methods cannot be assessed when applying the criteria and methods of empirical natural sciences. Despite these controversies, Americans' confidence in the CAM-provided methods and techniques of treatment grew during the 1990s. This was due to the expert opinion of the working group appointed by the National Institutes of Health (NIH) in 1996, which recommended that more attention be paid to the use of non-conventional methods with a view to combating the HIV/AIDS epidemic. Similarly, permissive reactions were observable in the strategies of large insurance companies, which decided in the mid-1990s to refund medical expenses that their clients incurred when seeking help from non-conventional therapists (Ibid: 367). The response of the medical system at that time to CAM expansion was generally approving and favorable, with most doctors allowing such methods within specified limits. On the other hand, persons who were not physicians or medical students could not be members of some CAM-promoting organizations (this practice is obligatory for example in the American Holistic Medical Association). In Goldstein's studies another central issue was the attempt to explain the rapid development in popularity of alternative and complementary methods in the 1990s, considering they had been known in the US for over a century. Goldstein (as do we in reference to Poland in this book) sees two main reasons: changes occurring in social life and in transformations of contemporary medicine. The lasting dysfunction of biomedicine applies to its sociopsychological rather than technological aspects, such as arrogance, distance towards patients, disregard for their emotional needs and growing skepticism of patients towards the iatrogenic medical industry, which generates huge costs while failing to visibly reduce mortality from killer diseases. The continuing criticism of the 'biomedical empire' fuelled by influential US antimedical movements and patients' rights organizations resulted in diminished prestige of medicine and stronger criticism of it (Ibid: 369). An important question from the perspective of social sciences is whether and to what extent the CAM development will change the paradigms of contemporary medicine and move its boundaries further on so that it will include previously barely-tolerated or rejected methods of treatment. Is CAM a permanent social phenomenon or rather a fashionable trend promoted by the popular media, marketing and advertising? It is a fact that the CAM complex produces specific social and psychological phenomena but they have not yet been sufficiently verified by biomedicine and, more broadly, by contemporary natural sciences. Ecological and alterglobalist movements, ideas of the New Left, feminist demands, popularity of new religious movements and New Age ideology, and growing skepticism about biomedicine, which was partly caused by all the abovementioned factors, for the first time put doctors in a situation of real competition: this movement is not only *not* on the defensive but is also boldly entering the areas formerly reserved for medical professionals. As a result, medicine has been forced to develop and apply new strategies to remain functional and retain the ability to adapt. In the US in the period in question, medicine chose an approach of cooperation rather than conflict and struggle. Although we are observing this phenomenon in the making, there is no doubt that the development and social acceptance of CAM produced lasting changes in US society and led to transformations in the whole system of healthcare. Michael Goldstein's position demonstrates that, over the last twenty years, a spontaneous social grass-roots movement for granting equal rights to CAM has arisen in the United States. It was public pressure that forced the Federal Authorities to establish the Office of Alternative Medicine at the National Institutes of Health. There is no doubt therefore that the complex of social, cultural or even political phenomena produced by CAM expansion should be the object of systematic sociological inquiry.

M. Goldstein's studies are among those most cited in sociological literature on CAM. We will now see how this author's view evolved over the last several years (Goldstein 2000: 284-297). In his later research he studied reactions of medicine (transformations of the medical system, of doctor-patient interaction, medical institutions and medical professions) to the growing popularity of CAM. The starting point are the facts given by the Editors of the "Journal of American Medical Association", who recognized CAM as the third most important subject matter out of 86 discussed in the journal in the second half of the 1990s. We should add at the same time that in the survey conducted among JAMA readers (mainly doctors) CAM rated third out of 73 subjects regarded as important for the development of medicine (Ibid: 284). Goldstein emphasizes that in the mid-1970s such popularity was surprising to many American medical sociologists. For example, the second edition of the popular American handbook *The Handbook of Medical Sociology* of 1972 devoted only one short paragraph to this subject in the chapter entitled *Limited, Marginal and Quasi Practitioners* (Ibid). This was only a brief essay about the struggle of doctors and pharmacists against non-conventional therapists, when the problem of biomedical dominance and expansion appeared marginal at the time. The fourth edition of the same handbook omitted the subject altogether because its authors concluded that the phenomenon was merely historical. It was only in the 1980s and 1990s that American medical sociology again noticed the complex of problems produced by the growing social acceptance of CAM. In the mid-1990s it was recognized that CAM could be analyzed e.g. through a prism of the progressive process of institutionalization and formalization of 'other' medicine (it was observed that around CAM new institutions were established, training systems developed, specialist periodicals founded, achievements certified, efficacy assessments recorded etc). It was also emphasized that an interesting research perspective might emerge from analysis of public reactions to CAM expansion (the establishment of Federal institutions for non-conventional medicine, evolution of the US Supreme Court decisions, or CAM-induced changes in commercial insurance systems) Another set of subjects is the description and interpretation of changes in the medical system as a result of the emergence of a new offer on the healthcare provision market. Goldstein maintains that all these circumstances make sociological research on CAM of increasing importance (Ibid: 285).

The key point in studies on the subject in question is the discussion of differences between evidence-based medicine and non-medical healing systems (e.g. CAM). Goldstein's definition of CAM in his studies is based on the following differences between the two traditions of treatment:

1. CAM is not taught at major medical schools.
2. The grounds for the functioning of such methods cannot be explained within the laws and rules generally respected by biomedicine.

In his book Goldstein also presents the most important features of CAM methods:

a) Subscribing to holistic ideas; consequently we take into consideration, at the same time and to an even extent, psychical (spiritual) and social elements in explaining health- and illness-related phenomena; pathological mechanisms are unique in each patient; greater interest is taken in the patient during treatment than in a particular disease. These features are especially important in US society, which highly values uniqueness and individualism of the human being.
b) The principle of interpenetration of mind, body and soul as the foundation of CAM; this feature accounts for the high social acceptance of non-conventional methods, while it is criticized by representatives of 'orthodox biomedicine'. CAM also emphasizes the significance of faith and the spiritual as factors which are the source of health. Surveys conducted on American national samples (Time/CNN, 1996; Gallup Poll, 1997) stress the immense role of religious factors in US society. For most Americans, faith and personal prayer is a factor that

increases chances of recovery and convalescence. Thus, the values professed by American society and CAM priorities largely overlap.

c) The majority of Americans believe that, by practicing CAM, they have an opportunity to improve their mental condition and enhance the potential for wellness. The founders of CAM also believe that health is something more than simply absence of illness; the system stresses the individual, subjective dimension of health and the fact that anyone, regardless of their physical condition, can feel well and define their goals and priorities in this field. From the sociological standpoint it is also important that CAM's philosophy of health is consistent with the main characteristics of the American lifestyle and system of values.
d) Vitalism: the concept of life as energy flow. In the majority of holistic CAM systems the central term is 'energy', its character, flow and potential (chiropractic, Ayurveda, traditional Chinese medicine, and the like). Evidence–based medicine almost entirely ignores and disregards this constituent, so significant in the ordinary American's interpretation of health and illness.
e) The element that distinguishes biomedicine from CAM to the greatest extent is views on the essence of the healing process. Unconventional healing requires the patient's active cooperation during the treatment process, joint responsibility for a therapy, recognition of joint definitions of health and illness, and close patient-healer relationships ('the main reason for healing is love) (Ibid: 286-287). We should add that various social movements and ideologies redefine the concept of healing in their own way, most often accepting the CAM approach (New Age, ecologism, the New Left, gay rights movement, etc.).

In Goldstein's views (at different stages of his research work) there is a recurrent theme of professionalization of the social movement that developed around CAM. We will return to the subject once again. Professionalization in the CAM domain manifests itself in different ways: building of organizational infrastructure (e.g. the American Holistic Medical Association, American Association of Holistic Nurses), the entry of chiropractic and osteopathy into the network of US medical institutions, or the establishment of the National Institutes of Health Office of Alternative Medicine. Despite these changes and transformations, Goldstein emphasizes, the acceptance of CAM by the ordinary physician is not very high. The months-long discussion in the "New England Journal of Medicine" did not culminate in a radical change of attitudes towards non-conventional methods: most doctors remained skeptical or expressed ambivalent opinions. Critics repeated once again that at the end of the twentieth century and after the year 2000 many methodologically correct studies had been conducted to assess the efficacy of the best-known non-conventional methods and it turned out that many such methods and techniques of treatment either could not be scientifically verified or yielded negative results when tested. On the other hand, ordinary clients utilizing services of 'other' medicine are not particularly interested in reports on the subject, and if they indeed seek information, they do so via the Internet, taking part in discussion forums or using Wikipedia (some sites devoted to alternative medicine register over 90 thousand visits per day in the US). What are the forecasts for CAM then? Goldstein asserts they are good – its driving force is the continuing acceptance and trust of patients (clients) for over 15 years. This increases the economic capacity of these methods: the sick, and more and more frequently, the healthy who seek ways to enhance their wellness potential through CAM, usually make parallel use of both types of medicine at the same time. The change in the picture of diseases indicated by social epidemiology – the growing number of patients suffering from sociopsychosomatic, geriatric and chronic diseases – provides an opportunity for the existence and development of complementary methods in the twenty-first century. We will look once again at the reaction of medical sociology to social problems produced by CAM. As has been said earlier, in the mid-1990s many American medical sociologists viewed the CAM complex with reservations as a phenomenon diverging from the standards accepted in modern societies (medicalization, professionalization of medical services, dominant position of biomedicine); the problem was regarded as deviant and foreign. The direction of discussion at that time (as was the case in Poland) tended more towards labeling non-medical methods rather than trying to carry out a more in-depth analysis. The popularity of the methods was attributed to a fashion for 'irrational' ideas; it was explained that there were special 'cultural niches' in society that were filled by non-conventional views on health and illness. At this point the CAM offer was allegedly targeted at insolvent and uninsured members of ethnic and religious minorities (including illegal immigrants, e.g. in California). The forecasts that interpreted the CAM movement as a temporary transient fashion did not come true. That is why at present, Goldstein believes, the sociology of health and illness should devote more room to analyzing this complex of phenomena and processes. Studies have to show CAM in the broad context of micro-, meso- and macrosocial transformations. The second point of reference is the changes and transformations of the contemporary medical system (comprehensively presented by S. Nettleton as seven factor groups that make up biomedicine, to which we will return further on in this subchapter). According to Goldstein, medical sociology can and must continue investigations into CAM and include them into its mainstream inquiries.

Apart from the earlier views of A. C. Twaddle and R. M. Hessler, and of M. Goldstein, longitudinal studies on 'the other current of medicine' were carried out by William C. Cockerham, who devoted an extensive chapter to the phenomenon in the next editions of his handbook *Medical Sociology* (Cockerham 2004: 167 et seq.). He asserts that his investigations show a general trend towards gradual convergence of evidence-based medicine with some methods and techniques of treatment that were previously situated on the borderline between medicine and non-medicine, a good example being osteopathy. Cockerham repeats that the method (and its specific 'philosophy of treatment') was regarded as charlatanry by doctors as late as sixty years ago. Proponents of 'osteopathic manipulations' are currently taking effective legal and administrative measures in order to gradually include osteopathy into mainstream medicine. A specialist national institution was established to represent and lobby for this method of treatment (American Osteopathic Association), a professional training system was introduced (including doctoral programs), many agencies were set up in particular states to monitor the quality of work of such therapists, osteopathy was registered as part of the American Medical Association (AMO), and osteopaths (osteopathic physicians) are treated as certified specialists in adjunctive therapy in orthopedics and traumatology of the motor organ (Ibid:168). Cockerham's figures show that, in 2000, there were 44,605 osteopathic physicians in the US, which constituted 55% of the whole professional group. Like Goldstein, Cockerham attempted to define CAM as practices **generally not used** by physicians [*my emphasis*, W. P.]. Another characteristic of these methods is that their practical usefulness and safety standards have not been verified, also we do not know whether these methods help or do harm or whether they are neutral to the course of physiological processes (in which case they would be ineffective from the biomedical standpoint). The author emphasizes that another characteristic is that they are mainly based on subjective testimonies by satisfied patients (Ibid: 169) (the same syndrome was noted in my own studies on the Kashpirovsky phenomenon. Like Goldstein, Cockerham points out a paradox relating to the patients' positive attitude to CAM – this is a kind of advance confidence. Both authors give a similar diagnosis that insufficient importance was attached by medical sociology to non-conventional methods (this is not that there were too few sociological studies - in 1995-2005 as many as several hundred were conducted but rather that the quality of research projects implemented was not satisfactory) (Ibid: 170). Cockerham's conception also stresses the elements of change in lifestyle regarding health and illness. American patients are more and more educated (through the Internet), creative and self-confident, as well as taking the initiative and control in health matters; they are also increasingly responsible and value their own autonomy in this field. They are also the people who consciously experiment with their own health, trying out diverse conventional and non-conventional therapies while treating the same or different diseases. In the US we can distinguish several patient categories, who utilize the US we can distinguish several patient categories, who utilize CAM for various reasons. Some are members of the upper and middle classes who wish to be trendy by using fashionable treatments (New Age Medicine); at the same time they also use conventional practices even if they are only partly satisfied with them. The most frequent methods are Ayurveda, traditional Chinese medicine, and homeopathy. The second group comprises persons with a lower-class background who use these treatments for religious reasons, due to cultural affinity and because of the comparatively low cost of treatment (Ibid: 170, 176). A large group of non-conventional practices has increasingly diversified over the last decade. As has been shown above, osteopathy, as the least controversial, was practically absorbed by medicine (observe that the price was the loss of its special 'philosophy of treatment'). Towards other treatment traditions (naturopathy or, recently, homeopathy) medicine still has unfriendly or ambivalent attitudes: (they are **not generally accepted** by the medical profession [*my emphasis*, W. P.], Cockerham 2004: 183). The popularity of these methods in society, Cockerham believes, generally stems from the fact that non-conventional therapists can fulfill emotional and sociopsychological needs of today's patients better than physicians. To sum up, we can conclude that the more the patient's important needs are not be satisfied by biomedicine, the greater the popularity of and trust in CAM treatments will be. Of course, there are no simple relationships: various mediating factors play a role here (this relationship certainly does not obey the simple physical rule of communicating vessels).

A kind of unifying brackets that join together the old and recent studies on the sociology of non-medical healing systems is the handbook *The Sociology of Health,* ***Healing*** [*my emphasis* W. P.] *and Illness* (2006). Observe, firstly, that the term healing was used in the title of a sociomedical monograph for the first time, which, as Cockerham predicted, symbolizes the growing importance of these issues (Weiss and Lonnquist 2006: 219-243). Its authors adopted the same system of problem presentation as Goldstein's book did when discussing differences between CAM and EBM, characterizing the most popular treatment techniques (chiropractic, osteopathy, acupuncture, faith healing, and folk medical systems of selected ethnic groups), but new research themes also appear here, which we will emphasize. At the beginning of the handbook we read that CAM does not have proven standards of effectiveness and predictable safety of the treatments provided. Evidence-based medicine emphasizes these deficiencies but this is also a fact that it is not exclusively the struggle for scientific truth on its part but first of all the struggle for power, cultural hegemony and its own economic interests (Ibid; 220). The book also provides new information from the "National Health Interview Survey" of 2006 on the range of CAM utilization in the US. The survey shows that 36% of adult Americans use some forms of non-conventional treatment from time to time or regularly (Ibid: 221). If we added to this group those who use prayers or practice all kinds of 'megavitamin' treatments, the percentage of patients utilizing such methods would rise to 62%. It should be stressed that, each year, Americans spend more money on non-conventional methods than on biomedicine (Ibid). Like Goldstein, Weiss and Lonnquist accentuate the complementary rather than alternative model of use of non-medical methods, which is termed the dual model of medical care. They also emphasize psychological aspects, pointing out that the healer can often create a more intimate, warmer atmosphere of interaction, following the rule of more words, closer relationship and more sympathy. This variant of course requires the healer to devote far more time to his patients (the healer-patient interaction is on average four times as long as the analogous physician-patient relation) (Ibid: 223). In countries with a market system of health services provision, which prefer pluralism and respect freedom of choice, one cannot arbitrarily impose or force a particular treatment option on people; yet on the other hand, each citizen has the right to reliable, accurate and objective information (even critical) about the methods that s/he chooses. There is still no such information about some CAM methods.

The foregoing section has presented the main currents in sociological research on complementary and alternative medicine; the most representative and most cited interpretations chosen were those by R. M. Hessler and A. C. Twaddle, M. Goldstein, W. C. Cockerham, and G. L. Weiss and L. E. Lonnquist. The studies were conducted according to a similar research pattern; that is why certain repetitions were unavoidable in this presentation. The continuing popularity of CAM cannot be viewed as surprising because this kind of 'other' medicine is deeply embedded in the American system of values and culture. On the other hand, the ordinary consumer of health services tends to be better informed about the deficiencies, imperfections and even threats involved when utilizing biomedicine. This 'black side of medicine' is today widely known owing to consumer movements and initiatives for patients' rights, and due to better, speedier and more complete access to information on health and illness, which influences people's behavior in these conditions. When forecasting future trends in the American health services market, one of the best-known medical sociologists J. McKinlay predicts that, by 2015, non-conventional medicine provision will be a permanent health-related offer, especially with regard to such treatment methods and techniques as chiropractic, naturopathy and acupuncture (McKinlay 2006).

We will now look at the subject of the sociology of non-medical healing systems from the standpoint of European sociomedical thought. As before, we will ignore contributory texts and reports but will focus on comprehensive presentations in the classic handbooks of our discipline. One of these is the book by Sara Nettleton, *The Sociology of Health and Illness* (Nettleton 1996: 290-214). This volume contains a subchapter entirely devoted to alternative medicine and a sociological interpretation of this social phenomenon. The text is especially interesting for us because it applies to social and cultural realities in Europe. Like the authors quoted above, Nettleton stresses that the methods outside of biomedicine are nothing new in the United Kingdom: the change relates only to the current scale of this social phenomenon. The history of medicine provides many examples of the development of medical bungling in the nineteenth century. At that time the majority of the population was cut off, mainly for economic reasons, from professional medicine, its quality being not much higher than the methods of bunglers. Under such circumstances, some health- and disease-related needs were fulfilled through traditional folk medical systems and self-treatment. It was only in the first two decades of the twentieth century that the foundations of professional healthcare developed and gradually began to influence the health of ordinary people. The establishment of the National Health Service was a genuine turning point when bureaucratic, centralized, and government–funded biomedicine dissociated itself from non-medicine (Ibid: 210). During the period of development of biomedicine between the 1940s and the 1970s, 'other medicine' was not noticeable and existed on the periphery of the professional medical system. The situation began to change, Nettleton writes, in the last twenty years. At present everything indicates that we are dealing with the syndrome of mutually determining factors: social interest produces mass popularity of CAM and prompts people to use it; consequently patients have more treatment experience, which intensifies social interest, and the circle closes. The biomedical stance towards CAM is evolving: it is clearly being forced by public pressure to treat CAM as a partner, and there is public opposition to discrimination against its methods. Like all the above-cited authors, Nettleton attaches great importance to proper terminology enabling precise description of the complex of issues in question. In British medical sociology the terms 'unorthodox medicine', or 'holistic', 'non-conventional', 'alternative' and complementary' medicine are often used interchangeably, which only compounds the chaos. There are authors, however, who decidedly prefer particular terminology. For example, the sociologist M. Saks is in favor of the term 'alternative medicine' because he believes that this criterion clearly defines the relations of 'other' medicine with EBM. The term 'complementary medicine' is an ill-considered one because, Saks maintains, homeopathy and its assumptions, for example, are entirely inconsistent with the canons of allopathic medicine. The well-known student of CAM, U. Sharma, in turn finds 'complementary medicine' highly suitable because the term symbolizes the possibility of convergence between two traditions of treatment. Like the American scholars, Nettleton emphasizes that it is difficult to determine the scale of public popularity of such methods in the United Kingdom since there are very few representative studies on the subject. A study of consumer preferences conducted by the British Medical Association (BMA) shows that one out of four patients undergoing treatment in the UK utilizes some form of CAM. A survey carried out as part of the Social Trends Project suggests in turn that this ratio is 1: 10. The report stresses that by far the most popular treatments are homeopathy and osteopathy. It is also difficult to calculate exactly the number of practicing healers. Estimates say that the ratio may be 12 therapists per 100 thousand people (Ibid: 211). Another problem in focus was the question about the social reasons for the popularity of CAM. Nettleton emphasizes the problems related to market laws and healthcare economics. Present-day governments are increasingly withdrawing from detailed regulation of the health services system, hoping for the optimal character of market regulations; similarly, the number of provisions concerning the way CAM functions in the United Kingdom are gradually being limited. Other students of the phenomenon, e.g. K. Bakx, seek the reason for acceptance of non-conventional treatment methods in the sphere of culture and ideology: this is, on the one hand, a crisis of faith in activities based on science and high technologies and, on the other hand, the effect of counterculture phenomena, where the use of non-conventional methods symbolizes one's own (self-creative) lifestyle and is proof of one's independence and practice of fashionable, pro-ecological behaviors. People, especially the Leftist-minded, who are critical of 'medical empires', also maintain that the choice of CAM is a public expression of a no-confidence vote against technochemical medicine while the use of self-treatment demonstrates conscious choice and refusal to yield to marketing pressure by pharmaceutical corporations. Like the previously discussed results of American research, the British analyses show that the overwhelming majority of clients of non-conventional healthcare services treat such methods as complementary to conventional medicine and visit doctors' offices for parallel treatment (Ibid: 211). Since the UK medical market is increasingly turning into a consumer's market, the chances for further development of non-conventional medicine on the threshold of the twenty-first century are high. Institutional medicine tries to approach the CAM phenomenon in the most adaptive way possible. As early as 1988 British physicians had set up a Working Group, which published the first report on the relations between EBM and CAM. The document reiterated in particular the qualitative differences between evidence-based medicine and its imitations (doctrines 'embracing superstition, magic and the supernatural'). In the report the medical system creates its image as a guarantor of public health quality, taking care of the patient's safety and suggesting that use of treatment techniques of unproven efficacy violates safety standards. That is why, before the patient consciously chooses a treatment option, s/he should obtain complete and competent information about each group of treatments. Another report, this time supported by the British Medical Association, introduced the definition of good practice, which will protect the patient, in the formal-legal sense, against, for example, prolonged treatment for profit-seeking reasons, undue influence by the healer causing patient to terminate treatment by the doctor, etc. The report imposes formal requirements on all non-conventional methods available on the market: the establishment of formal organizational structures associating healers of a particular kind; keeping of accurate registers of members; introduction of the system of training and certification of qualifications; creation of an ethical code and observance of it; and the necessity to conduct systematic research on the efficacy of individual treatment methods (Ibid: 213).

To sum up, Sarah Nettleton described economic, social and cultural changes that constitute the background for treatment methods and techniques developing in the UK outside of institutional technochemical medicine. The author characterized and interpreted the main ways in which the medical system reacted to the expansion of 'other' medicine, with its phases defined by the terms 'open hostility' and 'selective cooperation'. She also pointed out the progressive institutionalization of the CAM system, and the formalization of relations between non-conventional healthcare and evidence-based medicine. (Ibid: 214).

A complementary presentation of problems related to the 'sociology of non-medical healing systems' can be found in the publications by the co-founder of classic medical sociology, Judith Shuval. It was to this scholar that the European Society of Health and Medical Sociology (ESHMS) granted an award in 2006 *inter alia* for studies on CAM (Shuval 2006). The choice by the ESHMS authorities of this subject as the summing up of the 11th ESHMS Congress seems to show the importance of the problems among those studied by contemporary medical sociology (Ibid). In her speech Shuval focused on methodological questions and taxonomic problems (many definitions based on different criteria and inconsistent quality of research on CAM.). We should add that it was the problems of terms and definitions and the structure of internal non-medical methods that were the priority in my investigations, being a serious methodological challenge at the same time. Shuval presented the changing attitude of institutions and medical professions towards non-conventional methods, and described the main ideological currents within CAM, having discussed in detail etiological problems, diagnostic methods, applied variants of prevention and, finally, the views related to treatment philosophy. Like other authors, she listed the characteristics of EBM: being based on empirical grounds, use of standard statistical techniques and methodological rules, rationality as the criterion for deciding what is true and what is false, and acceptance of paradigms generally adopted in sciences. Shuval stresses that when compared with EBM, various theories of healing reveal all their defects. Their strength lies, however, in that they easily fit into the context of trendy holistic and ecological views, and good relations with patients. We can see clearly that the expansion of 'other' medicine into the area of the medical system in Europe is associated with outpatient care rather than with clinical medicine, which does not intend to open itself to CAM (similarly, clinicians are more critical of CAM than family doctors are) (Ibid).

In the 1990s the same author made a synthesis of earlier sociological studies on non-conventional medicine (Shuval 1992: 116-121). She analyzed the models of relations between biomedical structures and CAM. She found that in Europe there are two basic integration models: market-oriented, aiming at the fulfillment of all patient (client) needs, and the system of 'bureaucratic government regulations', functioning in most EU countries (Giarelli 2006:87). In the overwhelming majority of European countries, CAM provision has the character of services parallel to mainstream biomedicine because intensive care units and medical procedure centers do not admit healers to the treatment process practically anywhere in Europe. Similarly, in most EU countries, expenses incurred by patients treated by healers are not refunded by health insurance systems. In Poland and Western Europe there are two kinds of healers: traditional representatives of folk medical systems, and modern 'healing managers', who set up commercial health consortia, use advanced advertising and public relations techniques, practice in large urban areas, and use the Internet, etc. Shuval also tried to describe the social context of CAM in the multi-ethnic Israeli society: when explaining the mechanisms of confidence in non-conventional methods, she emphasized the 'cultural closeness' of the healer and the patient, which appears when the healer uses religious elements and appeals to strong emotions (Shuval 1992: 118 et seq.). When the patient so wishes, it is possible for a healer and a physician to make a joint diagnosis, although this applies chiefly to homeopathy and osteopathy (Ibid: 120).

We will try to sum up the results of research on non-conventional methods conducted by European medical sociologists. At the beginning of this chapter we discussed the connections between Polish and British sociologies of health and illness (Ostrowska 2004: 31 et seq.). Generally speaking, the feature of a good research project is to fit the CAM phenomenon into the context of sociomedical studies or, even more broadly, that of general sociology (as did A. Giddens in his well-known handbook). The research task thus formulated enables analysis of the extent of social popularity of such methods, reasons for public acceptance of CAM, social effects of the emergence of alternative methods on the health services market, the description of social relations between the non-conventional and biomedical systems, characteristics of healer-patient relations, the analysis of the impact of CAM's presence on the functioning of medical institutions and the medical profession, and health insurance systems' reactions to frequent patient utilization of non-medical methods. As the earlier chapters indicate, the non-medical healing systems may be shown from the perspective of a physician, patient and healer, and from the standpoint of the system of social policy (an extremely interesting prospect of sociological studies on non-medical healing was shown by Ursula Sharma and Sarah Cant (Albrecht et al. 2003: 426-439). An important concept, which places the 'healing phenomenon' in the broader sociological context, is the process of 'medicalization' and 'demedicalization'. This complicated complex of factors with its own dynamics took a different course in the countries of advanced capitalism than in post-socialist societies.[25] This process, characteristic of the latter half of the twentieth century, meant the expansion of biomedicine in political, legal, and economic spheres (and in the sphere of dominant paradigms in natural sciences). The system gradually subordinated to itself and appropriated the social sphere around the concepts such as health, illness, treatment, prevention, rehabilitation and health promotion, etc. The power and formal and informal influences of biomedicine have accumulated and expanded; as a result it impacts on more and more aspects of ordinary peoples' lives and their families' lives (microsocial level), through the functioning of government institutions and agencies, the Parliament and the legal system (mesosocial level) and, finally, the state's policy, where one can (or most often cannot) notice the influences of all kinds of biomedical lobbies (macrosocial level). Under these circumstances, medical treatment, taking medicines, and controlling the condition of health in medical institutions are defined and forced upon us as the only culturally accepted manner of behavior. And conversely, failure to utilize biomedical offers (or limited utilization thereof), for example by choosing non-medical healing systems is becoming proof and symbol of civilizational backwardness and therapeutic nihilism, i.e. a reprehensible, careless and imprudent behavior. In this way, commercial, biotechnical and profit-seeking medicine creates a special system of punishments and awards, applies mechanisms of public control, and imposes, more or less directly, a 'medicocentric orientation' and conformism upon a large portion of health market clients. Since the mid-1970s there have been discussions and disputes in the Western world on the limits of 'medical usurpation' in the areas of such clinical disciplines as gynecology and obstetrics, genetics, psychiatry and plastic surgery (even the techniques of 'colonization of the human body' by biomedicine were recognized as classic in the sociology of health and illness). It

---

25 Cf. different definitions of medicalization, e.g. Sokołowska 1986: 224-227, or classical Western interpretation by P. Conrad in Bird et al. 2000; 322-325.

is a kind of paradox that medical expansion and usurpation are taking place when we know perfectly well that most of our health- and illness-related needs are realized outside of medicine, e.g. as part of self-treatment, while the medical system itself has a comparatively negligible impact on society's health condition (Armstrong 2003: 24-35). Therefore, a significant manifestation of medicalization is to define problems that have formerly remained outside of 'the control and power of physicians', and are now under their exclusive supervision (pregnancy, labor, puerperium, states of ill-being, etc.). Medicine first defines a new phenomenon as a problem, then arouses the client's fear and a sense of threat, and finally offers a 'rational' and 'modern' solution in the form of medical intervention, or the use of pharmacotherapy. We can trace these mechanisms precisely, observing the 'rise of new diseases' – ADHD (attention deficit hyperactivity disorder), PMS (premenstrual syndrome), CFS (chronic fatigue syndrome), etc. (Conrad 2000: 322). The 'reverse' of the phenomenon in question is demedicalization. We can assume that the symbolic beginning was the American Psychiatric Association's decision to stop defining homosexuality as a disease, which happened in 1973 (Ibid: 323). Another symbol was the introduction in the mid-1970s of social medicine and epidemiology into public health, followed by the introduction of various versions of holistic conceptions into clinical disciplines. It was these new ecological-social conceptions emphasizing the role of cultural, civilizational, economic and psychological factors that redefined the limits of medicine, trying to partly diminish the area of its influence. Those changes, *inter alia*, in the ways of defining health-related problems as 'medical' and 'non-medical' paved the way for the non-professional mode of treatment (self-treatment, therapeutic practices of healers). The media-publicized new views on 'the philosophy of holistic medicine' also encouraged ordinary people to take over some of physicians' competences in the area of prevention, diagnosis and therapy. Thus, at present there are two parallel ways of 'coping with illness' and two 'medicines', competing to some extent but also complementary. After the long exclusive monopoly of biomedicine, in the countries of the Euro-American culture, during the last thirty years it has not only been doctors who have treated patients, and it has not only been in medical institutions that the therapeutic process has taken place. Consequently, we are dealing with both the process of demedicalization and deprofessionalization of healthcare (Cant and Sharma 2003: 426-427). As we noted earlier, at the meeting point of medicine and 'non-medicine' certain treatment methods and techniques emerged, which had the status of being allied to biomedicine without fully being medicine. Therapists who use them usually work together with physicians, often in medical institutions, although their legal and formal status as 'paramedical professions' is regulated differently in the EU countries. Western societies, more and more pluralist in terms of ethnicity, religion, culture and world-views, are willing to recognize free choice of treatment techniques as an element of lifestyle and the citizen's natural law. Popularization via the Internet and electronic media of the pro-health lifestyle, and even the cult of health (healthism), endeavors to achieve wellness/well-being, alternative ways of healthcare and health conservation, and opens the way to non-physicians who assert that they will take care of the good condition of the client's body in a better, less expensive and more effective way. In the symbolic quadrangle defining the framework of this analysis – patients, healers, physicians and State institutions (social policy) - it is the former who force changes in the adopted ways of treatment, which is evidenced by the fact that, on average, one third of Europeans who sought help when ill had or have experience with the use of non-medical treatments (Ibid: 427). Non-medical treatment is practiced in organizations such as self-help groups, consumer groups, informal support networks, and in families. At the same time some medical school graduates, encouraged by the permissive approach of the medical system and by public acceptance of non-conventional methods, are beginning first to take an interest in such treatment techniques and are then applying them as an exclusive or complementary way of performing the 'social role of physician'. As the previously discussed studies show, such ways of treatment are preferred mainly by women and middle-aged persons with a comparatively high financial status and education, who choose a pro-health lifestyle and often have negative experience with institutional biomedicine. Persons in this group are also 'selective consumers' of medicine and non-medical ways of treatment, who utilize both systems depending on subjectively defined health needs. More ad more often, patients in this group themselves design therapy strategies, consulting or not consulting them with the attending physician. A constituent of such decisions is an attempt to calculate a profit-and-loss balance by considering such parameters as the price of service, side effects risk, and possible refund of expenses by an insurance company. An important element is also the opinion on the quality of patient-physician or patient-healer interaction (we should remember that, for example, a conversation between patient and healer starting homeopathic treatment lasts over an hour on average). Extensive and lengthy contact with the patient, thorough and joint discussion of the symptoms, collective assessment of treatment results, and adoption of often the same 'holistic-ecological' vision of treatment all make the patient trust and believe in the non-conventional therapist and his/her healing techniques. The patient feels that s/he is treated as an important expert on health and illness, his/her interaction with the healer is on equal terms and symmetrical, and there is practically no cultural distance because the healer is frequently treated both as an expert and a friend. The healer is interested in the patient's lifestyle and working conditions, or his/her family situation. The role of therapists very often overlaps with the responsibilities of health promoter and health auditor. This is how the well-known bioenergy therapist Zbyszek Nowak is described by his patients. Currently, in the overwhelming majority of EU countries (including Poland) non-medical services are offered only by private practitioners, the expenses not being refunded by health insurance. It would be interesting to find out how the 'social role of healer' and the status of CAM might change were these methods (as a large portion of patients would wish) to be provided in National Health Service centers and the expenses for alternative treatments to be refunded. Thus, out of a vast array of diverse health options competing for the attention of the increasingly demanding client (whether ill or healthy), it is the consumer who chooses, on the basis of many subjective criteria, what is best for the treatment of his/her disease at a particular stage of its progression. Such choices often vary, and they are inconsistent and unstable; in a sense they stem from both the features of the service recipient and the character of growing competition on the health/illness market. The shape of the medical system is impacted by civic and consumer movements, and by the patients' rights movement, which demand demonopolization of health services, liberalization, reduction of costs of the functioning of the healthcare system, and partial separation of medicine from State institutions, to which it has clung. It is difficult to judge precisely whether discussions on these problems will increase the chances of non-medical healing systems' development, although many analyses indicate that the era of biomedical monopoly on health service provision ended at the threshold of the twenty-first century.

While presenting the state of research on the sociology of non-medical healing systems, we have discussed studies conducted in the Polish and Western sociology of health and illness. We should not, however, omit the texts published for many years in the prestigious international sociomedical journal "Social Science and Medicine". It is obviously impossible (or even unnecessary) to analyze all materials on the subject since this book deals with the Polish context of non-medical healing systems. I will therefore seek to present and comment on the main research currents that have appeared in the journal since 2000, laying emphasis on social phenomena, facts and processes that may help us to understand the social context in which 'other medicine' is functioning in Poland.[26]

26 The issues of non-medical treatment systems are also discussed *inter alia* in the journal "Sociology of Health and Illness". See an interesting article by K. A. Hirschkorn, *Exclusive versus everyday forms of professional knowledge: legitimacy claims in conventional and alternative medicine*, 28,5, 2006: 533-557. The article - an analysis on the borderline of medical sociology and sociology compares the EBM knowledge with diversified everyday knowledge forms on health and illness, on which CAM is based.

For example, remarks by K. A. Hirschkorn (2006, 28, 5: 533-557) confirm, as I noted in the previous chapters, the legitimacy of the thesis about qualitative differences between CAM and the information/knowledge underlying the activities and identity of evidence-based medicine (EBM) i.e. based on generally accepted standard paradigms of science, on verifiable and repeatable methodology, statistical techniques enabling registry of results of clinical tests and basic research, and on collection and reasonable evaluation of the assembled scientific evidence, etc. Despite many attempts to reconcile biomedicine with the healing systems based on everyday knowledge forms, even if the two forms have coexisted side by side for many years, they still tend to repel rather than attract each other (homeopathic medicines in Poland are almost entirely prescribed by the few practicing homeopaths).[27]

We will now discuss the perspectives of sociological studies on CAM, taking into account the abovementioned four points of reference: patients, healers (CAM representatives), physicians (working within EBM), and State authorities (pursuing specific policies towards EBM and CAM). In the present book we use and justify the need to introduce the term **sociology of non-medical healing systems** to cover the whole of research carried out by social scientists on the methods outside of institutional biomedicine. We should note that a closely similar term was used by English sociologists Philip Tovey and Jon Adams in 2003 (2003, 56: 1469-1480). As we have declared, the first point of reference for the following state of sociological research on CAM presented in "Social Science and Medicine" will be reports discussing patients' attitude to CAM, those outside the Euro-American cultural sphere (from Asia, South American, Africa, and Oceania) having been disregarded. The research covers the period after 2000 but, in a few cases, earlier studies will be discussed because their results seem especially significant. In this group the oldest, comparatively speaking, is the Canadian study conducted in 1994-1995 on a random sample of patients using the five most popular non-conventional methods in that country: naturopathy, Reiki, chiropractic, acupuncture, and traditional Chinese medicine

27 See the analyses of similar themes: D. Mechanic, *Medical Sociology. A Selective View* (1968: 91-94). Similar differences between the then forms of EBM and CAM were pointed out by R. M. Coe, who emphasizes that, for example, folk medicine uses 'basically different explanations' for the etiology of most diseases; the knowledge of lay people is esoteric: it is a type of reasoning without criticism, based on rigid customs, traditions and unchanging views of local therapists. In these interpretations, any individual enjoying prestige and respect in a local community can declare him/herself a healer and try to heal people, as the knowledge s/he refers to is commonly known and available to anyone ('folk medicine is literary medicine of the people) (Coe 1970: 124-157).

(TCM). The study was carried out using an extensive interview questionnaire (Kelner and Wellman 1997, 45: 203-212). This research was one of the first to show that clients on the pluralist health services market selectively choose and 'mix' diverse CAM methods and techniques. Very often these are changing fashions influenced by the topical media information; patients mix biomedical and non-conventional healing practices. Typical users of CAM services are young or middle-aged members of middle class, with a comparatively high level of education. The predominant group was freelance professionals and white-collar workers, most of the clients being born Canadians of Anglo-Saxon origin. Respondents who used such services exclusively were asked why they did not utilize treatment offered by family doctors (Ibid: 206). Four main reasons for the choice of CAM were established: subjective faith in greater efficacy of CAM treatments; earlier negative experience associated with treatment of one's diseases by institutional biomedicine; fear of side effects after pharmacological therapy; negative assessment of the physician-patient interaction (Ibid: 204). For comparison, we will juxtapose these results with those of the later project also carried out in Canada in 2000. These were based on the results of from in-depth free-form interviews (digitally recorded); the subjects were HIV carriers. Interviews were conducted with the support of the City of Toronto authorities (Community AIDS Treatment Information Exchange). Extensive knowledge was obtained about individual 'treatment strategies' used by patients (Pawluch et al. 2000, 51: 151-264). It was found that most patients consciously limit the use of institutional medicine, choosing the way of 'holistic healing'. This group of patients feared first of all the adverse effects of chemotherapy – the basis of biotechnical medicine. By comparison, CAM methods appeared to be more friendly, ecological and natural. Those surveyed also stressed that healers offered more convincing strategies for overcoming the effects of diseases. In their comments, the authors of the survey emphasized that on the whole Canadian patients are becoming increasingly skeptical about and disillusioned with medicine and science in general. Complementary and alternative methods aroused more optimism, reduced stress more effectively and allowed the patient to 'understand' the ongoing disease more fully (Ibid: 262). Methodologically similar ('illness narratives') were the sociological studies on patients with a diagnosed HIV carrier status in Australia, which were meant to show 'the subjective world of experience of patients with a severe, incurable disease'. One of the objectives was also to analyze in depth the mechanisms of choosing complementary methods from the individual perspective of patients usually treated with biochemical methods, who sought better, they believed, therapeutic solutions to help them cope with HIV/AIDS effects (Ezzy 2000, 50: 605-617). The analysis covered 45 patients with diagnosed HIV, who were staying at therapy centers in Melbourne,

Sydney, and Brisbane. The methodology used permitted exact reconstruction of the subjective picture of experiencing particular stages of the progressive disease, and setting these feelings in time – in the past, present or the future. The patients subjectively felt that complementary methods were psychologically closer; while deeper and longer contact with the healer enhanced, they believed, their subjective wellness, making them more optimistic and hopeful, and allowing them to be more effectively motivated to fight the disease (Ibid: 616). Another example is the sociological survey of preferences of patients who choose conventional biomedicine as treatment for one disease, and use CAM strategies for coping with others (Connor 2004, 59: 1695-1705). L. Connor's study emphasizes the rapidly growing public popularity of and trust in 'other medicine' in Australia after 2000. Surveys show that, in recent years in this country, the monopoly of biomedicine on health- and illness-related services has been broken and progressive deprofessionalization and demonopolization in the health services market are taking place although, as Connor stresses, government institutions and agencies do not support the CAM market. What bodes well for the future of CAM is the current fashion for such strategies for coping with disease, the support of popular media, refunds of CAM treatment costs by some private insurance companies, an ageing population, the rising frequency of chronic and psychosomatic diseases, and increasingly great patient acceptance of the holistic approach in health and illness (Ibid; 1703). Comparatively few studies reported in "Social Science and Medicine" are concerned with self-treatment, which is why one of them will be discussed here (Stevenson et al. 2003, 57: 513-527). Its authors observe that the introduction of new communication technologies and techniques of disseminating knowledge about health and illness led to the rapidly growing popularity and general spread of self-treatment. The article defined self-treatment as a manner of lay (non-scientific, non-professional and non-specialist) actions and knowledge, in which illness is first defined, the degree of threat to health is determined and the earliest measures taken to eliminate it (Ibid; 513).'Ordinary people' spontaneously choose between different methods of diagnosis and treatment and define remedies they trust. As part of such strategies, apart from knowledge provided by the professional sector, they turn to information available in the folk sector, using methods that are both closer to biomedicine (osteopathy) and those in opposition to it (faith healing). The offer of the non-conventional medicine sector is more and more easily available, owing for example to Internet sales (Ibid: 525). Changes occurring recently in the UK (deregulation of the health services market, healthism, the impact of educational programs of the 'your health is in your hands' type, etc.) will, Stevenson et al. believe, lead in the distant future to the rise of the new 'medicine without physician' in certain areas of healthcare. In our earlier discussion we repeatedly emphasized that one of the factors contributing to the development of complementary medicine was the multiethnic character of Western societies. Another element that prompts patients to utilize non-conventional methods is the chronic character of diseases, which is the main reason for constantly seeking help (Kakai et al. 2903, 56: 851-862). The pluralist and multiethnic American society is a good observation field to watch social reactions to non-conventional ways of treatment. The study in question analyzed the attitude of different ethnic groups to CAM (native Hawaiians, persons of Japanese origins, white Americans). It showed the role of the factor of 'cultural identification' in choosing different treatment strategies. The researchers were also interested in such factors as patients' individual beliefs and views on the etiology and character of cancers, the chances of treating them with conventional and non-conventional methods, and confidence in CAM and in EBM methods. It turned out that in all the ethnic groups studied, which functioned in what the authors termed 'the highly technological society', important sources of information about the choice of conventional or non-conventional treatment methods for cancer patients were Internet forums, medical information bulletins, popular science magazines, also available on-line information passed on via direct contact, talks in patients' own families, with close friends and acquaintances, and consultations with members of ethnic minorities who had similar health problems (Ibid: 851-853).

Another element that defines the framework of our analysis is **healers** who represent and practice within the CAM system. One of the best-known treatment methods available on the medical services market for over a century and having especially privileged relations with biomedicine is chiropractic. In many Western countries it is also one of the most institutionalized forms of non-conventional medicine (Villanueva-Russel 2005, 60: 545-561). In her article, Y. Villanueva-Russel defines CAM and describes relations between non-medical healing systems and institutional medicine. The latter was extremely important for chiropractic as its point of reference (Ibid: 545). For several dozen years chiropractic and its eminent representatives consistently tried to have their profession institutionalized and the status of this method legitimated as allied with biomedicine. A very interesting special question is the attempt to reconcile 'the esoteric principle of vitalism' with medicine based on evidence and positivist and empirical principles (Ibid: 558). Chiropractic is facing the problem of defining its identity: in keeping with the canon of its own 'healing strategy' it should be, in accordance with the assumptions of its founder, D. D. Palmer, science, art and philosophy. Y. Villanueva-Russel writes that the objective set for present-day chiropractic is to reliably determine which part of it can be retained and developed without going against the paradigm of natural sciences, and which has to be eliminated as a price for the alliance with biomedicine (Ibid: 559). A similar theme (professionalization) may concern another treatment technique close to medicine (although it is not part of it in most Western countries) i.e. acupuncture (Baer et al. 1998, 46: 533-537). This paper by American medical sociologists gives an interesting presentation of the professionalization of acupuncture in the US, placing this phenomenon in the broader social context of cultural and civilization changes on the one hand, and transformations taking place within the medical system on the other. The authors stress that at the end of the twentieth and the beginning of the twenty-first centuries new, pluralist, holistic, and heterogeneous medicine has been emerging in the United States. In a broader context, we have to examine the changing position of acupuncture, especially in California, where almost half of the US licensed acupuncture therapists practice this method. It is in this state, the authors believe, that new trends and tendencies develop which are then gradually recognized in the whole country. It is here that the numbers of New Age followers increase fast, recognition of Oriental religions and philosophies grows, and influential feminist centers and ecological movements operate. The authors repeat that the acupuncture version adjusted to Western realities was formed in Los Angeles in 1981 (Ibid: 533). The social response of medicine to the popularity of acupuncturists took several different forms: reactionary extremity, conservative opposition, liberal support, progressive support, and the attitude, which the authors called 'medical heresy' (Ibid). Mainstream medicine is generally favorably inclined towards the technique itself. By contrast, it is skeptical about the philosophy of the treatment from which acupuncture derives. The process of institutionalizing this healing orientation went in two directions: one trend consisted in demanding that medical doctors practicing acupuncture be allowed to use it without restriction in biomedicine; the other insisted that non-physician acupuncturists be granted as many rights and privileges as possible. The lobbying institution for both groups was the American Academy of Acupuncture and Oriental Medicine (AAAOM). This organization coordinated promotion, information and propaganda campaigns. For example, the Accreditation Commission for Acupuncture and Oriental Medicine was established as a body responsible for assessing and certifying acupuncturists; training and research institutions and those devoted to other Oriental healing traditions were also set up. As a result, by the late 1980s more than 500 acupuncturists/non-physicians already had the right to practice in the State of California (Ibid: 534). Similar legal and administrative provisions, favorable to this treatment method, were introduced by Florida, Hawaii, Montana, New Jersey, and New York (now in 28 states). In California, some insurance companies recognize acupuncture as part of biomedicine. The Baer et al. study suggests that the main reason for the popularity of acupuncture is patient dissatisfaction with the quality of some medical services, iatrogenicity in medicine, and awareness that this method is comparatively safe and inexpensive. An additional asset is that the method is believed to be effective in treating pain in chronic diseases. A new opportunity for acupuncture may be the attempt to reform the US healthcare system (cost reduction). Under such a plan, inexpensive and effective methods may be preferred (Ibid: 536).

The next constituent of our presentation of the state of research on CAM is **physicians** as part of evidence-based medicine (EBM). We will begin by briefly discussing an especially interesting analysis which covers the largest group in the profession: general practitioners (GPs). The study in question surveyed the attitudes and opinions of this professional group towards CAM. The main factor, which differentiated opinions, was previous experience with methods of 'other medicine'. Those GPs who had encountered such methods in practice and regarded them as part of emergent holistic medicine showed a more permissive attitude while others, who had either had no experience or a negative experience, e.g. on account of the low efficacy of the methods, expressed skeptical or even critical opinions in the survey (Easthope et al. 2000, 51: 1555-1561). The authors point out that almost all GPs surveyed had definite opinions on CAM because, over the last twenty years, non-conventional treatment methods have become a common element of social reality. Easthope et al. assert that 49% of the population in Western countries is estimated to use some CAM forms (including self-treatment) regularly or from time to time (Ibid: 1555). At the same time one in five doctors surveyed reported that they had heard detailed accounts of CAM practices from their patients. The article states that it is difficult to estimate the actual scale of practice of non-conventional methods in Western countries as different studies use diverse terminology and classify some methods as alternative while the same treatment techniques (e.g. osteopathy) are counted as official medicine in other surveys. In the survey in question, the main criterion for distinguishing CAM from EBM is the fact that the former is not taught in the overwhelming majority of medical schools and, consequently, is not part of the canon of medical knowledge (Ibid: 1556). Despite the prevalent skepticism stemming from the belief of the physicians polled that these methods have no scientific value, some of the respondents saw certain virtues of CAM, which were termed as complementary to mainstream medicine. Particularly acceptable were those treatment techniques that were free from mystical and magical elements (e.g. acupuncture in its Western version, i.e. separated from the context of traditional Chinese philosophy). Of 467 GPs surveyed, most of them believed that their critical opinions would not significantly matter because the healthcare system evolves towards the consumer-oriented market, where patient (client) preferences will play a fundamental role, with the patients frequently choosing CAM. The authors conclude that, regardless of personal opinions on 'other medicine', most of the GP respondents accepted the permanent presence of non-conventional methods on the health services market. Some believe that they should adapt to the new conditions and use such methods in their practice (this most often applied to acupuncture and osteopathy), while others think they should cooperate with non-conventional therapists. The report also emphasizes that, on the whole, the degree of CAM acceptance by general practitioners is significantly higher than among clinicians. We can add that this is small wonder since sociomedical studies in many countries show that almost 40% of the problems with which patients come to GPs are sociopsychological rather than biomedical. If we assume that the essence of non-conventional treatments is 'amateur socio- and psychotherapy' and use of the placebo effect, we should not be amazed that a portion of general practitioners have a generally positive attitude towards CAM. The proof of this permissive attitude is that some portion of respondents suggested the need to include 'paramedical methods', chiefly acupuncture, chiropractic and osteopathy, in the future professional training of medical doctors. The same respondents believe that, should circumstances arise, under which conventional medicine would be ineffective, they would refer their patients to 'safe' therapists practicing 'paramedicine' (Ibid: 1569). We will continue our discussion of surveys of the basic physician category – GPs - and present an interesting Canadian project (Verhoff and Sutherland 1995, 41: 511-515). The project used an extensive survey questionnaire to be completed by 200 randomly selected general practitioners. Most of them (65%) had already known of their patients utilizing methods of this type; consequently, they had definite views on the subject. Using their own self-assessment criteria, the GP respondents found acupuncture, hypnosis and chiropractic the most effective methods in treating chronic pain conditions and in relieving the effects of chronic diseases (Ibid: 511). The report points out that CAM methods were accepted by patients in Canada at precisely that time and, if we apply a very broad definition of CAM (including herbal therapies), 20% of persons with health problems admitted utilizing such methods. A large portion of patients, the authors stress, ignored the fact that these methods did not meet basic scientific criteria required by the science of health and illness. The article states that, over the last twenty years, CAM has freed itself from 'centuries-old ethnic and cultural isolation'; it had been previously practiced for centuries in Canada by many Indian tribes as a form of ethnic and folk medicine. From the mid-1990s onwards the Canadian Medical Association (CMA) and provincial federal governments attached increasingly greater importance to research on the efficacy of CAM methods, especially treatment techniques that are highly popular with patients (acupuncture, chiropractic, hypnosis). 16% of Canadian physicians polled said they had already had personal experience of practicing hypnosis and acupuncture (Ibid). As in the studies discussed here, the main recommendations to use these types of methods were chronic pain complaints, asthmatic diseases, and problems with addiction to psychoactive drugs (Ibid: 513). The widespread nature of these ailments in the ageing Canadian society made the respondents conclude that, when taking decisions on whether to utilize CAM, they would need a regular supply of information on the efficacy and safety of methods offered by 'other' medicine. The doctors stressed that they had to know what methods a patient could safely use and in what health situations they a patient could safely attend Referring to the results obtained, the authors predict that, the more psychosomatic the nature of present-day diseases, the more frequently patients will use the methods that, in their subjective judgment, will bring relief (even if momentary), support and wellbeing (whether objective or subjective) (Ibid: 514).

As has been said earlier, one of the most popular treatments, which is counted among alternative methods in some countries while in others it exists on the borderline of medicine and CAM, and elsewhere it is practiced as part of medicine, is acupuncture. In New Zealand sociomedical surveys were conducted on the changing status of acupuncture and, as a result of long-lasting professionalization processes, a professional category emerged in that country: medical acupuncturists (Dew 2000, 50: 1785-1795). For many years acupuncture, as an integral part of traditional Chinese medicine (TCM) was criticized for being incompatible with the fundamental principles of the medical paradigm in clinical disciplines (this method was most sharply criticized by neurosurgery) (Ibid:1787). Physicians were warned against using or even tolerating this treatment technique, which was considered dangerous to patients. After several years of disputes, certain forms of this method of therapy were eventually recognized, culminating in the establishment of the Acupuncture Association of New Zealand in 1975. Discussion on the status of acupuncture and medical acupuncturists (of whom a large group have MD degrees) now concerns three basic issues: the possibility of precisely assessing the efficacy of such methods by means of today's biomedical criteria; the scientific status of acupuncture (opponents point out that it is still a method that does not meet standard criteria of science – 'acupuncture is pseudoscientific'); and the assessment of the market status of the method so popular with patients. Thus, despite its availability in many medical centers, the position of acupuncture and medical acupuncturists is still the subject of public dispute despite the passage of time, and medical acupuncturists describe themselves as deviant insiders (Ibid: 1793-1794).

To finish the presentation of this subject, we will discuss one more piece of research regarded as classic in the sociology of non-medical healing systems, in which multiethnic Israeli society was studied. The survey deserves presentation not only because it was prepared by classical medical sociologists (Bernstein and Shuval) but also because it is part of a long-term research project on CAM and was carried out on a large sample of 2030 Israeli patients (Bernstein and Shuval 1997, 44: 1341-1348). In their project the two authors emphasize that 6% of the population surveyed practice various forms of CAM (Ibid: 1341). The Israel survey shows, as do many other studies cited from different countries, that the main reason why patients sought a non-conventional therapist's help was their subjective judgment that the efficacy of EBM treatment was low. In the same project Bernstein and Shuval also interviewed family doctors (primary care physicians). This group of respondents was skeptical and critical of CAM; doctors believed that the overwhelming majority of results obtained by healers could be explained primarily by the placebo effect. In their overall assessment of CAM these respondents were divided: from supporting the opinion that alternative methods are clever deception and fraud or scientific bluff to favorable opinions on 'other medicine' – that patients should always be offered some kind of help in illness (Ibid: 1345). In the sample surveyed, no physician used alternative (complementary) methods of treatment but some of them stated hat they would be willing to refer their patients to such therapists under certain circumstances if they concluded that it was the only remaining possibility of help left. Those who regarded medicine as both a biomedical and psychosomatic discipline considered themselves to be more tolerant towards non-conventional medicine ('If a patient asks, and says he believes it will help, and I believe that the problem is in large part psychosocial I don't oppose') (Ibid). We should emphasize that most physicians saw no serious dangers in patient utilization of CAM, perhaps because in the same survey a large portion of patients did not inform their doctors about such treatments. Physicians generally said that potential threats existed not in complementary methods as such but might be associated with poorly trained therapists. Another weakness of CAM is that all the different methods and techniques of treatment cannot be verified using standard biomedical criteria. Bernstein and Shuval stress that the future of CAM in Israel may be the practicing of some of CAM methods under a physician's supervision in medical institutions. They also suggested that a Ministry of Health agency be set up, which would conduct continuing research (including sociological) on the character, effectiveness and forms of, and forecasts on, CAM (Ibid; 1346).

Observations on the role of central medical institutions in relation to CAM will allow us to examine the policies of government authorities in selected European countries towards 'non-conventional medicine' and its practitioners because it is the State administration authorities that take decisions, for example, on the legal status of 'other medicine'. We will begin with general remarks: in the classic sociology of health and illness, medicine is treated as a system that is an integral part of the larger whole of the social and civilizational supersystem. As early as the turn of the nineteenth century, in Western European countries many medical institutions became the object of government interest. The growing range of political, economic, demographic and even military interests resulted in the increased supervision by governments of the functioning of medicine as a formalized system. An element of this supervision was greater subordination of the medical profession to central government institutions. In the 1940s and 1950s there was a strong tendency to partly 'nationalize' medicine, e.g. by establishing national health service organizations (Bizoń 1976: 121-131). Rapid and deep changes that have taken place in the social and civilizational supersystem since the mid-twentieth century have activated special defense mechanisms in medicine, which will protect it against excessive public supervision. E. Freidson described various relational models determining relationships between State and medicine. In the free-market model, for example, based on the right to free competition, non-medical healing systems compete for the client's recognition and preferences with biomedicine on equal terms. Under this system the healthcare purchaser has to make independent and autonomous decisions about which offer s/he finds optimal. In the specialist model it is the government and central authorities that assess, ration and certify diverse healthcare offers and qualify some of them to enter the market, while rejecting others. In this variant almost the whole monopoly on the 'sale of health services' belongs to the medical doctor (Freidson 1976: 157-158). Freidson also described another model (a bureaucratic one), which increased the role of legal, organizational and political regulations by central authorities over ways of satisfying the needs in health and illness (Ibid: 168-169). The author suggested the solutions in the 'consumer model' as the optimal ways of solving health problems: this model protects the system against the extremes of the specialist and bureaucratic models. The optimal solution emphasizes the active role of patients as the subjects of the treatment process, and stresses their autonomy but also full responsibility for their decisions. These features of the patient should be taken into consideration not only by the doctor with whom s/he has direct contact but also by the medical system as a whole. Since the time when Freidson made his analysis, relations between the medical system and government healthcare institutions have certainly changed considerably; however, in the majority of developed countries government institutions still control and correct the healthcare market in various ways and to differing extents (Cockerham 2004: 313-341 and 343-367). A good example of the controlling and regulating function by the modern State and government agencies is the monitoring of and supervision of the spontaneously developing diverse forms of 'other medicine'. The earlier sections of my study described similar problems in different contexts, referring mainly to Polish and

American realities and to materials published in "Social Science in Medicine". Here is an interesting example from the Netherlands, where the government was the first in Europe to pass new legislative solutions regulating the formal and legal status of non-conventional therapies and their relations with institutional biomedicine (Schepers and Hermans 1999, 48: 343-351). The Dutch government had been trying to define the legal status of CAM for a long time; the Dutch Parliament passed the Individual Health Care Professions Bill, which replaced earlier formal solutions and brought to an end the monopoly of the Dutch medical profession on the provision of health- and illness-related services (Ibid: 343). Earlier prohibitions and requirements applying to CAM were repealed, which made the Dutch system a model of liberal approach. Doctors' control over the phenomena of health and illness was restricted, which was in keeping with a general tendency to deprofessionalize and demedicalize the system of healthcare provision. In the theory of medical sociology the 'neo-Weberian approach' is, Schepers and Hermans maintain, a good perspective from which to analyze mutual relations between biomedicine and non-conventional healing systems (Ibid: 344). Previously, in the nineteenth century, the authorities of the Kingdom of Netherlands strengthened the position of medicine by means of parliamentary Acts (1818, 1865). It was only in the latter half of the twentieth century that three main arguments caused the system to gradually open up to changes, taking the client's (patient's) needs into consideration to a greater extent. The first cause was the rapid development of consumer movements and organizations fighting for patients' rights. Second, demands were growing for the new law to define the term 'medical practice' in a more open manner and give patients a change to utilize the services of licensed healers, guaranteeing they would not use charlatans' methods. Third, there was a call to increase the number of paramedical specializations and determine their status, competence and responsibilities. Over the last decade in Europe we have witnessed two standard procedures regarding the regulations in force. One applies in Scandinavia and the Netherlands, where anyone who has fulfilled liberally defined criteria can offer their services on the healthcare market (except of the highly specialist kinds reserved exclusively for physicians); the other is binding in Southern European countries and in France, Belgium, and Luxemburg, where the principal role in the provision of health- and illness-related services is played by medical school graduates. To sum up, the Dutch studies showed transformations taking place in the medical services market, where it is the consumer market that actually functions in some countries; consequently, this broke the monopoly of biomedicine and physicians on healthcare services (1993-1998). In the Netherlands, for example, various CAM practitioners have been able, since 1998, to apply for government subsidies for the development of their methods; this strengthens the position of both methods and their practitioners. At the same time the number of Dutch physicians practicing non-conventional methods (usually the least controversial) or cooperating with healers has been steadily growing. The response of patients has been, in turn, to make parallel use of conventional biomedical methods and complementary techniques (Ibid: 350; and Baer (a) 2010: 73-399).

To recapitulate diverse CAM-related themes discussed in "Social Science and Medicine" in the last decade and a half, we can conclude that there are four essential elements that organize the course of our presentation. These elements make a special quadrangle defined by the terms:

- Patients (their attitude to CAM, assessment of efficacy, selection criteria, etc.).
- Healers, who represent the CAM system (problems of professionalization and institutionalization, relations with patients and physicians, etc.).
- Physicians (representing biomedicine, evidence-based medicine, their opinions of CAM, attitude to healers, etc.).
- Government authorities (State agencies, legislation concerning CAM, administrative control over non-conventional methods and therapists practicing them, centrally coordinated studies on CAM efficacy, etc.).

We have presented sociomedical studies published in the journal "Social Science and Medicine" in an attempt to compare the results of Polish studies with similar projects realized in the Euro-American cultural sphere. This comparison prompts a conclusion that most of the works discussed are of more or less contributory character. An exception is these longitudinal studies on complementary medicine conducted by the Judith Shuval team; however, their analyses partly apply to specific cultural and social realities in Israel. The text by P. Tovey and J. Adams (2003) merits separate attention: they use *inter alia* the term 'a sociology of complementary and alternative medicine', which is close to 'sociology of non-medical healing systems', which I have used since 1998.

The history of research on CAM presented by the dozen-odd authors cited here shows that the number of such projects has systematically grown since the mid-1990s although they are highly diversified in their methodological and theoretical approaches (we should note interesting studies based on qualitative methods).

As we said earlier, the constant research theme present in the analyses in the sociology of health and illness is the problem of the range of public interest in CAM as a whole and the popularity of individual methods and techniques that make up 'complementary and alternative medicine'. The methods recognized by patients and doctors as the least controversial - acupuncture, osteopathy and chiropractic - turned out to be the most trusted and acceptable. By contrast, the public was most skeptical about therapeutic techniques in which the effects of treatment were difficult to measure while their character is regarded by physicians as a kind of manipulation of the patient (non-conventional hypnotic methods, faith healing). It is interesting to note the prevalent form of use of preferred non-conventional methods; most of them are practiced in parallel with treatment by institutional biomedicine. There is a growing tendency to 'mix' selected treatments. Patients may seek non-conventional techniques for some of their ailments, and they may visit the doctor's office to treat others in the same period; comparatively often, patients do not inform their physician about CAM utilization.

If we tried to offer a sociodemographic description of a typical patient group using non-conventional methods, it would turn out that the dominant subjects were middle- and upper-class women, aged 40-50 years, with a high or comparatively high socioeconomic status, who live in large metropolitan areas or on their outskirts. By contrast, traditional folk medicine (one can see this in the multiethnic American society) is gaining recognition among the impoverished and poorly-educated population of ethnic minority origin, first-generation immigrants who arrived from Asian, African and Latin American countries; very often they are persons without residence permits and health insurance.

The sociologists who contributed to "Social Science and Medicine" were also interested in why patients opted for non-conventional treatment methods. Reports show that the recurrent motives in the reasons syndrome were as follows: a subjective sense of dissatisfaction and discomfort in contacts with physicians and institutional medicine, especially the critical assessment of physician-patient interaction; fear of side effects when using various diagnostic and therapeutic techniques provided by technochemical medicine with a simultaneous conviction that CAM is comparatively safe; economic reasons, i.e. the inexpensive offer of non-conventional medicine; finally, acceptance of a holistic approach to treatment, which, patients maintain, is more often adopted by healers than by physicians. Studies also show that patients are aware of the limitations of non-medical healing systems, which is why they prefer this offer in treating chronic diseases of psychosomatic etiology or chronic pain conditions. At the same time reports indicate that there are more and more people believe that non-conventional methods and the therapists who use them are more effective in providing support and enhancing the patient's subjective satisfaction with the treatment process. Proponents of CAM are satisfied with the fact that, on the pluralist healthcare market, they can consciously choose the type of health services that they deem optimal in treating a specific disease at a specific moment. A highly significant factor that increases interest in CAM is the new social communication techniques widely available in developed countries – especially the Internet, which shows scores of thousands of information items on non-conventional methods.

Another point of reference we have adopted was the healers (representatives of CAM system). The studies cited above showed first of all the interesting process of institutionalization and professionalization of the 'social role of healers' and the 'healing industry' as a whole. Since the mid-1990s healers in the developed Western countries have persistently striven first to legalize the health services that they provide; they have then sought the status of a full-rights auxiliary profession in relation to the medical profession (osteopathy, chiropractic, acupuncture). These attempts have succeeded in that some government agencies have taken on the role of institutions that certified and verified the quality of services offered by selected CAM methods. Thus, the State has taken on the role of guaranteeing the safety and efficacy of treatment methods or techniques (in the Netherlands and Scandinavian countries). At the same time, non-conventional therapists have set up their own lobbying and educational institutions, and even independent research centers, whose task is to assess the efficacy of some CAM methods. A significant element of 'institutional recognition' was the decision by some private insurance companies to refund treatment costs incurred by CAM clients.

The goals of the healing lobby are to obtain public funds to finance their own organizational development and research on CAM, to prohibit any discrimination (legal and institutional) against non-conventional methods, and to provide opportunities for large-scale advertising of such healing techniques, treating them as fully complementary and alternative to institutional mainstream biomedicine. In particular, the lobby sought the possibility of practicing such methods in out- and inpatient health service centers. One group of Western European countries (the Netherlands and Scandinavian countries) appears to opt for such solutions while others (such as the UK) want to first analyze objective research on the safety and verified efficacy of CAM before they make final decisions; still others (e.g. Italy) are at the stage of parliamentary discussions on the status of non-conventional medicine. It is highly probable that analyses of this type conducted using standard biomedical methods will yield negative results. In these circumstances the use of qualitative methods (free-form interview, personal documents analysis, narrative analysis, and participant observation) may show the picture of the true value of these methods as perceived by patients: the degree and type of satisfied instrumental and expressive needs, the kind of quality of relations with the healer, subjective factors determining faith in a therapy's success, the mechanism of feeling wellness and wellbeing, and the like. This conclusion is legitimate, it seems, in the context of the Western studies discussed above, in which the above-mentioned methodological approach was applied. It is also significant from the perspective of the choice of research method described in the present book.

The next link in the analysis of the sociology of non-medical healing systems is physicians, who represent institutional biomedicine (EBM). The literature analyzed in this subchapter shows the position of physicians who generally tend to have more and more favorable attitudes towards the CAM system and CAM practitioners although these methods have not been confirmed for efficacy and do not meet standard safety criteria. It should be emphasized that general practitioners are more friendly towards and tolerant of non-conventional methods than clinicians. In the case of the two physician categories, of high importance for their attitude towards 'other medicine' were prior contacts with this form of treatment and their subjective assessment of such experience. Positive impressions had a generally positive effect on subsequent opinions on the subject. The methods that the surveyed doctors trusted most (which was repeatedly emphasized) were the least controversial from the standpoint of biomedical paradigms: those whose practitioners that had formally or informally cooperated with biomedicine for years (osteopathy, chiropractic, and acupuncture). In some research reports the doctors surveyed emphasized that their attitude to CAM was also influenced by fashions promoted by the media and PR campaigns commissioned by lobbyist centers working for non-conventional therapists (this is clearly exemplified by the fact that public opinion has been swayed in favor of homeopathy). The opinions of physicians were also influenced (it is difficult to say to what extent) by the fashion for a 'holistic approach' not only to health and illness but also to ecological problems, lifestyle, etc. Studies show that the medical community accepted the thought that the growing plurality on the health services market results in the free choice of treatment options by the patient, who selects, by his subjective criteria, some or other therapy methods that suit him/her best. In a dozen-odd countries (e.g. US, Australia, New Zealand) specialists with the required licenses have appeared, who, while not being physicians, practice within official medical institutions; they are medical acupuncturists. The physicians' attitude to CAM tends to be increasingly selective (the same mechanism as in patient opinions). Methods uncontroversial from the standpoint of biomedical criteria are rather 'domesticated' and tolerated although they are far from being completely approved, while treatment techniques to which (rightly or wrongly) a mystical or magical character is attributed (faith healing, touch for health, non-conventional hypnosis versions) are criticized, marginalized or totally ignored.

Finally, a brief remark on the fourth element of the present analysis: the attitudes of governments (State authorities) to CAM. The studies discussed above show highly diverse attitudes of the authorities in individual countries to non-conventional methods – from intransigent hostility (the United Kingdom) to almost complete acceptance (the Netherlands). There is also a group of countries which have carried on discussions (often for many years) on the optimal attitude towards non-medical healing systems (Italy). Here, there is a clash between various lobbies and interest groups which represent both biomedicine and CAM. The results of disputes and public debates are difficult to forecast. However, it is true that, for first time in several decades, the monopoly of doctors and medicine on the provision of health- and illness-related services has been shaken and subsequently broken. It is difficult to forecast the further course of events but it is also interesting to ask whether consumer pressure for greater availability of non-conventional services will continue or whether new facts, for example the recently disclosed reports showing the true, negligible effectiveness of homeopathy, will discourage some patients contemplating the optimal mode of treatment and who have not yet used healer services from utilization of non-conventional, alternative methods. Much will also depend on the reaction of central EU institutions supervising and controlling the health market: whether decisions and regulations concerning CAM will be implemented to apply to all EU member countries or whether these questions will depend on decisions taken by individual Community members.

2.3. Other Research Perspectives (Medical Anthropology, History of Medicine, Clinical Medicine)

2.3.1. Medical Anthropology

Classic definitions of the sociology of health and illness are indicative of the broad range and varied character of studies conducted in this discipline. This characteristic is a result of *inter alia* the kind of phenomena that are of interest to sociologists specializing in this field. The concepts of health, illness and medicine (defined as knowledge and the system of practical actions) are situated in a varied and historically changing domain. The complexity and variability of social, psychological, cultural, economic, demographic and even physiological phenomena, which medical sociology has to study and refer to, make this subdiscipline especially suitable for analyzing areas on the borderline between different research fields, and for cooperation with other related disciplines as illustrated, for example, by the remarks by Weiss and Lonnquist (2006: 1-2). These two authors emphasize that medical sociologists must cooperate with all kinds of physicians, psychologists, anthropologists, medical historians, political scientists, demographers and, more and more frequently, with geneticists and bioethicists (Ibid: 4). Such classic themes as, for example, relations between the social environment and health and illness bring our discipline closer to social epidemiology; studies on the patient's social role and the experiencing of illness bring it closer to psychology; analyses of the effect of categories - age, gender, marital status - on health and illness bring it closer to demography; finally, the study of the role of cultural factors in CAM utilization brings it closer to anthropology (Cockerham 2004: 13-39, 40-71, 72-93).

It is the last of those disciplines – anthropology of health, illness and medicine – that seems to be especially relevant to those concerned with the sociology of non-medical healing systems. We will therefore try to look closely at this anthropological subdiscipline and its relations with the sociology of health and illness seen from the perspective of studies conducted on the past and present-day methods of non-conventional healing systems (see Piątkowski and Płonka-Syroka 2008). Sol Levine, when discussing the status of sociology of health and illness stressed that it should be integrated with its 'parallel sister disciplines' and that multidisciplinary studies needed to be conducted. P. Conrad, on the other hand, pointed out a close relationship between anthropology and medical sociology: *Parallel Play in Medical Anthropology and Medical Sociology* (Bird et al.2000: 377). B. J. Good and M. J. Delvecchio-Good described the historical development of medical anthropology from the projects by classics of the discipline, C. Leslie and A. Kleinman, to modern studies on biotechnologies, cultural determinants of mental health, and on patient experience of mental diseases (Ibid: 379-85). For his part, Robert T. Trotter emphasized the role of culture as a causative factor of social behaviors of individuals and human groups. Fundamental values and their hierarchies as derivatives of internalized culture determine behavioral patterns in human communities. Culture shapes emotions and shows how to express them; it influences one's kind of lifestyle, allowing us to communicate with other people and build permanent relations in small groups based on social bonds (see R. T. Trotter 2003: 210-211). Trotter's observations can be applied to the phenomena of health and illness examined in the broad cultural context: it is this area of interest that characterizes both medical sociology and medical anthropology. The latter – usually defined as a scientific discipline whose subject may be generally described as convictions and practices associated with health and illness in their broad socio-cultural context – is now a well-established subdiscipline of cultural/social anthropology (D. Penkala-Gawęcka 2008: 219). D. Penkala-Gawęcka wrote many times on the evolution of Polish medical anthropology (1995, 78: 169-191; 2006 1 (8): 153-162). The issues of health and illness were present in the studies on cultural anthropology practically from the first, already historical inquiries. Initially, the healing practices of 'exotic peoples' were the object of study, which then gradually covered folk medical systems functioning in Western Europe. From the latter half of the nineteenth century, beliefs associated with health and illness began to be interpreted according to the evolutionist paradigm as unscientific and irrational; these were beliefs that should disappear in modern societies developing on the basis of science and technology (Penkala-Gawęcka 2008: 220). Today's medical anthropology is a clearly defined subdiscipline with its own scientific identity, and is a very interesting partner to the sociology of health and illness. Similar methodological and theoretical foundations of both disciplines make it easier to conduct joint research and compare their results (studies on health and illness in the phenomenological depiction, interpretive orientations, etc). A. Kleinman, a co-founder of anthropology of health and illness, suggested for example that medicine be studied taking into account signs, values and behavioral patterns on the basis of the terms 'illness' (convictions about causes of illnesses, experience of symptoms and behavioral patterns associated with illness), 'disease' (the syndrome of pathological and functional changes), and sickness (illness treated in a general sense) (Ibid: 229). Also of great interest to the sociologist of health and illness is the model of explanation of this concept as presented by Kleinman, which covers interpretations of etiology, symptoms, paraphysiology, the course of illness and the treatment process. B. Good and A. Gaines, representatives of the interpretive approach, tried to capture the temporal variability of semantic configuration of illness under the influence of socio-cultural and political transformations (Ibid: 231). Both anthropology and medical sociology tend to conduct interdisciplinary studies. This natural, as it were, tendency to cooperate stems, as has been shown above, from both the similarity of core theories and similar methodologies (qualitative studies) and from the use of a number of identical concepts and terms. Medical anthropologist D. Penkala-Gawęcka writes of these affinities: 'Undoubtedly, medical sociology is closest to medical anthropology. More and more frequently they not only call each other "sister disciplines" out of courtesy, but also take advantage of their theoretical conceptions, the scope of their research being similar, especially as far as studies on socio-cultural determinants of biomedicine or on doctor-patient communication are concerned. They often tackle the problems of progressive medicalization, sociologists and anthropologists being interested, out of many general and detailed issues, in how certain conditions regarded as undesirable and threatening the social order, are labeled illnesses' (Ibid: 234). She concludes her remarks on the intensifying connections between medical anthropology and the sociology of health and illness as follows: 'One may hope that already deep-rooted in the Polish system of science, medical sociology, whose representatives are beginning to appreciate medical anthropology as a complementary or even parallel discipline, will meet it more and more frequently to mutual advantage as part of various interdisciplinary projects' (Ibid: 241). We attempt here to present a brief argumentation for the need to take into consideration the most important results of studies on non-medical healing systems conducted in the field of anthropology of health and illness. The representative of social sciences will find the emphasis on 'cultural interpretation' especially interesting because this research perspective is explored comparatively rarely in Polish medical sociology (Ostrowska 1999). In its research into peasant (i.e. farmer) communities this discipline studies folk medical systems (of interest to us), whereas it devotes considerable room to present-day forms of healing when describing town communities (Mach 1998, 1: 41). We should therefore look at the selection of classic studies conducted in recent years by medical anthropologists and highlight especially those findings and research conclusions that apply to the less known aspects of the functioning of non-medical healing systems in Poland. We will begin with a brief presentation of Danuta Tylkowa's studies (referred to further on in this book) on the folk medical system in south-eastern Poland (Tylkowa 1989). From the standpoint of the goal of my book, the most interesting theme is one indicated as 'the present', which Tylkowa used in the title of her study. We will first quote the definition of 'ethnomedicine' followed in the study: '[…] ethnomedicine is a department of medical anthropology which deals with problems associated with the health and illness of village communities and the population from outside of the Western cultural circle' (Ibid: 7). Tylkowa stresses that 'folk medical knowledge is the object of interdisciplinary research', which is explored by '[…] medical doctors, biologists, pharmacologists, and specialists in related domains, that is sociologists […]' (Ibid:8). Folk medical knowledge was one of those departments of rural culture that ethnologists (ethnographers) found highly interesting. The presented studies took a wide historical perspective into account: 'The investigations cover the period from the turn of the nineteenth and twentieth centuries. It is still remembered by the oldest inhabitants of the villages investigated, which allows us to try and define the degree of vitality of traditional elements in the **currently functioning** medical system in this area [*my emphasis*, W. P.]' (Ibid: 9). Danuta Tylkowa analyzes etiological views, diagnostic methods, preventive measures and treatments characteristic of folk medicine (Beskid Żywiecki, Beskid Śląski and Beskid Sądecki regions). As in the study by Bejnarowicz discussed earlier, a number of interviews were conducted with folk therapists (bone-setters, village midwives, herbalists), with persons who were not folk practitioners but provided medical advice to their families and neighbors, and with those who used the services of non-professional medicine (Ibid: 110). At the parallel level, interviews were conducted with physicians and other healthcare personnel who provided professional medical services in the area investigated. The methods of interview questionnaire and participant observation were used (studies were completed in the late 1980s and published in 1989). The portion of results of longitudinal analyses by D. Tylkowa that may interest the sociologist of non-medical healing systems can be reduced to the following major points:

1) Ethnomedical analysis, like earlier sociomedical studies, demonstrated the progressive reduction and disappearance of the impact of mystical-magical elements on the interpretation of phenomena related to health and illness (no beliefs in the magical effect of trees and herbs on the rise of illness and in the pathogenic influence of animals, etc.). On the other hand, interviews unearthed opinions of respondents who mentioned the importance of magic and spells. Tylkowa writes, 'During the field work the explanation of the causes of illness in the form of *scarowany*, meaning someone on whom a spell was cast, was not infrequent' (Ibid: 22).
2) Despite social, cultural, moral and economic transformations, the report emphasizes the strong role of tradition and its influence on cultivation of certain folk medical practices. Tylkowa asserts *inter alia* that, 'The power of tradition in this field of health care is demonstrated by the fact that even now, despite far greater opportunities to utilize the services of medical doctors, village inhabitants often seek the help of village bone-setters, especially those who continue formerly popular specializations' (Ibid: 34).
3) The studies show that the traditional approach (opinions, beliefs, behaviors) overlaps with new ways of thinking on health and illness, due to the development of science, access to mass culture, and contacts with medical professions. As a result, '[…] irrational elements still intermingled with rational views' (Ibid: 98).
4) In the 1980s it was observed that under the influence of the growing role of the medical system '[…] more and more frequently recommendations of medical doctors were preferred both in prevention and in treatment. However, this process was not uniform and went differently within the communities studied […]' (Ibid: 100). The persistence of traditional contents associated with health and illness (health awareness, attitudes, needs, behaviors) '[…] characterized the older generation, especially women, while the prevalence of scientifically grounded information was usually reported in the younger generation' (Ibid: 101).
5) In the summing up of her field studies G. Tylkowa points out that 'When assessing in general the changes taking place currently in folk medicine […] in Poland we can say that they are characterized by a growing tendency for patients to use the help and care of medical doctors, which is largely made possible by the dense network of national health service centers in the villages investigated […] It should be stressed, however, that – which has already been said – folk medical practices are still a living phenomenon […]

> The fact that recognition for some folk medicine practitioners did not diminish even when the population of the villages investigated had an opportunity to use the services of the official healthcare centers, seems to indicate that in the opinions of **most inhabitants** [*my emphasis*, W. P.] the therapeutic activities of the practitioners were characterized by sufficient instrumental competence, especially in the case of those conditions with which academic medicine was believed to be unsuccessful' (Ibid: 106-107).

Longitudinal research as part of medical ethnology/anthropology (by D. Tylkowa, A. Paluch, D. Penkala-Gawęcka) show that folk medicine, despite changes and transformations taking place during the revolution in civilization, is still present in the Polish country villages, and folk therapists (albeit to a limited extent) offer diagnostic, medical and preventive help, which is approved not only by local village communities but also by people from the outside, e.g. some inhabitants of large cities who come specially to undergo 'natural' treatment by village specialists in health and illness. The growing popularity of traditional forms of folk medical systems is indicated by recent journalistic reports. For example, in the Podlasie [Podlachia, north-eastern Poland] region, in the area of the villages of Orla, Morze, Grabowiec, Parcewo, Dubicze Cerkiewne, and Szernie, south east of Bielsko Podlaskie, at least more than a dozen persons practice the casting of healing spells and preventing illnesses. Old women who perform these practices use religious elements (icons, the Bible and crosses) and material objects (candles, linen cloth, wax, and flax) to drive away 'evil powers'. The treatment technique consists in saying a prayer while a ball of flax burns over the patient's head, which is wrapped in a piece of linen cloth. If the remains of the burnt plant fly upwards, it is a good sign; if they fall down on the patient's head, this means bad luck: misfortune is near. Therapeutic recommendations include the need to eat sugar and chalk, which allegedly improve sight acuity. These women (*szeptuchy* – witches, psychics) think that the unfavorable opinions about them are spread by the local Orthodox priests who earn money administering funeral rites while the *szeptuchy* prolong people's lives by healing them. These traditional village therapists do not take money for their services, although the clients customarily leave twenty zloty on the table. Evil spells cast by other people, 'bad nerves', 'fears/ghosts' are driven out of the patient's body by means of instruments associated with the worship of saints (invocations to angels and archangels); very often the Bible is put on the patient's head as a symbolic gesture. After the prayer has been said, the patient is given dry bread, sugar, a bottle of holy water and poppy seed. The water should be drunk, the bread should be eaten out of sight of the family at home and the seed should be spilled in the place where the patient expects trouble. The patient must not smoke or wash for three days.

Some young family members of these folk therapists are ashamed of what their grandmothers do and do not believe in the effectiveness of the practiced rites. The therapists, on the other hand, emphasize that the gift of healing was given them by God (which is why they cannot treat animals, for example). They believe that they are most effective when treating nervous diseases. The therapeutic techniques applied by the *szeptuchy* of Podlasie contain almost all the elements of the social roles of traditional folk doctors, the overwhelming majority of the elements not having changed for several decades (Frankowska 2008, 4: 116-121). Another example of an anthropological approach to the study of non-conventional treatment methods was the project carried out in a small town in Wielkopolska [Great Poland] province (Penkala-Gawęcka 1991, 74: 43-54). Penkala-Gawęcka explains the origin of the social popularity of non-medical healing systems in Poland in the mid-1970s, emphasizing the role of such charismatic healers as C. Harris, Rev. C. Klimuszko or S. Nardelli. Non-conventional treatment methods were promoted in earlier years *inter alia* by Professor Z. Garnuszewski (acupuncture) and Professor A. Ożarowski (herbal medicine). A separate position, Penkala-Gawęcka believes, should be granted to the non-conventional therapist A.M. Kashpirovsky. She maintains that the media career of this healer in the early 1990s was a significant factor that enhanced public interest in non-conventional therapies (Ibid: 44). An important element that accelerated the fashion for utilization of non-conventional treatment methods was the appearance on the market of commercial magazines presenting these types of treatment (e.g. "Szaman [Shaman]", "Uzdrawiacz [Healer]", and "Nie z tej Ziemi [Out of This World]"). D. Penkala-Gawęcka observes that the rising popularity of these activities around health and illness did not produce a wave of scientific publications on the subject, the works by M. Sokołowska, L. Stomma and W. Piątkowski being an exception (Ibid: 45). An interesting section of D. Penkala-Gawęcka's article is the description of results obtained by the team of medical ethnologists/anthropologists during their fieldwork in the small town of Ślesin. There are few such studies in Poland, which is why their results are worth presenting. The report emphasizes the persistent popularity of home medicine (self-treatment) practiced in the circle of family and neighbors, and of therapies offered by 'professional healers'. Like the earlier studies by D. Tylkowa, this report also distinguished elements of everyday etiological, diagnostic and therapeutic knowledge for the purpose of description of non-medical healing systems. Moreover, in all these sections material factors and mystical-magical factors (spells/charms) were identified, the former being more expanded. Respondents stressed that, in the past, one encountered many witches who could cast spells but now there are none. Penkala-Gawęcka presents descriptions of 'culturally determined' illnesses, i.e. without biomedically classified equivalents, such as 'breaking', 'overswaying', 'tearing-off', 'stabbing' and 'the shifted vein'. Some terms used by respondents referred to the everyday name of an illness and at the same time to its cause. Among plant medicinal agents (herbs), female respondents (informants were elderly women) preferred chamomile, linden, peppermint, and linseed. Therapeutic products were still collected by the individual practitioner but some of them were also bought in pharmacies. Some of those surveyed were regarded by others as the persons who were able to better treat typical frequent illnesses (they were said to have acquired this knowledge from their mothers and grandmothers). They provided help to their neighbors, families and close friends. The Ślesin study report also points out that, in the immediate vicinity of this town, there were no persons who practiced non-professional treatment services as their occupation. Of other self-treatment methods, cupping (formerly also cutting to remove bad blood) was highly popular; leeches were also used not long ago to treat high blood pressure; for kidney pains, patients wrapped cat pelts around them or applied ant infusion made with methyl alcohol. Informants also mentioned therapeutic remedies that were no longer used: drinking dog's fat for tuberculosis or using human urine to treat frostbite. The report draws attention to the changing fashions, often caused by the media reporting on allegedly 'miraculous medicinal products', e.g. 'milk-grown Chinese mushroom' recommended for stomach diseases, 'Japanese crystals' grown on water with raisins to treat liver ailments, or 'amber infusions' for general health and as a natural cure. Many people also played videocassettes with recorded 'health sessions' by A. Kashpirovsky. The study conclusions emphasize that the informants were highly satisfied with such televised forms of treatment, stressing that 'it was better than operations and poisoning with medicines' – 'even if it doesn't help, it certainly won't do any harm' (Ibid: 49). However, there were those who emphasized that the treatment helped them personally to get rid of the illnesses they suffered from (infertility, rheumatoid pains, heart conditions, etc.). As has been said earlier, the popularity of mystical-magical elements is dwindling but some of their relic forms can be found in preventive behaviors: red ribbons tied on fences or on a child's bed, rare but still-found cases of incensing in cases of toothache when herbs are burnt, having been first blessed on the octave of Corpus Christi (Ibid: 50). Most of the Ślesin inhabitants questioned believed in the efficacy of the intercession of the Heavenly Mother of Licheń sanctuary, but the necessary condition for healing was profound faith and ardent prayer. The Ślesin parish congregation also believed in the healing power of St. Valentine (in the local church there is a picture of the saint). Prayers to this saint were said to effectively help treat epilepsy, with respondents insisting that there had been much 'miraculous healing' in this area due to the intercession of this saint. Local experts in the curative method called 'measuring' comprised several female inhabitants of the town – elderly women who specialized in providing help to infants and babies. 'Measuring' is practiced in the cases of 'breaking oneself', the symptoms being fever, crying, and vomiting. Physicians diagnosed such symptoms as bronchitis while the women folk doctors were convinced that the 'real' cause was the 'shifting of bones in the backbone', which could cause a humpback. This treatment can be practiced in three different ways, *inter alia* by measuring the child's body with a cotton scarf. First the distance between elbows with the arms outstretched is measured, then the same scarf is used to check whether the distance measured is equal to the circumference of the child's chest: if the circumference is larger, the child is 'broken'. Treatment consists of pulling the child's arms with the scarf so as to eliminate the difference. This technique is generally believed to be more effective than the doctor's procedures. Interestingly enough, the popularity of the method and belief in its efficacy produces a growing number of women who claim that they practice efficient 'measuring'. Some informants recalled the local 'dynasty of chiropractors', for example Matusz of Konin, who was said to be highly effective and allegedly had more successes than physicians in the neighborhood (Ibid: 52). In the vicinity of the town there were also several bioenergy therapists who combined this method with radiesthesia and herbal medicine. To sum up, we can say that the field studies conducted by the Poznań team of medical anthropologists allow us to determine the range of popularity of self-treatment, folk medical systems and healing practices popular in a small town in Wielkopolska province. Self-treatment turned out to be most popular, including the locally practiced methods of 'measuring'. Folk medicine was represented mainly by chiropractors, while the local healers produced 'living and dead water' and practiced bioenergy therapy. There were no reports of persons in this area providing non-conventional treatment methods in a professional capacity and treating this occupation as the main way of earning a living. Those surveyed usually regarded their healing practices as an additional source of income. It should be stressed that the local population assessed non-conventional methods as a good complement to biomedicine. Penkala-Gawęcka emphasized that non-medical healthcare in the area investigated underwent dynamic changes, with the old 'etiological and therapy theories' of folk doctors coexisting with new ones publicized by the media (chiefly by the TV at that time).

The foregoing presentation discussed the most typical and popular treatment methods in a small town. When speaking of the rising popularity of non-conventional medical systems observable all over Poland, a student of the phenomenon, Z. Libera writes: 'Patients trust folk doctors more than physicians. One testimony of a cured person, not confirmed by anything, is enough. Health recoveries publicized by the press are treated skeptically by the majority of physicians, who most often come into conflict with healers. None of the doctors with high degrees could do anything about it. The wave of folk medical/quack practices is sweeping across the country at a lightning speed' (Libera 2003: 9). He also cites the cases of so-called simple, common people (giving the example of Stanisław K., a farm laborer) announcing that they had 'a miraculous revelation' which, from that moment on, enabled them to treat all illnesses with a guarantee of complete success. Soon, the 'healing practice' brings financial success and changes their previous life. A primitive house with the adjoining cattle barn is replaced by a huge mansion, the destination of mass pilgrimages by many patients. Today Stanisław K. is willing to treat all diseases (including tumors), and when some patients do not feel better despite repeated visits, the folk doctor explains the failure as decreed by God: 'Heavenly Mother so willed' (Ibid: 9). In conclusion, the author points out that a folk doctor is an integral part of folk culture, which no longer exists in its classic form but leaves traces of its presence in modern culture. Consequently, we can no longer speak of 'folk medicine' as it was described by nineteenth and early twentieth century ethnography/ethnology. Poorly educated people now living in country villages and small towns can only '[…] more or less resemble the folk doctor of the "backward and ignorant people" but they are not one […] However, without this historical figure it is difficult to understand "present-day folk medical practices" and thereby present-day "folk doctors" (Ibid: 247). Libera also maintains that, in order to describe and explain the unprecedented popularity of non-conventional medicine, it is necessary to conduct a broad range of studies as part of the anthropology of the present. Another expert in folk medical systems, D. Penkala-Gawęcka, in turn asserts that ethnological literature on this problem in the post-WWII period usually described either a selected treatment technique or studied various strategies for fighting one particular disease; therefore there were hardly any comprehensive analyses (Penkala-Gawęcka 1995, 78; 175). As has been said above, one of the most important and interesting problems from the standpoint of sociology and anthropology is the analysis of the effect of modernization processes (in the spheres of culture, education, technology, and ways of communication) on the shape, character and functions of folk medical systems/folk medicine. It is still relevant to ask the oft-repeated question to what extent do changes in civilization ('modernity coming to the countryside') and the well-established presence and availability of medical institutions and medical professionals bring about the collapse of the traditional healing system, and does it still exist at least in the relic form as in many areas in Podlasie region? To what extent do the present-day folk practitioners still operating in small local communities resemble previous specialists 'knowledgeable about illnesses' and to what extent are they better or worse counterparts of urban 'businessmen-healers' who use public relations specialists to promote themselves, have their own advertising web pages, and publish the results of their 'studies' on the efficacy of their methods in specialist healers' periodicals? Should the term 'village folk doctor/ practitioner' be replaced by another name, and if so – by what? Without fear of contradiction we can say that field research conducted by medical ethnologists as far back as the early 1990s (Penkala-Gawęcka and others) proves that folk medical practices have survived, albeit in various changing forms, because many analyses show that this domain of culture tends to **change at a slower pace than others** [*my emphasis*, W. P.]. We can therefore fully agree with Penkala-Gawęcka that, '[…] folk medicine is not so much disappearing as fundamentally transforming' (Ibid: 177). Adam Paluch maintains that folk medicine, an integral part of cultural reality, should be the object of systematic ethnological analyses carried out not from the perspective of scientistic approach, where interesting phenomena are evaluated using empirical criteria, but in such a way that we might '[…] explain the reality investigated, understand its sense, discovering the truth about it in hidden structures and in codes and archetypes unseen by the naked eye […]' (Paluch: 1998, 5: 20). Since the present book presents the results of my own studies based on the application of 'soft' research methods in analyzing the collected personal documents, I closely espouse the approach defined here as constructivist-interpretive, the more so, given that the use of natural-science rationality criteria to interpret the mystical-magical and religious elements, so important in the folk medical systems, appears entirely pointless (Górny 1996, 2: 19-20). As I have written earlier, apart from classic field studies and theoretical discussion on the folk medical systems (folk medicine) practiced in villages and small towns, the object of analysis by present-day anthropology is the description and interpretation of various urban forms of non-conventional medical systems and the phenomena surrounding this domain (astrology, fortune-telling, magic and the occult) (Libera 2003: 247). In those studies ethnologists try to establish the cultural causes of the growing popularity of CAM in Euro-American urban civilization. Scholars usually regard these phenomena as part of the growing popularity of holistic medicine or fascination with oriental medicine. In such cases the choice of treatment option is an element of the broader choice of 'alternative lifestyle' and the way of perceiving the present (Tomaszewska 2004, 1/2: 86).

A. Tomaszewska observes that the perspective adopted in ethnology indicates the inevitable crisis of Western neoliberal civilization, manifested *inter alia* in the disintegration of two fundamental elements of Western man's thinking: Christian religion and modern science which are fading in importance as unquestionable authorities. She advances the thesis that the intensifying manifestations of cultural destabilization are indirect proof of the growing public interest in alternative medicine (Ibid: 92). CAM is a symbol of the new times and new thinking based on intuition and reference to syncretic culture, and to eclectic non-European treatment practices adopted for the needs of Western man. Its popularity seems to be partly founded here on the contrast between Western rationality and oriental esotericism because it is in CAM that emphasis is placed on the intuitive, the emotional and the non-material. That is why therapies of this kind will provide a chance to cleanse oneself of the 'dirt of Western civilization', 'evil energy' and bad emotions stemming from the system-imposed competition between people (Ibid: 94). Tomaszewska also conducted a survey of healers which shows that according to non-conventional therapists almost all their patients come to CAM offices after lengthy and unsuccessful courses of treatment in medical institutions. CAM therapists also believe that many clients do not believe in the efficacy of alternative methods but want to be convinced that they have tried all possible treatment strategies. Tomaszewska analyzed separate elements of the CAM system: its language level, patient-healer interaction, therapeutic measures and rituals, patients' ideas of the character of 'alternative' methods etc. Invoking J. Kmita's theory of culture, she distinguished within 'alternative medicine' the technical-utilitarian practices (character of treatment and ways of action upon the patient's body) and symbolic practices (language, ways of communication, or worldview assumptions). These symbolic elements make up a characteristic 'healer's worldview' based *inter alia* on acceptance of holism, of the existence of relationship between the universe, man and nature – the network of complex symbolic elements that overlap with one another and intermingle. In Tomaszewska' view some treatment methods practiced in the West and based on thaumaturgical foundations tend towards 'evolutionary' magic while also introducing new values indicating that civilization based on science has its limits and is not fully effective. In this interpretation, Western civilization is unable to answer many significant questions that trouble many contemporary people. Tomaszewska writes, '[...] The increasingly evident crisis of Western culture, including science, can no longer be denied; the emerging void is filled with contents associated with the emotional side of man, his [...] spirituality, religiousness, mental needs: all these are offered by New Age movements and natural medicine (Tomaszewska 2004, 1/2 : 110). As I have said above, a significant research theme of 'anthropology of the present' is work on describing new forms of magic and superstition. Within this context that appeared the theme concerning the attitude of the clergy towards magical elements present in views directly relating to health and illness (Jaźwiecka-Bujalska 2000: 103-116). Other studies were oriented towards examining present-day fortune-telling and the esoteric services market, treated by contemporary anthropologists as a manifestation of the revival of magical behaviors in Polish society. In this interpretation the rising interest in occult practices is the indirect result of changing fashions in the 'ideas market'. K. Kość, the author of the studies, observes, 'What was attributed not long ago to the uneducated class is today becoming a privilege of the elite members: actors, show business stars, politicians and other opinion-making professions' (Kość 2004, 2 (48): 4). When discussing the reasons for the growing popularity of magical practices, emphasis is placed on the broader context of the phenomenon: emancipation and increased independence, loosening of social bonds, and the emergence (e.g. as a result of emigration) of large numbers of people alienated and suffering from the 'lonely in the crowd syndrome'. Anthropologists are also taking an interest in the phenomena not yet sufficiently investigated: hypnosis, psychokinesis, telepathy, and clairvoyance; it may be interesting to examine the phenomenon of 'various pseudosciences' more and more concerned with health and illness (Ibid: 9). Demands are mounting for the institutionalization of pseudoscience, which leads to the establishment of bioenergy laboratories, non-conventional medicine institutes, and research laboratories for the study of natural therapies, iridology, magnetotherapy, radiesthesia and macrobiotics. A whole market is forming around the institutional structure that organizes Health and Marvels Fairs, Natural Medicine festivals, etc. Since the early 1990s magazines (usually monthlies) have been published that promote individual 'eminent healers' or 'miraculous treatment methods' (usually this is more or less covert self-advertising published in such magazines as "Uzdrawiacz [Healer]", "Czwarty Wymiar [The Fourth Dimension]", "Nie z tej ziemi [Out of this World]", "Wróżka [Fortune-teller]"). According to figures cited by Kość, in the late 1990s in Warsaw alone about 300 people professionally earned their living in 'the magic business'. In conclusion, in her view the acceptance by present-day mass culture of even the most fanciful and incredible information and the growing faith of some part of society in the supernatural, extrasensory powers and their impact on human life, including health and illness, mean that '[…] at present one can observe harmonious and symbiotic coexistence of rational, scientific judgments with irrational and magical ones, of astrological manipulations with [..] astronomical observations, and fortune-telling practices using psychological principles. As we can suspect, this is one of the effects of the growing feeling of uncertainty, threat and alienation of the individual in the modern world' (Ibid: 19). Other authors describing similar cultural phenomena, also partially related to health and illness, characterize the syndrome of features of present-day culture by using the term 'present-day instant mysticism' (Śliwiński 2004: 167-175). P. J. Sliwiński analyzed the assumptions, 'ideology' and goals set by the organizers of Natural Medicine Festivals. These events take the form of large commercial undertakings and serve, as the leaflets claim, to enable direct contact between healers and their clients. Under such conditions therapists allegedly guarantee safe and professional services and present their certified achievements. Śliwiński pointed out the pseudoscientific jargon of pamphlets, posters and leaflets handed out. Festivals resemble today's town fairs where, along with the bioenergy stands, there are stalls selling sheep wool products, carpet cleaning liquids, cosmetics, charms, amulets, crystals with allegedly 'healing properties' as well as tarot cards, etc. (Ibid: 170). All manner of fortune-tellers set up their stands next to radiesthetists, and those representatives of a mail order radiesthetic company, which advertises computer-generated 'oberon diagnosis'. Therapists attach great significance to their appearance in order to look as much like doctors as possible (white coats, badges with 'doctor of holistic medicine'), these people use quasi-scientific language, trying to sound competent and trustworthy. The Fair's customers, in turn, behave as if they were shopping at the market – haggling over prices, exchanging information about novel treatments and medicinal products, and arguing with the therapists. During lectures, talks and meetings with patients, advertising announcements can be heard constantly. P. J. Śliwiński treats the phenomenon as some kind of 'instant mysticism', which in turn is part of a broader phenomenon of so-called 'city religion' oriented towards satisfying the needs of the modern urban middle class who are 'tired of life', or relieving the syndrome of urban loneliness. Śliwiński believes that the development of studies on 'city religion' is a significant element in the exploration of new forms of city religiousness (Ibid: 174, and Kowalczewska 2001: 81-90).

Summing up this section of our discussion on selected trends in studies conducted by ethnology/anthropology on health and illness, we can say that medical sociology and anthropology investigate similar areas of social reality from different but complementary perspectives. Because of this feature, the two disciplines are recognized as 'sister domains of science'. Both study the effect of cultural phenomena on social life, also explaining those associated with health and illness. A distinct evolution in research by medical anthropology is noticeable: from research work focusing on medical practices of primitive peoples to studies on diverse forms of present-day CAM conducted in Euro-American societies. Projects currently being implemented in the two disciplines are very close due to the adoption of similar methodological assumptions (e.g. qualitative methods), similar theoretical conceptions (e.g. phenomenological basis), and the use of almost identical taxonomies. Classic ethnological/anthropological studies described changes in the folk medical systems in local communities during modernization transformations (Burszta, Tylkowa, Paluch, and others) and, since the mid-1990s, the present-day forms of healing practiced in large cities (Kowalczewska, Kość, Śliwiński, Tomaszewska). Research studies on traditional folk medicine described and interpreted transformations that occurred as a result of modernization processes: elimination of traditional village midwives (old women), and disappearance of mystical-magical elements in diagnostics and treatment; however, there are still enclaves where traditional folk practitioners are still popular, e.g. *szeptuchy* [local witches] in Podlasie region in the Bielsko Podlaskie area. Ethnological investigations carried out in the early 1990s in the small town of Ślesin (Wielkopolska province) allowed the researchers to thoroughly describe forms of home treatment/self-treatment practiced by people who did not call themselves healers but enjoyed such recognition among their families and neighbors. These people practiced healing on an ad hoc basis exclusively at the request of their close relatives and friends and expected no remuneration for their service. These studies also demonstrated the significant role of religious elements in non-professional therapies (Penkala-Gawęcka). Research undertaken by medical anthropology showed cases of 'transformation' of the folk practitioner into a 'businessman-bioenergy therapist', who used enthusiastic testimonies of some of his patients to expand highly-paid therapeutic services (Libera). Medical anthropology also emphasizes, as demonstrated by the foregoing example, that today there is no longer any traditional local community or folk culture in the previously-known forms and manifestations; consequently, there is no longer a classic folk medicine provided by folk practitioners (we encounter instead its commercial imitations). All village therapists increasingly resemble town healers; it is suggested (Paluch) that the optimal research approach when exploring the phenomena of health and illness is a 'constructivist-interpretive' perspective making it possible to discover the whole hidden sense and logic of the treatment process and permitting us to understand the phenomena of health and illness in their cultural context. Another perspective is defined by the anthropology of the present (Libera), allowing us to describe and interpret all kinds of phenomena around health and illness. These are, for example, modern forms of magic, the occult and the esoteric, and fortune-telling and astrology. They are becoming increasingly popular in urban communities – studies of this type place non-professional help in health and illness in the context of occult practices (Kość). Another factor that increases interest from ordinary people in this kind of healthcare provision is the popularity of such practices among politicians, media and celebrities. In this context 'instant urban mysticism' is described; this also offers psychotronic services, bioenergy therapies, and the like. The syndrome of health- and illness-related phenomena is treated as an element of new religious orientations, the so-called 'city religion', which is part of non-traditional forms of urban religiousness (P. J. Śliwinski).

2.3.2. History of Medicine

Historical aspects appear repeatedly in various contexts in this book, whether in the description of the history of research on non-medical healing systems in Poland or in the characteristics of the approach to problems that can be termed sociological-historical. Without examining in detail the relationship between sociology and history (there are still disputes about whether history can be considered a social science), we can simply observe that knowing history in its social dimension is one of the essential elements of self-identification of individuals and communities (Zamorski 1998: 276 et seq.). History and the historian frequently enter the domain of many related sciences, for example when investigating the structure and character of selected social groups they 'infringe on the sociologist's competence'. Similarly, studies in social history are based on the use of many elements of sociological knowledge (Ibid: 280). Discussion on similarities and differences has a long tradition. As B. Szacka writes, '[...] what distinguishes history from sociology is the individual's point of view. A historian asks about the causes of a war while a sociologist about the causes of wars as such' (Szacka 2003: 28). To mark the line of division between present-day historical and sociological interpretations is sometimes difficult and problematic. As I explain in the following sections, sociology has developed a so-called historical sociology, which uses data from the past for social analyses. In classic college handbooks of general sociology there are historically-oriented chapters which may concern for example the history of sociology as science, history of a specific sociological subdiscipline, or the evolution in time of a particular social idea (Ibid: 207 et seq., and J. Szacki 1998: 283-289). The canon of sociological readings includes *inter alia* Stefan Czarnowski's discussion of the social functions of history (Czarnowski 1995: 479-482). The same orientation also applies to the studies by Kazimierz Dobrowolski on the problems of historical background or to those by Nina Assorodobraj-Kula on the social activity of history (Dobrowolski 1981: 754-768, Assorodobraj-Kula 1981: 856-869). The role of historical themes in sociology was summed up concisely by P. Sztompka, who emphasized that, 'Every past event is connected not only chronologically but is also causally linked to present and future events. By reconstructing this necessary and correct sequence the sociologist discovers "laws of history"' (Sztompka 2002: 493).

This short introduction is intended to reinforce the idea that, if we want to fully know, describe and interpret the research orientation defined as 'the sociology of non-medical healing systems' we should characterize the studies in this area conducted after 1990 by medical historians. In the following sections we will confine ourselves to analyzing selected examples of such research work which, it seems, can be inspiring to the sociologist of health and illness. We will present mainly the results of research inquiries by Polish authors, with one conscious exception. We will be interested principally in books although sometimes we will present materials that appeared in serial publications (*Medycyna Nowożytna, Studia z Dziejów Kultury Zdrowotnej*).

The group of monographs entirely devoted to alternative medicine includes the book by Robert Jütte, first published in Germany in the mid-1990s (*Geschichte der alternativen Medizin*, in Poland in 2001). In the *Introduction* the author writes that alternative medicine is becoming part of the growing cultural trend towards creating 'alternative areas of individual decisions' in modern Western societies, which is why there are more and more frequent discussions on alternative energy, alternative food, alternative upbringing or alternative education (the idea of 'society without school'). Jütte also accentuates the essential significance of taxonomic stipulations for precise analysis of the complex of phenomena known as alternative and complementary medicine. From the historical perspective it is obvious that alternative healing methods could be spoken of only after the scientific canon of technochemical medicine had fully developed. Previously, for example in the nineteenth century, homeopathy or mesmerism did not differ much from what was offered by the then medical sciences. Jütte rightly emphasizes the fact that from the historian's point of view '[...] we will regard as alternative the modes of treatment that, in a particular medical culture, which is also subject to an evolutionary process, are, at a given time or for a longer period, more or less strongly **rejected by the prevalent medical mainstream** [*my emphasis*, W. P] because they challenge this dominant current partly or entirely, or aim at the direct and fundament change of the medical system' (Ibid: 19). In the meaning of this definition the classic alternative currents include: homeopathy, anthroposophic medicine and traditional folk naturotherapy. Jütte stresses a peculiar paradox: on the one hand, widespread and persistent interest in alternative methods and, on the other, a scant number of scientific publications on the subject. Against the broad historical background, he discusses the evolution of views on the conception of health and illness, which occurred in Germany in 1945-1995, pointing out the rising popularity of the term 'holistic medicine', which was introduced and popularized by Professor Werner Zabel from 1949. Since the 1960s there has been an increase in acceptance of 'alternative medicine' in the Federal Republic of Germany. Jütte attributed this to the effects of the 1968 student revolt and approval for the then emerging ecological movement represented by the influential Green Party of Germany (Ibid: 72-73). From the mid-1970s the pro-health movement developing in Germany also began to invoke traditional ways of treatment and folk medicine. In the 1980s the radical Left became increasingly involved in CAM promotion; on the other hand, 'other medicine', with the help of skilful advertising and marketing, more and more resembled 'medical business', to which it was supposed to be a characteristic alternative. The business side of CAM, unjustly disregarded in many research publications, is based on genuine foundations – the persistent popularity of non-conventional methods. The Allensbach (Germany) Institute's sociological studies in 1989 showed that 46% of adult Germans considered such therapies effective and 47% rather effective (Ibid: 77). As was found in earlier Western European and American studies, the higher the level of respondents, the greater the approval of non-conventional methods. An indirect manifestation of acceptance of and trust in CAM was the amount of expenditure on non-conventional medicinal products. In 1992 Germans spent about DM 2.3 billion on homeopathic and herbal medicines. Studies by Germany's Medical Chamber also determined the popularity of individual treatment techniques: for years homeopathy and naturo/phytotherapy as well as diverse forms of massage topped the lists (but not for example cupping). Jütte stresses that in German society, citizens demonstrate increasingly greater independence and initiative in matters of health and illness, which is recently the result of the availability of medical portals to millions of people, a wave of publications on CAM, and the Germans', especially the young and well-off, obsession with healthism. As in other Western countries (including Poland), the role of the promoter of non-conventional methods is played by the commercial media (women's magazines, hobbyist periodicals or tabloids). For example in her TV programs the healer Uriella claims that, by means of divine rays, she can treat any disease, even the incurable, such as advanced tumors or AIDS/HIV – her company makes the so-called 'althrum water', which self-charges with 'divine magnetism'. In Germany, healers established several hundred foundations and associations (e.g. the Fiat Lux Order) in order to promote the ideas of healing; some of those institutions were prosecuted by public prosecutors on charges of swindling money from seriously ill patients and their families. In the mid-1980s spiritual healers also began their activities, '[…] usually moving in pseudoscientific, esoteric or paramedical circles, and coming from all manner of middle-class professions' (Ibid: 128). Summing up the historical evolution of various types of *ausserschulische Therapie* [non-formal alternative therapies] not accepted by biomedicine, i. e. natural healing methods (herbal medicine, water treatments, heliotherapy), biodynamic treatment methods (homeopathy, anthroposophy), Oriental healing methods (acupuncture, Ayurveda), and methods based on religion and magic (mesmerism and spiritual healing), Jütte writes, 'Studies in medical ethnology and cultural sociology irrefutably demonstrated that it is first of all culturally determined beliefs that make people accept some ways and techniques of treatment, and reject others' (Ibid: 307). A significant role in the future position of

CAM methods will be played by European Union legislation. The Lannove amendment submitted to the European Parliament in Strasbourg stipulates that alternative methods are tolerated and admissible only in six EU countries. Interdisciplinary analyses of the CAM domain must necessarily involve historical sciences, biomedicine, ethnology and social sciences, Jütte concludes.

We will now present the Polish interpretation of the problems of non-conventional healing systems from the perspective of medical history (Brzeziński 2000: 406-427). In his university handbooks of medical history Tadeusz Brzeziński ascribes the rapidly growing popularity of treatment methods and techniques not accepted by the medical community to the body of features characteristic of modern medicine: reduction of health and illness phenomena exclusively to the pathophysiological dimension while disregarding sociopsychological aspects, and excessive technologization/technicization which leads to the patient feeling the reification and dehumanization of medicine, which in turn limits the efficacy of medical sciences, especially when dealing with the growing group of patients with chronic diseases. He also points out that medical sciences, like all natural sciences trying to rationalize the phenomena and processes that they investigate, reject that which they cannot explain logically; this also applies to dissident medical currents that are both long-established and highly popular with patients (Ibid: 406). Brzeziński emphasizes that '[…] both within medicine and outside of it there emerge or persist trends that derive directly from folk medicine […] – the natural medicine of the ancients, or that are based on more or less rational assumptions. To the former group I would assign all physiotherapy […] and natural healing modes derived from folk medicine; to the latter – so-called non-conventional medicine' (Ibid: 406-407). We should observe that when discussing some non-conventional treatment techniques, Brzeziński stresses that in several countries they function 'on the fringe of or even within medicine'. This applies, for example, to acupuncture despite the fact that '**no convincing scientific evidence has been published yet** [*my emphasis*, W. P.] that explains its therapeutic action […] Skeptics point to its exclusively psychotherapeutic effect, which they justify, *inter alia*, by the lack of positive results in children, who are not susceptible to this type of suggestion' (Ibid: 409-410). In his assessment of social phenomena 'surrounding' non-conventional ways of treatment from the standpoint of history of medicine, Brzeziński emphasizes that, 'We cannot reject the method applied with success in many cases (even if it was symptomatic or temporary) only because we do not understand how it works. By contrast, the danger lies in ignoring recommendations and contraindications and in the use of the fashion for […] non-conventional medicine for one's own gains, disregarding the patient's interest' (Ibid: 410). While describing the historical evolution of homeopathic doctrine created by Friedrich

Samuel Hahnemann (1755-1843), presented in the treatise *Organon der rationellen Heilkunde* (1810), he asserts, '[…] however, the reasoning of homeopaths does not take into account the fact that dosage or choice of medicines adopted in official medicine is based on **scientific evidence**, which is **absent** from most of the homeopathic treatment methods [*my emphasis*, W. P.]' (Ibid: 414). In his discussion of another non-conventional doctrine - iridodiagnostics - and in reference to the discoveries of its founder Ignaz von Peczely (1825-1901) and to the evolution of views on the subject until the present, Brzeziński points out that 'The eminent German anatomopathologist A. Birch-Hirschfeld found in autopsy examinations that the described marks on the iris are merely normal variants of its structure and they do not have any equivalents in organ changes. The medical historian argues that the lack of obvious evidence of the efficacy of non-conventional methods does not discourage their proponents or increase public skepticism. As has been repeatedly pointed out in the present book, for centuries healers have adduced subjective, favorable opinions about their methods given by some patients – this is what Mesmer and Hahnemann did, and so do today's 'businessmen - bioenergy therapists'. The bridge between the classic therapeutic techniques applied by F. A. Mesmer and present-day 'biotronic schools' was the achievements, little known in Poland, of the German doctor K. Trampler (died 1969), who put his patients in a mystical mood during mass session and then started to 'pass energy' (also over a distance). In 1955 he unexpectedly agreed to have the efficacy of his method verified by the Institute of Psychology and Mental Hygiene in Freiburg. Observations covered 538 people, mainly middle-class women aged 40-50. The effects obtained from this well-known and popular healer neared the *placebo effect*, i.e. the administration of an agent neutral to the patient who is convinced that this is an effective drug with potent action (Ibid: 421). The group of treatments outside of evidence-based medicine, extensively discussed by Tadeusz Brzeziński, shows that none of these methods (used for over 150 years in the cases of homeopathy and mesmerism) fulfilled the efficacy criteria established by medicine, although paradoxically the methods did not lose popularity with masses of their proponents.

Another example is J. Jeszke's monograph on medical history, based on the results of field investigations – this study is entirely devoted to the folk medical system in Wielkopolska province (from the early nineteenth century to the mid-1990s). As the author stresses in the *Introduction*, on the bases of available literature and numerous legacy sources (official documents, personal testimonies, etc.) it is possible to reconstruct the folk medical system as part of the traditional peasant culture, placing emphasis on the direction and mechanism of changes. The theoretical foundation of the presentation was the findings of the Poznań methodological school of studies on culture (Jeszke 1996: 5). In his project each particular problem associated with the folk medical system was discussed and presented in comparative terms in the periods of 1801-1918, 1919-1945, and after 1945. Jeszke was particularly interested in the folk names of diseases, etiology of diseases, folk diagnostics and folk medicines (Ibid: 37).From the sociological point of view the most interesting is the 'mechanism of changes' interpreted by the author. What then are the permanent elements in the folk medical system and what has been transformed? His conclusions can be reduced to several main points: the social role of the traditional folk practitioner disappears while, at the same time, local 'chiropractic dynasties' have been functioning for decades; they most often treat patients using one tried and tested treatment method (technique); the expansion of and access to medical professionals and institutions did not lead to the complete elimination of folk medicine despite gloomy forecasts. The studies show that an element of change (e.g. as compared with the interwar period recalled by the oldest informants) is the absence of fear of the use of biomedicine, which was still quite frequent in the 1990s. From the biomedical standpoint, there was also considerable increase in the extent of rationality in health- and illness-related behaviors. The author stresses that this tendency was forced not only by the external impact of medicine but also by changes occurring within the whole folk medical system. For example, elements that turned out to be ineffective in therapeutic treatment were eliminated. Jeszke also emphasizes the importance of pluralization processes in health behaviors – the patient can now choose different options: he/she can use self-treatment, choose healthcare provided by physicians and medical institutions, practice some other version of non-medical healing or, finally, can do nothing, waiting for the disease symptoms to disappear by themselves (Ibid: 110-111).

An example of a study devoted to non-conventional methods of treatment and written from the standpoint of medical history (and anthropology of knowledge) is the publication by B. Płonka-Syroka (2007) on mesmerism. She not only shows the historical evolution of this therapeutic doctrine by characterizing its transformations in 1773-1778, 1778-1792 and 1784-1815, but also analyzes the main reasons for the popularity of this already dissident method of treatment at that time, which offered patients simple, quick, effective and inexpensive forms of help in illness. Płonka-Syroka stresses that even to nineteenth-century academic medicine mesmerism was unacceptable because of its reference to mysterious knowledge, associations with astrology, and methodological shortcomings (Ibid: 5). Mesmeric techniques also influenced bioenergy therapy, currently popular in Poland, because they utilize both Mesmer's conceptions of cosmic fluid, touch healing '[...] and many formerly practiced methods of special positioning of the hand, and the mesmerizer's action upon the body of the patient being healed' (Ibid: 221). In the 1950s and 1960s mesmerism was also drawn upon by other schools of alternative medicine. Płonka-Syroka observes that all over Poland hundreds of doctors' offices and other centers offered classic mesmerization services. The objective of the historical interpretation was to show how the cultural context of that period influenced researchers' description and interpretation of states of mental dependence and submission between the person being hypnotized and the hypnotherapist. A detailed analysis of this relationship, the author believes, can provide knowledge about today's crisis in doctor-patient interaction. The achievements of 'post-mesmeric' thought may also be important for present-day psychotherapeutic techniques. For example, today's approach in this area challenges the patient's subordination to the therapist as infringing upon the subjectivity of the sick person (Ibid: 222). At present the patient can make joint decisions about the choice of treatment methods, the doctor-patient interaction becoming clearly democratized. An interesting topic of research in history is to forecast to what extent interpretations of hypnosis will draw upon the historical roots based in part in F. A. Mesmer's therapy system. The historical perspective in interpretations of non-conventional healing systems is also present in a number of papers that appeared in the serial publication *Studia z Dziejów Kultury Medycznej* [Studies in History of Medical Culture]. Part II of Volume V is titled *Medycyna niekonwencjonalna i komplementarna. Metody badań, teoria i praktyka* [Non-conventional and complementary medicine. Methods of research, theory and practice] (Płonka-Syroka 2002). Another example of a historical approach to description of non-medical healing systems is an attempt to characterize the phenomenon by comparison with the features of scientific medicine developed at the turn of the nineteenth century (Jagiełłowicz 2002). A. B. Jagiełłowicz states 'Conventional academic medicine, which arose in Western culture, is a compendium of knowledge about man, which covers three types of scientific activity: biological research in laboratories, technological clinical studies and clinical practice. The model of prevention, diagnostics and therapeutic treatment developed in the West in the nineteenth century. Its roots should be sought in seventeenth-century mechanistic philosophical systems inspired by the dual model of human nature (already defined in the Middle Ages). A categorical separation in philosophy of the two spheres of human existence - the spirit and the body – implied projection of the biologistic interpretation of human […] problems upon social pragmatics ' (Ibid: 147). Adopting the perspective of an ideas historian, Płonka-Syroka holds that one of the main reasons for acceptance of complementary medicine is the dysfunction of modern medical sciences. 'Old medicine' no longer has the features of efficacy and adaptability because it is based on the outdated neo-positivistic paradigm, a product of scientific thought at the turn of the nineteenth century. That is why the physician – a 'product' of the training system based on this paradigm – fails to sufficiently notice human individual needs during the treatment process, and the environmental determinants of health and illness (Ibid: 148).

The summation of those selected historical interpretations thematically linked with non-medical healing systems is the comprehensive study of the subject in question by Bożena Płonka-Syroka (2008). In the *Introduction* the author writes that human activities connected with diagnosing illnesses, establishing their etiology, and attempting to treat them were part of the basic domain of human cognitive activity, with which patterns of actions formed in long historical processes were associated. In the historian's (ethnologist's) theoretical approach to the study of non-medical healing systems (alternative medicine) it is important to adopt the abovementioned constructivist perspective based on the assumptions that defining health and illness has a historical and social character, it is a process changing in time and space, and it is relativized to patterns and values accepted in the culture investigated and to the culture's axiological order embracing the vision of the world regarded as natural in this culture (Ibid: 317). The adoption of the constructivist perspective as a research directive allows us to study, e.g. the within anthropology of wisdom, '[…] both academic medicine […] and so-called folk medicine/folk medical systems' (Ibid: 318). This theoretical-methodological perspective adopted by the historian of ideas enables us to perceive alternative medicine as a kind of socially molded ideology developed as a result of knowledge-making processes and accepted by members of a describable group (Ibid: 319).

Historical anthropology can characterize and interpret these types of phenomena by employing the methodology of studies on group consciousness determined by cognitive interests and epistemological foundations. The term 'alternative medicine' refers therefore to a conceptual standard opposing the consciousness and cognitive convention of the group against which this alternative manifests itself.

We can thus analyze two models of the 'alternative': one relates to folk systems of beliefs about illness; the other relates to views that arose within academic medicine but were competitive (dissident) with it. A good example is the doctrines developed at the turn of the eighteenth century – homeopathy and mesmerism - which were rejected by the medical community the moment they were founded. From the historical perspective, taking into account the context of its foundation, the efficacy of homeopathy, for example, can be assessed as a combined effect of the action of such factors as diet, drinking a lot of spring water, the results of rest, and the absence of fear of side effects of pharmacy drugs with potent action. However, the most essential element of efficacy is the occurrence of the *placebo effect*. A medical historian, like a sociologist, asks him/herself questions about the sources of popularity of dissident orientations, which have not been fully accepted by academic medicine for over two centuries. B. Płonka-Syroka stresses that, from the historical perspective, we can see clearly how great a role was played by such elements as 'client-oriented attitude': a good knowledge of the patient's needs associated with the process of being ill; deep and lasting relationship with the patient, effective realization of the patient's expressive needs; simple, appealing interpretations of the terms 'health', 'illness', and 'treatment'; uncomplicated therapeutic techniques; the impression induced by the therapist of the 'gentle' and safe action of the medicines used; consideration for the patient's worldview (including religious convictions) during treatment, and the stressing by the therapist of his/her good relations with the institutional church (Ibid: 337-338). Summing up the reflections on the advantage of studying the broadly understood history of medicine (historical anthropology) in the context of inquiries into the origin of 'other medicine', we will again ask the question: what does the adoption of a historical perspective contribute to sociological studies? Do historians treat the term 'non-medical healing systems' developed in sociology as consistent with their own standpoints? Recapitulating his own field studies in this domain, Jaromir Jeszke writes, 'This situation makes it possible to use in the historical perspective, albeit to a limited extent, the term 'non-medical healing systems' developed by Włodzimierz Piątkowski (Jeszke 1998: 64). Jeszke points out that the adoption of the sociological conceptual framework in the history of medical sciences requires that we constantly define temporally variable contents that were associated with the term 'medicine' in a given historical period. The fact that historians usually avoid contrasting the terms 'medicine' and 'healing(medical) systems may also be a problem'. Acceptance of the sociomedical approach and recognition of the terminology in the present book (non-medical healing systems divided into self-treatment, folk medical systems, and practices of present-day healers) is thus possible if the historian adopts the following assumptions:

A) The objective of studies is only the dissident currents or those remaining 'for ages' outside of biomedicine, which emerged after the healthcare system based on the 'anatomopathological paradigm' was formed (the period of the last 150 years).
B) The investigated treatment methods and techniques regarded as 'non-medical' must be in clear opposition to biomedical assumptions or at least raise serious doubts and controversies among physicians.
C) The methods in question should never be accepted by medical sciences.

Jeszke also points out that non-medical healing systems, despite being rejected by medicine (or perhaps because of this?), enjoyed substantial public recognition as far back as the early eighteenth century. As medical history describes and interprets dynamic changes occurring within medicine and within the trends outside of it, the term non-medical should be applied to all manner of philosophies and treatment techniques which, despite the march of time, have not been recognized by physicians as scientific. Therefore, a useful device for describing the character of dissident medical orientations is to include only those healing conceptions which have permanently remained outside biomedicine from the moment they arose and fully developed. Those healing conceptions are based on the views on health and illness and the treatment process (a different approach to etiology, prevention, diagnostics and therapy) that can in no way be reconciled with the universally binding doctrines of medicine (a natural science). In this interpretation, mesmerism and homeopathy, which never gained scientific status, will be regarded here as parascientific. A similar status seems to have been given, intentionally or not, to bioenergy therapy, which draws upon mesmerism and attempts to be 'an imitation of medicine'. All these currents - mesmerism, homeopathy and recently, bioenergy therapy in its present form - are characterized by 'continually unfulfilled aspirations for being scientific'. It should also be stressed that, from the standpoint of medical history, apart from dissident currents originating from medicine but developed in opposition to it (mesmerism, homeopathy), in the nineteenth century there emerged conceptions of ordinary, common origin also popular among city dwellers, such as V. Priessnitz's and S. Kneipp's hydrotherapies. These conceptions were based on the use of folk wisdom, observations of nature and commonsense thinking, and they never aspired to be called medicine. A distinct current is the classic, peasant folk medicine, which always remained outside of medicine over the last two centuries and was separated from this science by the 'cultural, mental and technological gap'. It should of course be added that from the mid-nineteenth century to the present day, the modes of treatment practiced by non-professional therapists who lived in the country and most often treated members of their families and close friends, always included some elements of transformed and distorted medical wisdom and selected elements of other methods of non-conventional medical systems practiced in large cities or, for example, now presented in the media. As has been emphasized in the earlier parts, ethnological studies show that the folk medical system (like the whole area of cultural reality) undergoes changes, modifications and transformations but the previously presented reports from Podlasie (2008) demonstrate that, among the ageing and increasingly ailing present-day rural population, there is still room for traditional therapists attracting hundreds (or perhaps thousands) of patients who believe in the qualifications, skills and efficacy of *szeptuny* – sorcerers/therapists. It should be pointed out that, as Jeszke emphasizes, despite qualitative differences between medicine and non-medicine the attitude of physicians and medical institutions to non-medical healing systems is no longer as explicitly critical as it still was in the 1960s. At present, we ought rather to speak of skepticism or selective tolerance. This may be the effect of the increasingly felt collapse of universally binding cultural canons, which leads to relativization of assessments and judgments (Jeszke 1993: 83-119). Such hesitant attitudes are also observable in university handbooks of medical sociology, where non-conventional methods were once classified as sectarian, then as doctrines of the past, and recently as natural and non-conventional methods of treatment. We are thus dealing with a paradoxical situation where, on the one hand, we are witnessing huge technological progress in modern clinical sciences, resulting in the growing qualitative differences between medicine and non-medicine while, on the other hand, the assessments and opinions on non-medical healing systems are curiously lenient and tolerant. We will discuss the causes of this state of affairs in the next section of this chapter.

2.3.3. Clinical Medicine

From the earliest development of sociology of health and illness, medical sciences were its significant point of reference. The discovery of social determinants of the most frequent diseases (socioetiology), interest in their sociological consequences, ascertainment of non-biological factors influencing the course of diseases (chronic, sociopsychosomatic) and cultural determinants of health are only selected examples of mutual relations between sociology and medicine (including clinical medicine). Sociological knowledge allows the physician to precisely understand and define the terms 'health' and 'illness'. It also explains the functioning of medical institutions and the medical system, make it easy to optimally determine physician-patient relations, and gives a complete picture of such fundamental phenomena as health awareness, attitudes towards health, and health needs; finally it explains social regularities governing the rules of behavior in health and illness (Tobiasz-Adamczyk 1999: 305-309; Weiss and Lonnquist 2006: 12-33). B. Uramowska-Żyto, when analyzing the character of medical knowledge, referred to T. Kuhn's conception of the essence of 'normal science'. Medicine as normal science has many features that are the foundation of its practical activities. It has to examine facts that broaden and enhance its efficacy, compare facts with theory, show such classes of phenomena where conformity between facts and theory can be proven and finally, collect information that provides details of pragmatic theories and specifies their scope (Uramowska-Żyto 1980: 35-36). Describing the essence of medical sciences, M. Sokołowska observed: 'Modern medicine has a scientific orientation. Consequently, it excludes magical and religious explanations of health, illness, life and death from its orbit (Sokołowska 1980: 235). The modern Western sociology of health and illness stresses that, despite the shortcomings of medicine as science, the medical model is still the dominant scientific manner of interpreting phenomena occurring in the human organism and their determinants. No other kind of criticism of biotechnical medicine, even one with theoretical ambitions, has yet produced an alternative way of describing physiological processes (compare for example the description of the biomedical explanation of health and illness in Gabe et al. 2006: 125-129). It appears therefore that if we want to analyze the non-medical **healing systems** it is essential that we present the outlook on ways of treatment practiced most often by lay people, which have insufficient scientific grounds from the standpoint of clinical medicine. The beginning of physicians' persistent interest of physicians in problems of non-medical healing systems dates back to the early 1990s when, for example, the All-Polish Conference 'Medical Error' held a special panel discussion on 'paramedicine'. It was then that two key questions were asked, which would subsequently constitute the axis of interdisciplinary studies: 'Why do people utilize non-conventional medicine?' and 'Does the use of these services essentially decide the state of human health?' (Więckowska 1994, 51/12: 541-542). Disputes over the character of the 'parapsychological discipline' as some doctors termed it in the mid-1990s were further aggravated with the publication of the Polish version of J. Randi's book devoted *inter alia* to gangster practices called parapsychic surgery (Randi 1995: 29-51). Among others, he described and repeated in a BBC TV-filmed experiment the deceitful tricks used by Filipino and European healers, who attempted treatment by means of 'psychic powers'. Randi offered to pay one million US dollars to those healers who could prove that they had cured an illness formerly diagnosed by physicians as incurable and not automatically remissible, and that a person who had had a course of 'alternative treatments' was completely healed (Ibid: 49). When assessing the state of research on non-medical healing systems and the prospects of this approach to health and illness, clinicians stated that there was a progressive revival of 'treatment practices of the past centuries', among which they counted acupuncture, homeopathy and bioenergy therapy as derivative of mesmerism (Sterkowicz 2002, 9: 59-64). In his article S. Sterkowicz emphasizes that those alternative methods had a chance to develop in the nineteenth century, when scientific medicine did not actually exist in the full sense of the term, and any kind of speculation on health and illness was legitimate to some extent (e.g. the *placebo effect* was not known then). Like today, the opinion of patients was of great importance, as some of them felt better after these types of therapies and even considered themselves cured. A huge role in producing such positive impressions was played by the contact with a charismatic healer. When evaluating non-conventional methods from the standpoint of clinical medicine today, we notice the 'gross naivety' of explanations for the effects obtained (Ibid: 60). 'This happens probably because of the originality, mystery, proper publicity […] lack of criticism in a large group of patients' (Ibid). Clinicians stress that, on the one hand, no-one should be forbidden to freely spend their money on the kind of treatment they deem effective; on the other hand, however, this means violation of the law which accords the right to diagnose and treat illnesses solely to the physician. For example, no Polish bioenergy therapist has been validly sentenced by a Polish court for unlawful provision of medical services. Sterkowicz maintains that clinical medicine attempts to explain the 'logic of biochemical effects' of these types of treatments by referring to psychotherapeutic mechanisms. According to these theories, a sense can receive external information and pass it on to the midbrain, the hypothalamus that combines brain activities with the working of the organs, the amygdala being a special kind of 'assessment center'. The mediator in stimuli transmission is mediatory substances (neurotransmitters), one of them being phenylethylamine (PEA). When cells in the limbic system are saturated with dopamine, the patient may not feel tired. The patient's behaviors are thus controlled by chemical transmitters, e.g. a needle insertion by the acupuncturist produces endorphins neutralizing the feeling of pain. This mechanism may partly account for the alleviation of unpleasant symptoms of illness because a placebo releases, in a neurophysiologic way the feelings of weakness and pain, or 'enhances the potential of life powers'. In this meaning the effects obtained by healers are **exclusively** [*my emphasis*, W. P.] symptomatic management **rather than causal treatment** (Ibid: 62). This type of non-conventional measure brings temporary relief and produces a short sociopsychological effect but '[…] **it cannot eliminate the causes of illness** [*my emphasis*, W. P.] […] and this is where the greatest harmfulness of paramedicine lies' (Ibid).

Clinicians insist that a physician using paramedicine is less dangerous than a group of people lacking academic training because they cannot and do not utilize diagnostic methods while their management of patients, e.g. in the case of bioenergy therapy, delays contact with medicine and doctors, resulting in 20-25% of cancer patients delaying proper treatment by about eight months because of prior unsuccessful healing attempts by non-conventional therapists. Of lesser importance are the circumstances of therapy, i. e. whether we are dealing with conscious deception for gain or whether the practitioners genuinely believe that they emit some kind of 'pantheist energy' (Ibid). From the formal-legal point of view a question arises: why did the Ministry of Labor enter the occupation of bioenergy therapist in the occupation register without consulting the Health Ministry on this, thereby violating the binding legal order (Law on the Profession of the Physician), and why did the Health Ministry not challenge such unlawful decisions? Similar actions should have been taken by the Supreme Medical Chamber (Ibid: 63). Stanisław Sterkowicz ends his discussion by emphasizing the promotional role of the commercial media in publicizing often sensational and unconfirmed information about the effects allegedly achieved by nonconventional therapists. Likewise, a detrimental role is played by serial programs broadcast by commercial TV companies, e.g. the *Ręce które leczą* [Hands that heal] program, which in fact constitute a kind of surreptitious advertising of businessmen-healers (Ibid: 64). Another kind of approach close to behavioral sciences is to look at the 'paramedicine phenomenon' from the standpoint of social psychiatry (Pilecki 1994, 5: 170-174). Social psychiatrists hold that the problem of investigating paramedicine should be treated in broad terms, from the perspective of analyses of social and cultural factors. M. Pilecki stresses that the optimal point of view should embrace the **sociological perspective** [*my emphasis*, W. P.]. That is why a separate subchapter is titled *Medycyna alternatywna – ujęcie socjologiczne* [Alternative Medicine – A Sociological Interpretation]. Using the W. Piątkowski classification, Pilecki distinguishes three kinds of non-medical healing systems: self-treatment, folk medical systems and therapeutic practices of healers (Ibid: 170-174). Unlike many publications on clinical medicine, he emphasizes that the sociological perspective allows the physician to understand social and cultural motives inducing people to utilize healers' services. Like S. Sterkowicz, this author also discusses hazards arising from the use of unconfirmed and unpredictable healing methods. He writes; 'Patients are persuaded by them [healers] to reduce the doses of or give up some drugs; especially during polypragmasia the unmentioned problem is also the effect of the healing methods applied by paratherapists on the health of their clients' (Ibid: 171). Cross-cultural psychiatry and psychology may be an interesting perspective enabling us to better understand the phenomenon of healing because the reaction of the patient exposed to intense stress can be examined in terms of his/her unconscious or conscious psychical needs and the therapist's actions aimed at satisfying them. A visit to a healer who uses non-conventional treatment methods is a kind of support provided most often in situations where the patient has not obtained the expected effective help, having first sought medical aid. The contact between the non-professional therapist and the patient can be interpreted in terms of 'non-specific psychotherapeutic effects' (Ibid). The point of view of cross-cultural psychiatry also makes it possible to reconstruct the world image offered to the patient by the therapist and to explain the mechanism describing the force of interpersonal relationships. In the healers' preferred image of the world, spiritual energy interpenetrates with the world of matter, and illness is treated as a kind of disorder of biopsychosocial balance while the healer's position is unique, exceptional, exempt from criticism, and undisputable. That is why a therapy session has its script, dynamism and drama with its own accumulation, the patient being the subject of the healer's actions. In this kind of contact there are simply no incurable diseases as the healer can eliminate their 'real' causes and bring the organism to the state of balance and finally, to the state of health. Therefore psychiatry, as a discipline of clinical medicine, makes it possible to understand the characteristic 'cultural relativity of etiology and therapeutic methods' (Ibid: 172). Pilecki says: 'Paramedicine is a great challenge to psychotherapy, prompting the latter to seek deeper grounding in the scientific paradigm' (Ibid.). The psychiatric interpretation of paramedicine may refer *inter alia* to the views of Freud and Jung and to the application of A. Kępiński's 'information metabolism theory'. The adoption of the perspective of clinical psychiatry permits us to find that for example stress induced by illness is a factor disturbing rationality (both of thinking and decisions); it is then that the kind of reasoning that is called irrational (prelogical) appears. In the clinical psychiatrist's view, the stable popularity enjoyed by non-conventional treatments in Poland, Europe and throughout the world, poses questions to medicine that should persuade it to analyze the reasons why the expressive needs and expectations of the patients are negligibly satisfied during contact with the physician. This special way of interpretation of non-medical healing systems by social psychiatry ends with a conclusion: 'Alternative medicine, however, often rejects illness and death as degeneration. It creates a delusion of human omnipotence. Such an approach can never be accepted by physicians' (Ibid: 174).

As has been said before, one of the few clinical disciplines that systematically attempted to evaluate non-conventional healing methods from the early 1980s is oncology. We will therefore examine selected examples of such analyses and present their conclusions. M. Pawlicki of the Jagiellonian University Medical College's Institute of Oncology Chemotherapy Clinic has carried out systematic analyses of the phenomenon of non-conventional healthcare for over thirty years. In oncology, complementary and alternative medicine (CAM) is usually defined as action that has an effect on the patient's health by means of measures and methods **generally not accepted** [*my emphasis*, W. P.] and not used by physicians. In clinical oncology it is commonly assumed that these measures may have an effect on the patient's psyche and some of them may even bring momentary relief in the case of vegetative conditions. It is difficult to assess this kind of treatment; it may be regarded as neutral activities or may be positively received by patients without serious organic diseases but with strong faith in the efficacy of the methods employed. It may, however, produce measurable damage caused by a wrongly selected therapeutic agent (e.g. in the treatment of diabetes), or deterioration of health as a result of improper chiropractic procedures, etc. From the standpoint of clinical oncology the highest danger is the substantial delay in commencing specialist treatment (on average, in 26% of patients with diagnosed tumors) (Pawlicki 1997, 1: 14-17). At the same time Pawlicki emphasizes that 'positive reports on non-conventional medicine **do not come from scientific publications. Specialist studies are few and do not yield encouraging results** [*my emphasis*, W. P.]' (Ibid: 15). From the patient's point of view these methods seem attractive as they appear not unforced, non-invasive, non-traumatic and without visible undesirable elements. By contrast, oncology offers mutilating surgery, unpleasant chemotherapy, lengthy hospital treatment, etc. Non-conventional therapists devote much time and attention to their patients, establishing deep emotional contact with them, showing interest in their personal problems, and offering comparatively inexpensive procedures to which they themselves attribute high efficacy. An additional popularity-enhancing factor is the very favorable media accounts; the flood of information presented in pamphlets without reviews, published by the interested party, i. e. non-conventional therapists, and wide availability of periodicals affiliated with Healers' Associations. These magazines in fact contain surreptitious advertising materials, and also present pseudo-assessments of the promoted healing methods, the opinions being far from reliable, accurate and objective (Ibid: 16). Positive opinions by patients about better health condition should be accounted for by the use of suggestion and the effect of the therapist's optimistic opinions. On the other hand, oncologists meet with cooperation on the part of some bioenergy therapists who refer their patients to oncological clinics if they suspect that those visiting their offices may suffer from cancerous conditions, which they cannot cure (Ibid: 18).

Professor Pawlicki's team also monitored the utilization of non-conventional healing methods by cancer patients (Pawlicki 1999, 1: 31-33). The studies were undertaken to discover the extent to which the use of non-conventional methods of treatment could influence the fates of the patients and the five-year survival rates (Ibid: 31). The investigation showed that one in four patients who started specialist treatment had previously engaged in non-conventional therapy, which delayed clinical procedures on average by four to six months. In 1997/1998 the delay covered as much as 27% of reporting patients, which meant that in a considerable number of cases causal treatment **was no longer possible** [*my emphasis*, W. P.] (Ibid.) It should be added that financial losses incurred by the family would have been substantial especially with the use of diverse, and hence very expensive drugs. From the standpoint of clinical oncology, most of the obtained results (of non-conventional therapy) approximate the *placebo effect* (Ibid: 32). Oncologists register patients who use various non-medical healing methods: bioenergy therapy, chiropractic treatment, treatment with illegal pseudo-drugs, diet methods, self-treatment, herbal medicine, amulets and talismans. The author of these studies believes that some of non-conventional therapists could be invited to cooperate in order to assist with palliative and hospice treatment. On the other hand, a large-scale information campaign should be launched in order to educate patients on the risk of seeking treatment from non-physicians and on the consequent hazards. The media should be also persuaded to provide reliable and objective information about alternative medicine (Ibid: 33). Analyzing the advantages and disadvantages of non-conventional healing systems, oncologist M. Pawlicki asserts that the advantages cover the possibility of controlled or uncontrolled *placebo effect*, a complementary role in augmenting clinical treatment, lower therapy costs and low risk of side effects. The risk factors are uncontrolled occurrence of adverse effects (during treatment with peat, with kerosene, and the use of antineoplastons), delay in receiving proper treatment, and psychological dependence on the healer, which may make it difficult to terminate therapy.

Studies on the range of risk in the treatment using non-conventional methods were also conducted by the Medical University of Gdansk Department of Palliative Medicine (Majewska et al. 1999, 5: 45-49). The aim of the study was to learn the views of patients in the terminal stages of cancerous disease on the efficacy of and their personal preferences for alternative medicine. The survey covered 44 subjects (22 men and 22 women) who used hospice care at home; the patents were at the stage of infiltration and metastases to many organs. The average age of the patients was 63.6 years. 75% of those surveyed believed that alternative medicine was effective to a different degree, while 25% of the informants were of the opposite opinion. The higher the level of the patient's education, the higher the level of approval of non-conventional healing methods (in the group with higher and secondary education 90.9% of the subjects considered such methods effective), while 67.0% of those surveyed were of the opinion that such methods could be effective in treating tumors. The most effective therapeutic techniques named by the patients were herbal medicine (46.3%) and bioenergy therapy (27.2%). The patients tried to determine the main reason for the popularity of non-conventional medicine, which, they concluded, was the inefficacy of biomedical therapies. 44% of subjects had direct experience of non-medical treatments, 20% of them still practicing such measures (Ibid: 46-47).

This theme is summed up by the study conducted by Professor M. Pawlicki's team, aimed at establishing the main causes of delays in the commencement of oncological treatment by a group of 204 patients with malignant tumors. Since the year 2000, 9% of the patients admitted by the Institute of Oncology in Krakow delayed seeking biomedical treatment (12 months on average); these delays were caused by their utilization of non-conventional treatments. As compared with the analysis carried out in 1987/1988 it turned out that, although patients used non-conventional therapies less often, the duration of delays in seeking specialist treatment increased (Pawlicki and Rysz-Postawa 2001, 5: 494-498). Recent reports in clinical oncology suggest that the popularity of non-conventional methods remains high among patients with such diagnoses. The use of non-conventional healing methods may sometimes be treated as a kind of care enhancing life quality, reducing stress, and optimizing mechanisms of coping with discomfort or improving adjustment to the situation of deteriorating health or the process of dying (Krasuska et al. 2003, 2, LVIII: 418-498). To recapitulate, reports of clinical oncology suggest that, although the actual healing role of non-conventional treatments has yet to be proved, the efficacy of these therapies should be systematically monitored. The main reason why these procedures should not be ignored is that they are widely used by patients with tumors. The problem has as much a biomedical as a psychosocial dimension (Marlicz 2003, 10: 277-279).

The analysis of the literature shows that treatment by means of non-conventional methods is also a subject of interest of gastroenterology, rheumatology, allergology, neurosurgery, rehabilitation and nursing sciences (Albrecht et al. 2001, 4: 311-313; Kolasiński 2001, 10: 213-241; Wielosz-Tokarzewska and Szczepański 2002, 4: 288-292; Górski 1996, 1(3): 168-171; Rutkowska et al. 2000, 14 (1): 17-21; Rutkowska et al. 2000, 8/9: 13-15; Lisowska 1995, 10: 21-22).

A separate theme of interest to the sociologist in this section of our presentation is the publications by medical doctors who have actively practiced non-conventional methods and have promoted them for years. We might add that there are eminent representatives of academic medicine who have had a liberal attitude to non conventional therapies. For example J. Aleksandrowicz stressed that some of these methods were close to medicine while others raised disputes and controversies, e.g. homeopathy (J. Aleksandrowicz 1990: 5-6). When assessing different methods of non-conventional natural medicine, it is emphasized that such methods cannot be used unrestrainedly, uncritically and at individual discretion. 'For that reason, prior to application of any procedure for therapeutic purposes in any condition or complaint, a specialist physician should be consulted […]' (Świrski, Ibid: 115). At the same time, when evaluating other branches of so-called alternative medicine, e.g. homeopathy, it is said that '[…] homeopathy still raises many controversies in the medical community. They concern both its healing efficacy and the principles upon which this current is based' (Rewerski, Ibid: 204). Advocates of homeopathy write: 'In order to successfully convince representatives of academic medicine of the efficacy of homeopathy, we would have to indisputably prove – by using specific methods –

the efficacy of homeopathic drugs [...] There are no such studies in pharmacological literature' (Ibid: 205). Summing up the general treatment efficacy in particular diseases, it is pointed out that 'Over the years in oncology not a single patient has been observed, in whom any objective improvement in the sense of inhibition of tumor growth has been found as a result of bioenergy therapies [...] there is enough ample material for these observations' (Pawlicki Ibid). Those physicians who support the practice of acupuncture attempt to argue that its value lies in the absence of side effects, the method being effective in treating pain complaints, relieving functional disorders of many organs, and in prevention. On the other hand, it is stressed that 'having no possibility of explaining all mechanisms of acupuncture should not prevent its application.' (Tomaszewski 1999, 94: 29). Doctors who use acupuncture believe that the main reason for its popularity and the popularity of similar methods is the deficit of medical services at the expected level and their high costs, which should prompt healthcare managers and physicians to provide CAM services in the same way as allopathic medicine (Woźniak et al. 2004 (1): 1150 et seq.) The cited doctors who actively promote acupuncture believe that knowledge of CAM methods and techniques is necessary for medical students and other healthcare personnel. Those who practice non-conventional methods define CAM as a set of '[...] medical health systems, procedures and products that **are not** [*my emphasis*, W. P.] recognized as a part of conventional medicine' (Ibid: 1151). Texts of this kind also introduce the term 'integrative medicine', which combines conventional medicine and CAM **with documented efficacy and efficiency** [*my emphasis*, W. P.] The foundation of this medicine is the use of 'natural, less invasive methods based on stimulation of self-treatment'. Proponents of such conceptions recommend that the teaching of teaching CAM be included in the curricula of medical studies. The main arguments for CAM are not so much the results of clinical studies as reference to public acceptance of these methods (Ibid: 1168). Supporters of acupuncture argue that the method can be attractive in treatments based on the application of pharmacology to chronic diseases: 'For acupuncture is a natural method based – as a healing factor – on the mobilization of the organism's vital forces to fight a disease, its capacity for self-regulation and self-regeneration' (Operacz 1997: 11-12). Acupuncture is based on the alleged action of **energy** [*my emphasis*, W. P.] Chi flowing through meridians and on the maintenance of balance between its opposing elements Yang and Yin; any obstruction in the energy flow or imbalance between Yang and Yin will result in the commencement of pathological changes in the human organism. Proponents of acupuncture stress that it is a scientific method and its mechanisms can be rationally explained (Ibid: 166). According to the promoter of this method in Poland, Professor Z. Garnuszewski, medicine is becoming more dehumanized, holistic views and the side effects of pharmacotherapy are increasingly being challenged, and there is the phenomenon of increasing drug dependence; thus, there is a greater need for methods of fighting illness 'without the agency of chemistry' (Garnuszewski 1996, 1: 25-28). When describing the efficacy and versatility of acupuncture, Garnuszewski suggests that it can be employed to treat HIV carriers (Ibid, 2: 120-121). Another non-conventional method that doctors sometimes use is homeopathy. Supporters of the method are convinced that there are strong relationships between homeopathy and acupuncture, one method characteristically complementing the other. The argument for such cooperation is the fact that they are complementarily used by patients who believe in the synergistic action of these techniques. One the other hand, even the advocates of both methods are aware that they are not accepted by the national healthcare service because they do have scientific grounds (Ibid: 331). Z. Garnuszewski therefore writes: 'It should be strongly emphasized, however, that although homeopathy **has not produced** [*my emphasis*, W. P.] reliable evidence of its efficacy, many experienced doctors talk about it with respect [...]' (Ibid). Doctors supporting homeopathy believe that this 'paramedical method', as they call it, stimulates the organism's own powers to fight illness, the task of homeopathic products being to 'back up the organism's immune system. The popularity of homeopathy also stems from inexpensive medicines and their availability, from being prevention-oriented, and from the creation of a treatment system open towards the patient' (Bielec 2001, 2: 10-12). Homeopaths themselves admit that attempts to test the method scientifically fail. Despite the belief that the method is safe 'we do not have a testable theory showing the mechanism of this therapy' (Riley et al. 2001, 4: 14). Homeopathic practitioners believe that the main reason why this treatment method is not accepted is that 'The conception and structures of thinking in conventional clinical studies **cannot be translated** [*my emphasis*, W.P.] onto the domain of homeopathy' (Albrecht 2002, 2: 13). That is why evidence-based medicine is 'neither anticipated nor expected in homeopathy' (Ibid: 13). Since 2002 the homeopathic community has also indicated other problems that restrict its development. The main formal barrier is legislative questions, which make it impossible or difficult to work in private practice in homeopathy offices because in the Polish Classification of Products and Services (2002) homeopathic physicians were excluded from the medical profession and transferred to the category of **paramedical** [*my emphasis* W. P.] service providers. Consequently, the list of VAT-exempt services **no longer includes** paramedical services, all homeopathy offices having been taxed at the 22% VAT rate (Mrozowska 2003, 3: 1). The main reason for these problems, the homeopathic community believes, is that homeopathy is treated like paramedicine rather than medicine. However, homeopaths state that there is only one university center in

Europe that conducts systematic studies in homeopathy (in Switzerland), and governments recognize homeopathy as an official method only in the UK, Rumania, Hungary, and in Belgium (Ibid: 2). Even homeopaths seem to feel the growing need to revise some canons of the concept. They concede that the so-called vital force is not related to the working of mechanisms of the immune system and apparatus; because this force is indeterminate and not substantiated by reliable evidence, it cannot be recognized as the reflection of the objective truth (Bożyk 2004, 2: 15). Homeopathic journals also contain examples of applications of these methods, one of them being 'the treatment of tumors with mistletoe'. The commentary reads, 'Mistletoe products are used to treat tumors as a supplement to three **basic** [*my emphasis*, W. P.] methods of tumor management such as surgeries, radiotherapy and or/chemotherapy […] The sooner we apply mistletoe therapy, the better results it will produce' (Raport 2004, 3: 24). What will homeopathy be like tomorrow? Will the number of patients believing in its efficacy continue to grow? Homeopathic doctors list the following problems that obstruct the development of this 'philosophy of healing': underestimation of the method by official healthcare providers; and lack of formal-legal regulations on the status of practitioners of homeopathic treatment methods. Advocates of the Hahnemann method report that 81% of Poles have heard about homeopathy and 30% use homeopathic treatments. We might add that the professional journal for healthcare managers, "Rynki Zdrowia" reports that homeopathic drugs accounted for less than 3% of the total amount of medicines sold in Poland in 2007. In the Polish circumstances the chief opponents of the method are representatives of academic medicine who demand *inter alia* that homeopathy-practicing doctors have their medical license revoked. In the statement of 15 April 2008 the Supreme Medical Council negatively judged the use by doctors of homeopathy and other alternative medicine methods, and condemned the tolerant attitude of some medical schools towards methods of unproven efficacy. Homeopaths maintain that this attitude prevents the teaching of homeopathy at medical universities (Sułkowski 2007, 3: 1-3). Despite the lack of legislative solutions and aversion of most medical organizations and associations, supporters of this current are optimistic, 'Homeopathy has good prospects before it [..], which depend on the efforts of its students; it will certainly change but it will always go forward because homeopathy is genuine' (Scimeca 2004, 4: 11).

To sum up, we can conclude the following:

Relations between medicine as knowledge plus a system of practices and social life define the basic area of activities of the sociology of health, illness and medicine.

The stance taken by representatives of clinical medicine towards non-conventional healthcare is especially important if we want to examine and understand relations between medicine and non-medicine.

Medicine as one of the fundamental natural sciences is based on scientifically documented knowledge (evidence-based medicine), which is collected and verified in a strictly specified way, by means of precisely defined, standard methods.

The axis of the foregoing medical publications of the 1990s until recently was an attempt to answer the question of why, despite great progress in the development of evidence-based methods of fighting against illness, so many patients yield to advertisements for methods publicized as inexpensive, painless, fast-working and highly effective. A question was also asked whether non-conventional methods can have a real effect on the patient's health condition.

From the standpoint of the history of medical sciences we can speak of the problem of non-medical healthcare only from the point when scientific medicine fully developed, i.e. from the first half of the twentieth century onwards.

Doctors point out that the main argument, which according to the healers, testifies to the high efficacy of their methods, is not the results of reliable clinical tests and studies (there are none) but the sociological, as it were, argument: the quoting of opinions of some 'satisfied patients'.

According to the view of medical circles that are critical of CAM, additional factors enhancing the popularity of healers are the permanent favorable support by the commercial media, and contravention of the Law on the Profession of Physician.

The main danger of patient utilization of non-conventional healing methods is delays in the commencement of proper treatment (with tumors the average delay may be as long as eight months).

The approach of social psychiatry (cited above) tries to establish the cultural reasons why patients prefer non-conventional medicine.

One of the few disciplines of clinical medicine that conducts systematic research on non-conventional healing methods is oncology. Clinical oncology emphasizes that there is not a single documented case of a patient being cured as a result of CAM utilization. Most of the effects obtained by healers that can be felt by the patient are the results of the *placebo effect.* Some oncologists, however, see a chance of cooperation with selected healers as part of terminal and palliative care.

A distinct, interesting theme is the analysis of opinions of doctors – supporters of non-conventional methods, mainly acupuncturists and homeopaths. As an argument for the efficacy of their healing techniques the latter produce carefully collected 'opinions of their own clients', patients being sometimes encouraged to write such testimonials.

Most non-conventional therapists maintain that the efficacy of their methods cannot be assessed using standard measures applied in academic medicine; on the other hand, the evaluation techniques that they propose are not accepted by clinical medicine. In these circumstances qualitative differences between medicine and non-medicine persist and even intensify.

PART TWO

POLISH FOLK MEDICAL SYSTEMS AND SELF-TREATMENT – CONTINUITY AND CHANGE

1. Sociomedical Studies on Folk Medical Systems and Village Self-Treatment. Problems and Controversies

The results of sociological studies conducted twenty years ago that most social needs caused by illness are realized **outside of** professional healthcare institutions, *inter alia* as part of self-treatment, folk medical systems, family and self-help groups (Sokołowska 1986; Freidson 1976; 157-158; Gottschalk-Olsen 1990: 3-5; and part III of this book 1.3 and 1.4; see also Senior and Viveash 1998: 12-13; and Nettleton 2009: 217-221). In the past this applied to most illnesses, now usually to sociopsychosomatic diseases, most frequent with a comparatively mild course and good prognosis. It should be remembered that the most popular and universal system offering help with the elimination of illness was (and still is in some non-urbanized Asian and African countries) folk medical systems. The role of folk medicine is largely determined by the percentage of the rural population in a given country. In Poland this rate was and still is one of the highest in Europe (in the fourteenth century- 85%, in 1931 – 73%, in 1987 – 39.1 %, and in 2005 – 38.6%, figures after Statistical Yearbooks, "Rocznik" 2006: 207).

The still large size of the peasant class is one though not the only argument for the need to conduct interdisciplinary studies on the system of folk medicine treated as a cultural legacy of the past (Burszta 1967: 393-394). The importance and relevance of this suggestion is also confirmed by the fact that behaviors in illness among peasant families are still traditional to some extent despite the impact of long-term industrialization and urbanization processes, educational revolution and the influence of the media.[28] A manifestation of this tradition is for example the presence of non-professional village therapists among those providing help with illness. This tendency seems to persist (Tylkowa 1989:34-36).

In this part we will focus on selected methodological problems; their analysis may speed up the completion of research objectives, especially in social sciences.

In recent decades medical sociology was one of the fastest developing sociological subdisciplines. This is confirmed by the theoretical achieve-

28 Field studies by A. Bartoszek show that self-treatment, especially among elderly women (demographically old age in the country is female) is a popular and lasting manner of coping with illness, with 44% of the women surveyed using self-treatment (Bartoszek 2001; Piątkowski 1990:41).

ments of the discipline, the development of its own methodology, and by the number of publications. Weiss and Lonnquist (2006: 1-11), when listing the main research current of the discipline, point to alternative and complementary healing practices. When analyzing the bibliography of the discipline we can easily see that most research ideas were oriented to urbanized and technologically/organizationally advanced industrial societies. There are practically no sociomedical (even Western) publications concerned with illness categories and social behaviors accompanying illness in rural (peasant) families, which largely hinders the conceptualization of one's own research projects. Nor are there frames of reference, a tried and tested methodology, and traditions of comparative studies.

1.1. Difficulties in Defining Concepts and Terms

The analysis of Polish and Western sociological, sociomedical, ethnological, medical and historical publications on folk medical systems shows that in order to name the non-professional ways of helping with illness used in the rural areas, different authors use diverse terms, often treating them as synonymous; for example: quack medicine, folk medicine, folk medical practices, magical healing practices, traditional medicine, irrational medical systems, etc. (Sokołowska 1987, 1: 84 et seq.; Brylak 1970: 309 et seq.; Tylkowa 1989; Sokołowska 1986; Piątkowski 1991; 239-241; Jeszke 1996: 93-109; Penkala-Gawęcka 2006; 21-26). As we can easily see, many of these terms contain the word *medicine*. The term does not seem well-founded when applied to several dozen diverse methods and 'theories' of healing found in the Polish countryside in the past and at present. Village folk healing practices and at-home self-treatment differ from medicine in the same way as each commonsense, intuitive, trial-and-error activity differs from standards of natural science, which is methodologically correct, applies appropriate methods of medical statistics, uses taxonomy that makes it possible to describe the results of the cognitive process in exact and unambiguous terms, and recognizes as scientific only those propositions that have sufficient justification as the reliable application of repeated and verified research methodologies, etc. (remember that modern medicine is termed evidence-based medicine (EBM), taxonomy issues having been dealt with extensively in Part One of this book).

Rural folk medical systems do not fulfill the foregoing criteria of 'being science', hence it is more appropriate to define them with a term 'folk medical systems' rather than folk medicine.[29] Unlike medicine, in folk healthcare the principal role is played by the folk practitioner's intuition and his/her individual therapeutic and diagnostic experience, and knowledge of illness prevention and illness origin. Folk medical systems do not have a 'theoretical superstructure', the dominant one being the orientation towards therapeutic practice, and there is no tendency to record one's own results (especially negative). When analyzing the constituents of the 'social role of the folk practitioner' we can see clearly that many folk therapists regard their therapeutic proficiency as unique, mysterious, and reserved exclusively for chosen successors. Although in the late twentieth century there was a noticeable penetration of some elements of medical knowledge (usually incomplete and distorted) into the practices in question, in most cases the competence of folk therapists practically does not go beyond everyday 'practical wisdom of life'. What we have said about folk healing practices is only aimed at emphasizing the qualitative differences between natural sciences represented by medicine and the traditional, trial and error-based, practically oriented, intuitive folk medical system. I do not express my opinion here on the biochemical efficiency of this type of healthcare (it appears that no systematic clinical studies on the subject have been conducted to date in Poland). In sociological research we can base our studies on the patient's self-assessment of his/her health. The results of preliminary sociomedical investigations on the subjective assessment of health condition show that for example their patients believe that folk chiropractors produce good treatment results; the same holds true for the opinions on the effects of therapies offered by village herbalists. While assessing the instrumental qualifications of non-professional therapists we must not forget at the same time about iatrogenicity of technochemical medicine, the growing problem of side effects, etc. This subject has not been sufficiently studied yet (Więckowska 2002; 174-181). Analysis of the elements of patient – folk therapist interaction most often shows that the patient's contact with the therapist is good; patients respect the use of religious elements during treatment, and people speak approvingly of the use of natural therapeutic agents. Village illness specialists are usually closely associated with the local communities where they operate; it often happens that while they work as farmers they feel it their duty

29 This subject was discussed by ethnologists Z. Libera and D. Penkala-Gawęcka. Libera emphasizes that predictions by positivist-scienticist science that folk medical systems would be marginalized did not come true '[...] interest in what is usually called folk medicine does not grow weaker while it exhibits its vitality, which will not diminish with the successes of science and medicine (1995;7). See also the results of field studies on folk medical systems in Ślesin, where typical village healing methods used by local folk practitioners were described (Penkala-Gawęcka 1996: 153-156).

to help those suffering with illness (Piątkowski 1990; 19).[30] A significant methodological postulate is to develop consistent views on the structure of folk medical systems. The author gave his views in Part One of this book. This conception distinguished four integral interrelated parts in folk medical systems: a) knowledge of the causes of illnesses, divided into material and magical-mystical causes; b) knowledge of illness prevention, with distinction between material and mystical-magical ways; c) diagnostic knowledge, most extensive, distinguishing material and mystical-magical factors; d) therapeutic knowledge covering material means and ways of treatment (including folk pharmacy and surgery) and mystical-magical and psychological ones (Piątkowski 1990).

1.2. Degree of Source Credibility

We should mention another problem faced by those conducting sociological research on the folk medical system: i.e. having an incomplete and unrepresentative set of sources and information, which may lead to a distorted picture of the system. A similar danger lies in the fact that folk healthcare at the turn of the nineteenth century was described and assessed from the perspective of the 'intelligentsia informants': landowners, village teachers, priests, etc; it was studied more often by enthusiasts and lovers of so-called village folklore than by suitably qualified persons. It is equally difficult to assess the reliability of the picture of the folk medical system as described by doctors of that period (*Pamiętniki lekarzy* 1939). We should remember that despite a huge deficit of medical professionals even those few graduates of medical schools who worked in the rural areas found it extremely difficult to make a living from private practice alone. The memoirs of country doctors show that it was hard to overcome the cultural, customary and psychological barriers which separated them from the rural people. The factor that effectively cut the peasant off from hospitals and pharmacies was poverty in the countryside. The most dangerous rivals of physicians, however, were village folk therapists (dishonest competitors), quacks/frauds who took patients from them. Frustrations and justified bitterness at being defeated by 'ignorant and slovenly' quacks prevented medical doctors, it seems, from objectively evaluating the behaviors of village therapists. Another source that permitted at least partial reconstruction of the folk medical system during the inter-

30 In the 1990s, when managing two research projects analyzing the effects of grave forms of chronic diseases (hemophilia and infantile cerebral palsy) I asked in the interview questionnaires about utilization of non-medical healing systems, which turned out to be fairly popular . See Rokicka-Milewska 1992: 250; Piątkowski and Karski 1988, XIX, 3-4: 152.

war period is peasant memoirs. But it should be borne in mind here that the memoirs competition was not oriented towards the issues of illness; consequently, accounts concerning this subject were usually fragmentary, marginal and sectorial. We should also understand that only peasants who could read and write were able to enter the competition. For that reason these documents present only a very rough picture of ways of coping with illness in the Polish countryside in the nineteenth and early and mid-twentieth centuries.

After WWII, with the nationalization of healthcare provision, the criminal and administrative law began to radically combat folk healing practices. Books and propaganda pamphlets were published to deride and discredit traditional folk healing methods and those who used them (Radzicki 160: 42; Ostrowski 1954; Borkowski 1980: 21-27). The Parliament at that time passed the Law on the Physician's profession (1950) which stated that help with illness could be provided only by certified graduates of medical schools (Article 26, Law on the Profession of Physician of 28 October 1950). Consequently, there are practically no data on folk healthcare for the period 1945-1960. The situation began to change in the mid-1960s, when the first studies on folk treatment methods were conducted, chiefly in the field of ethnology. To date, there has been no systematic medical study on the subject in question although medieval medicine arose *inter alia* from folk knowledge about health and illness. We may hope that initiating a discussion on methodological problems will not only bring us closer to the objective, and undistorted picture of folk medical systems but will also make us aware of the complementary character of many disciplines which study these important problems. (The perspective of interdisciplinary studies was outlined by B. Kuźnicka 1989: 5-9; Z. Libera also proposed ethnological-sociological-historical studies of folk medical systems, 1995: 7-8).

1.3. "Irrationality" of Folk Medical Systems

It is commonly assumed that the folk medical system contained (and still contains) beliefs based on the conviction that that there are supernatural forces and relationships that can be invoked and controlled by means of specific incantations and acts performed in a strictly defined way. This may give man the power over phenomena that he cannot control with natural means (Libera 1989: 154). If we adopt this definition of magical acts, we can see clearly that they were performed only when man could not influence the surrounding phenomena in other ways, for example by acting on the organism using material elements. Material acts were therefore complemented with magical elements. This is illustrated, among other sources, in peasants' memoirs (*Pamiętniki chłopów*), which described folk healing practices in the interwar period (*Pamiętniki chłopów* 1935-1936).

The causes of illnesses could therefore be not only material factors (injuries, fractures, excessive effort) but also spells and charms; illness could be prevented not only by choosing a 'healthy' site on which to build a house or the right diet, but also by amulets and talismans; the kind of illness (or its origin) could be established not only by viewing urine, feces or blood, but also through revelation or clairvoyance, by casting spells and incantations which were used together with the administering of herbal medicines and bloodletting.

Many publications on folk healing practices arbitrarily classify individual elements of this system, distinguishing between 'rational' and 'irrational' factors. Sometimes a conviction is expressed that so-called irrationality of the folk medical system was (is) associated with low (or non-existent) educational level of village therapists, assuming that elements defined as irrational will disappear with the progress of education, wide access to the mass media, etc. We know today that none of the elements of this reasoning is entirely true, that accepting and professing views inconsistent with the valid paradigm of natural sciences is not the exclusive feature of rural communities where the level of knowledge is predominantly low. For example, in the USA the wave of interest in the occult and Satanism and the fashion for exorcisms is characteristic of the urban middle class – there is ample sociological literature on the subject. The above-cited ethnological studies carried out by Danuta Tylkowa in the Carpathian Mountains show that magical elements can still be observed in rural communities in southern Poland (Tylkowa 1989; Recent representative sociological studies show great interest in soothsaying, prophecies, astrology and horoscopes in Polish society *Czy Polacy są przesądni…* 2006). In the 1990s the permanence of these elements was confirmed in the studies by D. Penkala-Gawęcka and J. Jeszke (the latter wrote that his investigations and other sources indicated a very high percentage of irrational behaviors, including magical-religious; 1993, I, 1).

To 'the peasant', folk culture (and its integral part – the healing system) constituted a logical, compact and uniform whole. The more we know about the past and present views of rural inhabitants, the more convinced we are of the relativity of the terms 'rational – irrational'. We should remember that acts and measures which some scholars regard as irrational were performed by specific persons and in a strictly defined way. This required considerable specialist knowledge of places, time, colors, etc., the 'spiritual' elements intermingling during the treatment process with material procedures and measures, which was meant to increase the efficacy of the therapy. This is clearly observable for example during skull trepanation operations performed in the present South-African folk medical system (Meschig and Schadewaldt 1982, 4: 32). Another example is the belief in fire as the ancient, universal symbol of illness destruction, often regarded as a healing and purifying agent. In the folk medical systems in different cultural circles it is generally assumed that illness, as something real and material penetrating into the human body, is situated *inter alia* in nails and hair. A logical consequence of this belief is thus the practice of cutting and burning the patient's nails, and the rite of removing tangled hair, etc. A similar case is the universal recognition of the magical meaning of figures (e.g. '3' and its power), words and sounds. The understandable consequence of the idea of illness as a concrete material entering the human body is dozens of known methods of driving it away by means of prayers, dreadful shamanic paraphernalia, violent dancing rites, piercing shrieks - illness had to be frightened and then given a chance to 'depart', e.g. through a trepanation hole (Ibid: 33-34). Treatment will be strengthened by the patient's 'seeing' this departure, hence they are shown pieces of 'cancerous tissue' by present-day Philippine healers, or white worms, known in folk healing methods, that leave the body as a result of successful treatment (Meek 1979: 60-61; on the present-day magical elements in the Polish folk medical system, see Winnicka 2002, 40: 78-81). Illness could be also expelled, as it were, 'from the inside', by giving a herbal medicine with a strong bitter taste to discourage the illness from staying in the human body, or a product made of dried fragments of dread-inspiring animals (snakes, lizards, bats, frogs) intended to scare the illness away (Zieleniewski 1845: 5 et seq.). Illnesses also seemed to disappear after the letting of bad blood, vomiting, and the administering of sweat-inducing agents.

Even these selectively chosen examples permit a conclusion that the fairly frequent division into rational and irrational elements in folk healthcare is carried out by researchers adopting a reductionist and scienticist system of values. The analysis of personal documents from the interwar period and the dichotomous classification of elements of the folk medical system were not perceived and accepted by the village population or by folk therapists who treated the villagers. Both these parties regarded healing procedures as accurate, homogeneous, logically justified and giving hope of recovery.

1.4. The Role of Historical Themes in Sociological Studies on the Folk Medical System

An introduction to the problem of the role of historical interpretation in studies on the sociology of non-biomedical healing is the position represented by Jan Stanisław Bystroń, a sociologist and ethnologist. Bystroń not only applied a sociological-ethnological approach, extremely successful in exploring the phenomena related to 'other medicine' but was also a forerunner of historical sociology. He emphasizes that folk culture also covers traditional healing practices, which are its integral part (Piątkowski 1999, I, XXIV). The folk medical system is an important kind of perspective in the perception and interpretation of the external world surrounding the individual (Burszta 1967: 394-395). Folk culture, according to Bystroń, is a set of contents passed by word of mouth (Bystroń 1947, 1). In the conception of historical and sociological studies on folk culture the central category is the conception of authorities (including persons endowed with authority). We should note immediately that village therapists, having very limited treatment methods (chiefly natural therapy) and few possibilities of using therapeutic techniques, based their healing success on the skilful development and strengthening of their prestige and authority in a local community. The permanence and comparatively limited variability of traditional folk medical systems (e.g. 'folk surgery') can be fully understood with reference to the historical sociology of J. S. Bystroń. The folk medical systems, functioning in small, comparatively isolated communities, and being based on the internal authority of the elderly, conserved and petrified old techniques of treatment and ways of applying of natural healing agents. On the other hand, the 'transmission belt' passing new medical developments into the country was the church and church people (the priest, the organist and the sexton), it was they who performed advisory functions in matters of health and illness by promoting new terms and ideas (Ibid). Similarly, diagnostic, therapeutic, etiological and preventive views, and treatment techniques were influenced by the manor, the landowner, and his family. Gradually, from the end of the nineteenth century the attitude to health and illness began to be molded by new communities and institutions: towns and schools (Piątkowski 1990).

We can thus say that the historical perspective allows the medical sociologist to understand more thoroughly the social phenomena that he describes and interprets, which is why this interpretation was adopted in my own research, especially in the studies of self-treatment and folk medical systems (Libiszowska-Żółtkowska et al. 1998, I). In the sociological interpretation presented here a significant role is played by description of historically changing forms of non-biomedical healthcare (self-treatment, folk medical systems and healing practices) from the primitive period to the Middle Ages to the Renaissance and the Enlightenment. A separate theme in this discussion is concerned with phenomena associated with non-professional treatment methods applied in the nineteenth and the first half of the twentieth centuries. During that period the history of the struggle between academic medicine and healing botchers was described in Poland and in Europe.

The starting point of my sociomedical analyses was also the assumption that the issues of non-biomedical healing systems appear in the general historical context or in medical history. In the general historical perspective the social scientist can be interested in the studies of communities of different types, which are described from the standpoint of various health- and illness-related behaviors. This is the case with H. Eildermann, who describes types of political systems, religions and healing practices of primitive societies (Eildermann 1953).

Health behaviors related to primitive healing systems are presented in a similar way by L. H. Morgan, who discusses three stages of mankind's transition from wildness to civilization (Morgan 1887). Health behaviors associated with folk healthcare are described more often and more accurately from the perspective of the history of medicine. Classic examples are the presentations by W. Szumowski (1935) B. Seyda (1962), M. Zieleniewski, Z. Kuchowicz, T. Brzeziński (especially his chapter on natural and non-conventional healing methods, 2000: 406-427) and others.

Studies on non-biomedical healthcare were also conducted by sociologists from Maria Curie-Skłodowska University, Lublin, Poland, S. Kosiński and S. Tokarski, who also included a historical perspective in their investigations. Kosiński's work is concerned with social determinants of health behaviors of the rural population from a historical standpoint (1864-1980). Using historical sources he attempts to reconstruct health awareness and attitudes to health and illness among the peasant population. In the introduction to his studies covering *inter alia* folk medical systems Kosiński opposes the disparaging attitude, frequent in sociology, to historical sources and interpretations. He stresses that the modern approach of the two sciences is characterized by the attitude of convergence and mutual inspirations (Kosiński 1983). The author presents the evolution of systems of help with illness from traditional folk healthcare to professional medicine, describing in detail the types of village therapists: shepherds, illness charmers, village old women-midwives, etc. He points to cultural, economic and psychological barriers, which cut the rural population off from professional medicine, and he tries to explain the phenomenon of the high prestige of nineteenth-century village therapists, who did not have advanced treatment techniques at their disposal but had 'the right approach' to the patient and were trusted by the people. In his assessment of the interwar period and in the detailed description of the processes of cultural and civilization transformations (modernization, institutionalization) he emphasizes the continuing high position of folk therapists in non-urbanized areas (Ibid: 171). By contrast, when discussing the end of the 1940s and the early 1950s, Kosiński shows the growing processes of professionalization of healthcare and administrative methods of combating the then folk therapists.

Another presentation of the issue of non-biomedical healing systems from the sociological perspective with reference to historical sources is Stanisław Tokarski's analyses (Tokarski 1992). In his study he gives a sociomedical description of health conditions in the Polish countryside from 1918 to 1989. As in Kosiński's publications, the main source here is historical material. When discussing health behaviors of the rural population at the turn of the nineteenth century, Tokarski emphasizes and examines the social roles and positions of the then village therapists (Ibid: 33). He also describes in detail traditional folk methods of treatment used as part of self-treatment and folk healing practices from the late nineteenth to the mid-twentieth centuries.

To sum up, we can conclude that since the beginning of medical sociology in Poland, sociomedical investigations have to some extent used historical inspirations and materials (Sokołowska 1969). The authors of these studies (S. Kosiński, S. Tokarski) refer to historical examples, appreciate this perspective and are inspired by sociological-historical interpretations (Bejnarowicz 1969). There is no doubt, as J. Jeszke rightly observes, that studies on non-biomedical healing systems would not be possible without taking into consideration the historical analysis of the changing social context of the phenomenon. It is also interesting to note the temporally changing evolution of the biomedical attitude towards other 'non-academic methods of treatment' – from hostility and resistance to attempted convergence (the 1970s and 1980s) to again challenging their scientific character and to growing criticism. The sociomedical studies discussed here make historical aspects one of the main points of reference. As has been shown earlier, modern research into the 'sociology of non-biomedical healing systems' inspired by historical interpretations can successfully adopt new perspectives, for example those of cultural sociology or sociology of knowledge. Historical inspirations create interesting forecasts for future interdisciplinary studies on non-biomedical healing systems. In this way the analyses of 'that which was serve to understand that which is and to project that which will be'.

2. Health and Illness in Peasant Families. The Social Framework of Self-Treatment and Folk Medical Systems in the Twentieth Century

The peasant class occupied and still occupies the central position in the historically formed social structure. In comparison with Western European countries Poland stood out as having a high percentage of the rural population, for example this rate was 85% in the fourteenth century. Although the urban population increased during the following centuries, we should remember that a large number of town inhabitants were engaged in agriculture. During the interwar period peasants accounted for 73% of the total Polish population (after the general census of 1931). Despite rapid social changes occurring in the past half-century the rural population accounted for 38.6% of all Poles (see the figures in the preceding section). This is one of the highest rates in Europe.

We will assume here that industrialization, urbanization, migrations, the educational revolution and the impact of the media did not cause fundamental changes in behavioral patterns toward illness in some part of the peasant population. These behaviors are still traditional to some degree. The main cause seems to be the long-lasting and multifaceted disadvantage of the peasant population (some scholars insist that the element that preserves the traditional behaviors and attitudes to health and illness forms a large percentage of the rural population with low education; Wdowiak and Syczewska-Weber 2006, 3-3: 140-150). It is only partly determined by the characteristics of agricultural production in small family-operated farms, which was largely the result of Communist Poland's agricultural policies based on the ideological assumption of the declining character of the peasant class. The consequence of this fact was the poor life quality of a considerable portion of individual farm-operating families (as indicated by many studies, e.g. Dyjak 2005: 92). Living conditions, working conditions, income size, household equipment, access to culture, and the amount of free time are some of the dimensions of this disadvantage. It is also observable in the quality of health services in the country. In principle the standard of healthcare in town and country should be similar. However, the analysis of epidemiological data shows discriminative differences: only 10% of practicing physicians work in the country, statistics showing that many of them come to work there from town, whether large or small. Many rural health centers have only one doctor, there is an acute deficit of basic specialists (pediatricians, gynecologists, etc.), and there are few specialist physicians. Village health centers are underequipped (with a shortage of specialist - diagnostic or rehabilitation- medical appliances), while village pharmacies usually have a narrower range of products. Elderly people in the country who cannot afford a private consultation with a specialist or a paid visit to non-public healthcare institutions fall ill more often, are usually ill for longer and have more acute symptoms. The ever-increasing costs of medicines and visits to a faraway clinical hospitals are, for village inhabitants, formidable barriers to commencing treatment (studies show that the most frequent cause of not treating a child is lack of money; Lachowski 2001,7; 287).

These facts lead to the conclusion that traditional peasant behaviors towards illness are objectively determined by the long-lasting and continuing (at least partly) disadvantage of this class (some reports maintain that the rural population is the 'great loser in the systemic transformation'; Wdowiak and Syczewska-Weber 2006, 3-4: 147; Skrętowicz and Gorczyca 2005).

In the following section we will discuss the state of health of the peasant population, typical ways of 'coping with illness', the determinants of behaviors in illness at the macro-social level, also taking into account meso- and microsocial determinants, emphasizing customs associated with illness, behavioral patterns, ways of expressing emotion, and fatalism. We will stress the importance of cultural and religious elements, and accentuate the special role played by women in coping with illness by using self-treatment and folk healing methods.

2.1. State of Health of the Polish Rural Population

The state of health of the peasant population over the last hundred years was indisputably poor. This is demonstrated by all kinds of available documents, scattered official letters, statistics, and projects to improve the health of peasants, diaries and memoirs written both by peasants and by representatives of other social strata living in the countryside (mainly landowners, physicians and priests).

In the past, peasant families did not regard health as a value in itself. The low status of health was associated with the constant threat to it, the frailty of life and poverty which, as peasant diarists wrote, 'did not let one live'. Children were easily produced, soon to die and be forgotten. 'Plague, war, and famine' would decimate the village population for centuries, and these people were helpless in the face of epidemics and natural disasters. Deeply internalized religious faith made the peasant treat illness humbly as 'divine judgment'. It was believed that two large groups - children and old people - had 'the shortest path to the heaven', which is why hardly anyone cared about their state of health (Tulli 1983; and 1990: 155-186; Piątkowski 2000, VI, 1: 65-72). Emphasizing the poor state of health, a seventeenth-century doctor wrote, 'in our country, where the rural population account for 3/4 of general population, mortality being far higher […] than in many European countries, the health of peasants deserves special concern on our part' (Starowolski 1606).

For centuries, the greatest epidemiological danger was tuberculosis. In the period1920-1933, in Wielkopolska [Great Poland] province alone, about a thousand people died of it every year, most of them children and young people. Another infectious disease that occurred on a mass scale and threatened peasant families was typhoid fever. Interwar medical reports accentuate epidemics of this disease, which affected whole villages and lasted for months. Educational authorities of the time alerted State agencies, reporting that there was hardly an elementary school (especially in the Eastern Borderland) that did not suspend teaching activities during the school year, because most pupils were absent, having fallen ill with infectious diseases. Despite their efforts, in the interwar period the public agencies failed to eliminate endemic incidences of syphilis, malaria, or trachoma (Lewczuk 1989). Poland was one of the countries with the worst health indicators, e.g. infant mortality rate in the country was high, while the death rate among the rural population in the same period was the highest in Europe.

The collapse of the healthcare system during WWII, the extermination of almost seven thousand physicians, the destruction of the healthcare service infrastructure, and extremely bad living conditions made the epidemiological situation in the country during the war and immediately after it absolutely tragic. People frequently suffered from all kinds of typhoid diseases, diphtheria, and malaria (Kosiński and Tokarski 1987). It was only a better organization of epidemiological services in 1956-1958, the compulsory assignment of medical school graduates to the countryside, and better supplies of medicines that made it possible to lower incidence rates of typhus, diphtheria, whooping cough, brucellosis, and typhoid fever (Saldak 1964, 7: 253-262). First successes also came in the fight against tuberculosis and venereal diseases (syphilis, gonorrhea), from which the peasantry had suffered for ages. This was achieved through educational/information campaigns, general screening tests, isolation of sick persons, and immediate free treatment. The tuberculosis incidence rate fell from 290.4 per 100 thousand in 1957 to 61.0 in 1984 (Kosiński and Tokarski 1987).

In the 1970s and 1980s the influence of intense agricultural mechanization and chemization processes on the state of health of the rural population made itself felt. The urbanization process also contributed substantially to the transfer of certain patterns of urban lifestyle into the countryside. Health statistics increasingly often recorded such causes of diseases and deaths as acute poisonings and accidents. At the end of the 1960s and in the early 1970s we can observe, on the one hand, a gradual decrease in the infant mortality rate, and on the other, an increase in excess mortality of males of up to 40 years old. The causes of this phenomenon have not been fully explained despite a number of plausible hypotheses associating it with alcoholism, smoking, imprudent nutritional habits, people overburdening themselves with two jobs, migration of the biologically stronger individuals to towns, and the inferior quality of healthcare. Recent studies on the health of the rural population (2000-2006) point to a higher threat to health caused by poor living conditions and low incomes. The high level of social stress, low self-assessment of health, a large number of accidents in farming work, and prevalence of cardiovascular and osteoarticular diseases are the results of this socioetiology (Filip and Lenart 2007, 1; 19-24).

In typical agricultural provinces (in eastern Poland) the prevailing causes mortality in the early 1980s were malignant tumors and cardiovascular diseases. In the country, bronchial asthma, pulmonary emphysema and bronchitis were three times as likely to be the causes of deaths (Ibid). It should be emphasized that in the structure of causes of death among the rural population, indeterminate states prevailed twice as often as the specified causes – this applied to one in ten inhabitants of the country. The problem of causes and effects of iatrogenic errors seems especially significant because studies show that physicians from villages and small towns often make mistakes in treating mental diseases (26%), injuries and accidents (25%), gynecological diseases (10%) and others (Tuszkiewicz 1968; see also studies on disabilities in the country – Piątkowski and Ostrowska 1994).

In the 1980s the number of cases of tumors and cardiovascular diseases rose sharply in Polish rural areas. Out of 3.7 million people suffering from hypertension, more than half did not begin treatment, this group covering largely the peasant population (*Raporty o stanie zdrowia…* 1982). A new phenomenon was the rapid ageing of the rural population. In the period 1987-1988 the percentage of people of post-productive age reached 14.3% in non-urbanized areas (10.9 % in towns). In typical agricultural provinces the elderly persons accounted for almost 20% of the population (Dzun 1989, 6: 48; Wdowiak and Syczewska-Weber 2006, 3-4). In the countryside, the aged are often impoverished, alone and ailing. Studies by L. Ostrowski show that poverty affected about 20% of the rural population in the late 1980s. Out of the investigated group of the rural impoverished, 2% defined their health as good, 30% defined it as average, and 68% believed their state of health was bad. Only one third of the 'aged and impoverished' group were able to walk freely at home, 42% moved with difficulty outside the home, 18% had problems walking in their flat and 7% were bedridden. Surveys carried out by Lublin's Institute of Rural Health [also called Institute of Rural Medicine] (2003) emphasize that the structural factors that petrify poverty are the large percentage of small farms (up to 5 hectares), poor economic conditions of families with many children, and a high percentage of people earning their living from irregular work (Ostrowski 1989, 11: 67 et seq.; Bujak 2003, 9: 107-128).

The examination of morbidity and mortality rates in the rural population over the last thirty years shows the overlapping of previously occurring diseases (animal-transmitted, infectious, parasitic, bronchial asthma, rheumatoid changes, overburdening of the locomotion organ) and diseases of a new type (hypertension, tumors, poisonings, injuries, etc.).

2.2. Characteristics of Illness Behavior in Peasant Families

Statistical figures show that members of the rural population fall ill more often than urban inhabitants. We can also prove that people in the country suffer from illness 'in a different way' than in town, this difference having developed historically. Sociological, sociomedical, ethnological and medical studies, and historical investigations using statistical, official and personal documents relating to the last hundred years demonstrate that behaviors in illness in peasant families are comparatively stable. S. Lachowski's studies demonstrate for example the continuing significance of self-treatment in the country, especially when treating children (2001, 7: 293).

The traditional nature of value systems, behavioral patterns and social roles has many sources but is also undoubtedly associated with the family character of the farm and, to some extent, its autonomy. The role of educational level is also important. A low level of education is a factor that makes one impervious to changes: a very large number of peasant family members have only elementary or basic vocational education. Moreover, the character of farm work and its organization still partly prevent peasant families from fully participating in culture, thereby making it difficult for them to adopt biopositive health behaviors. Until the mid-twentieth century, positive attitudes among the rural population towards the medical professions and institutions were extremely rare. One of the main features of the peasant style of being ill was self-sufficiency in fighting illness. The proof of stable tradition in the peasant approach to illness is the occurrence of **still overlapping** mystical-magical and natural elements. Reporting on the results of recent ethnological studies on folk healthcare, D. Tylkowa wrote, 'Folk knowledge about the origin of illness still contained natural elements (getting overchilled, overexertion) and mystical-magical, although one could notice that therapeutic elements were somewhat reduced both as the effect of education and the impact of the media, through steadily growing trans-local contacts, including contacts with academic medicine. There is no doubt, however, that the work of village therapists continued to combine irrational elements with rational views' (Tylkowa 1989: 98). Her research shows that the main carriers of tradition and conservativeness in the approach to illness are old **uneducated rural women functioning as local experts in health matters** [*my emphasis* W. P.].

Another relic of peasant traditionalism is the low status of health and life in the hierarchy of values. An analysis of characteristic features of peasant culture shows the limited range and importance of actions 'for health' in order to prevent illness, detect it early and avoid behavior that increases the risk of falling ill. Difficulties in studying the value of health and attitudes to health in the peasant tradition lie *inter alia* in the fact that health is perceived as a normal, unchanging state, stemming from 'divine grace' and not directly related to one's biopositive or bionegative behavior. For centuries, the living conditions of peasant families were so bad (hunger, cold, overwork) that illness leading to death (and eternal life) might have seemed like salvation. In the early seventeenth century Sz. Starowolski wrote that it was essential that the Republic [i.e. Poland] saw to it that lords did not willfully kill their serfs, deprive them of their land or overburden them with heavy work (Starowolski 1606). An extreme example of people's disregard for health was the practice of self-mutilation (blinding, breaking limbs) in order to achieve a better position in the 'respectable profession' of beggar and comparatively improve their living standards (Tulli 1983).

In the twentieth century, a disturbing underestimation of the value of health was also observed in the country. This was manifested, *inter alia*, in failure to understand the essence of prevention and in disregard for illness prevention measures. I. Solarz, one of the founders of the Health Cooperative in Markowa, when asked why its articles of association did not include illness prevention, said that curing was spectacular whereas prevention efforts could not be seen (Solarz 1937). Recent nationwide studies on preventive behaviors of the rural population (2006) showed insufficient knowledge of health education and deficient preventive behaviors (Florek 2006, 2L 246-249).

A manifestation of tradition in satisfying health needs of the rural population is the continuing role of self-treatment and folk healthcare. D. Tylkowa wrote, '[...] traditional healthcare is still a living phenomenon, especially in the use of natural therapeutic products and utilization of folk therapist services, particularly orthopedic and herbal practitioners. The fact that recognition of some folk healthcare practitioners did not drop even when the village population surveyed had an opportunity to utilize official healthcare service centers, seems to indicate that, in the view of most inhabitants, their (the practitioners') healing activity was characterized by sufficient instrumental efficiency, especially with conditions, in which academic medicine was believed to fail' (Tylkowa 1989: 107, Piątkowski 1990).

Self-treatment is the oldest, simplest and most common form of fulfilling health needs in peasant families. It is applied when the help of a physician (or a village folk therapist) is regarded as unnecessary because diagnosis is not difficult while easily available home therapeutic agents are sufficient to fight illness. Self-treatment covers the knowledge of the causes of typical, most frequent diseases, preventive measures, and treatment. This knowledge derives from one's life experience, the experience of close family and friends, and from stereotypical information drawn from scientific medicine, both past and present, and from healers' practices. The character of self-treatment depends on the place of residence (town or country). In rural areas, self-treatment is often closer to folk healing methods. The roles of non-professional therapists in peasant families are performed by the patients, their immediate families and friends, and neighbors. The patient's actions to determine the state of their own health, establish the kind of ailment, find the right therapeutic agent and to cure themselves are realized in the family and that is why they can be termed 'home medicine' or home ways of treatment (Lachowski 2001, 7; 293 et seq.). The families perform among others the caring/protective function, providing their sick members with help and support. Behaviors in illness take the form of characteristic social roles. As a rule self-treatment is applied by parents and grandparents to their children and grandchildren; the younger and fitter family members also provide therapeutic help to the elderly and infirm members.

The existence of the folk medical system is proof of continuing traditionalism in the peasants coping with illness. Recent ethnological studies cited in Part One of this study indicate that folk medicine commands high respect among the rural population. This is a clearly distinct, coherent and closed system resulting from centuries-long isolation and self-sufficiency of the countryside. The overwhelming majority of folk therapists have a comparatively low level of education, and very little (if any) any knowledge of current medical science. They regard their healing expertise as reserved for them and keep it in utmost secrecy. A characteristic of the techniques and measures of the folk medical system is the use of resources of mineral, animal, human and plant origin.

2.3. Woman as A Home Therapist

Both now and in the past, most diseases that we encounter in everyday life are cases with well-known etiology, a mild course and good prognosis (Sokołowska 1986: 13-20). The treatment of these typical diseases is often the province of women: sisters, wives, mothers, and grandmothers. The role of women as therapists can be viewed from the institutional and non-institutional standpoint (S. Lachowski's studies show that during a child's illness s/he is most often treated and looked after by his/her mother, who utilizes self-treatment; 2001: 293).

Statistical figures show that large numbers of young women choose medical studies at medical school and schools of pharmacy, dentistry or nursing; after graduation they work in healthcare institutions (Cockerham 2004; 194-196; Thomas 2003: 80). This is a fairly obvious finding but, at the same time, little is known about the motivations of young women to choose medical professions or the causes of the unusual persistence of promedical orientation. We are not sure in what way these motivations differ from the reasons why young men choose those professions. A separate, and not less important problem is the effect of feminization on the character of social relations between doctor and patient, or the way of functioning by medical institutions, especially outpatient healthcare. It also appears that, without an in-depth knowledge of the effects caused by the 'distinct character' of women as the largest group of healthcare personnel, and knowledge of their special interest, needs and aspirations, it is not possible to make far-reaching changes in the healthcare system. The variants of reform of this system presented to date in Poland do not seem to take note of the results of feminization of medical professions.

The interesting and insufficiently studied problems associated with the woman's role as a professional therapist (physician, dental surgeon, pharmacists or nurse) are not the dominant theme of this discussion (Cockerham and Glasser (2001: 307-309). In the following section we will be particularly interested in how the women fulfill special social roles **outside of the system of professional medical services**; the first is the role of a home therapist who takes measures to eliminate illness as part of self-treatment, while the second is the **social role of a village folk therapist** with healing expertise which allows her to not only treat members of her own family but also offer help to other people: neighbors, friends, and inhabitants of her own or neighboring village.

2.3.1. Self-Treatment – the Role of Women

Self-treatment covers knowledge about the causes of the simplest, most typical and most frequent diseases, and about preventive and therapeutic agents. This knowledge is the generalization of one's own life experience, the experience of one's closest family and friends, and the stereotypical information drawn from scientific medicine, both past and present, and the therapeutic practices of healers. The most often used therapeutic measures and techniques include compresses, embrocations or use of pharmaceuticals at one's own discretion. The character of self-treatment depends, as has been said, on the place of residence: the patient's self-treatment in town tends to be closer to professional medicine, in the country – it is closer to folk medical systems (Jeszke 1996: 108)

For centuries the greatest skill and competence in matters of illness was attributed to women, especially mothers and grandmothers - Lachowski's report confirms the widespread utilization of self-treatment by rural women and confirms the role of women as treatment experts (Lachowski 2001; Tylkowa 1989: 97-98). Owing to the specific features of her physiology (menstruation, labor, puerperium), the woman has always been regarded as more competent in the matters of illness. The care and upbringing of the infant consolidated her experience and enriched medicinal knowledge. Women were the first to find different properties of herbal agents; they learned to distinguish between them and divide them according to the simplest rule into medicinal, edible and poisonous (Paluch 1989: 11-12). The woman-mother gradually became the adviser and caregiver to the young generation. Her competence, experience and practical wisdom were believed to increase with age, which is why old women enjoyed the highest prestige and respect in regards to child-rearing, health and illness. Mothers, grandmothers and godmothers, apart from being able to recognize ailments first, also had some store of knowledge about etiology and prevention, almost always decided which treatment method to choose, and took part in rehabilitation. They eagerly shared their opinions about and experience with illnesses. The substance of the social role fulfilled by women as part of self-treatment is made up of a number of instrumental acts. Their range varies, which is clearly noticeable when comparing the 1930s with the 1940s, 50s, 60s, 70s and 1980s. Apart from instrumental acts, a mother or grandmother as a home illness expert also performed many expressive actions: she calmed down the patient, comforted him/her, and sometimes influencing his/her mind, unintentionally showing self-confidence and consistent behavior (Danilkiewicz 1993; Bartoszek 2001: 76).

Male members of the patient's family (fathers, grandfathers) seldom assumed the roles of therapists. Their help was most often limited to allotting some part of the family income for treatment purposes, and taking on extra domestic responsibilities when women had to look after the patient. In *Pamiętniki lekarzy* [Memoirs of Physicians] (1939) there are descriptions of behaviors demonstrating the significance of help which women provided for one another in the case of illness: 'The family doctor, hastily called in, already finds a large group of helpful female neighbors, who are trying to save their friend. One is heating hot water bottles and puts them where she can, another is running to fetch cold water from the well and prepare heart and head compresses, still another rubbing kerosene over the patient's back and legs for want of other embrocation – in other word, quite a commotion' (*Pamiętniki lekarzy* 1939: 204). Mutual provision of help by women was spontaneous and immediate: they shared experiences, exchanged information and decided on the most effective ways of management and the best therapeutic agents. Performing the roles of home therapists, women most often met the patient's expectations of skills and competence, and of a definite and accepted attitude: that of kindness, compassion and selflessness.

In the latter half of the twentieth century industrialization and urbanization processes and population migration from the country to town brought about the decomposition of the rural and small-town lifestyles. One of the changes may have consisted in diminishing the range of neighborly help with illness as compared with the previous period. At same time, from the mid-1970s the WHO had already placed emphasis on increasing the competence of individual family members (especially women) in health matters, and new forms of 'home treatment and cooperation were promoted as part of self-help groups' (Robinson and Henry 1977: 1-3). Studies on health needs carried out as part, among other things, of self-treatment investigations by S. Śliwińska in the mid-1970s, showed that the woman continued to perform the role of 'home doctor'. The results also demonstrate that she is the first to recognize illness and almost always decides what to do. The continuing role of women as 'those who know better and more about illnesses' stems from the fact that they are more interested in their own health, utilize professional and unprofessional help with illness more often, and fall ill more frequently. Figures quoted by Śliwińska show for example that in 82% of cases, rural women undertook to treat illnesses that they diagnosed as 'well-known and mild' using their own tried and tested ways. They sought medical help, when they encountered cases defined as 'most serious'. These female respondents also maintained that they started treatment upon the appearance of painful complaints[31].

The results obtained in studies of self-treatment demonstrated *inter alia* that women attribute to themselves the highest competence in treating adults, and the lowest in looking after the newborns. The most popular therapeutic measures are cupping, all manner of compresses and embrocations. The once-popular practice of incensing has entirely disappeared, and is now being identified with magical-mystical practices. Women respondents listed about 90 healing agents that they used, and named about 60 known ways of treatment (Piątkowski 1990).

---

31 The studies by A. Bartoszek (2001) quoted above show that 44.7% of the surveyed village housewives used self-treatment while 24.7 % agree that these methods are tried and tested and effective. According to the CBOS report of 1998 52% of Poles use 'home ways of treatment', 5% using services of non-conventional therapists. Self-treatment is especially frequent among those who say they had difficulty in gaining access to a physician (this is the case in the country). CBOS 1998.

2.3.2. Woman in the Social Role of Folk Practitioner (Folk medical system)

A characteristic feature of the ways of being ill, especially in peasant families, is the fulfillment of some part of one's health needs as part of folk healthcare. It is a clearly distinct, closed system stemming from the centuries-long isolation and self-sufficiency of rural areas. Consequently, there arose one of the most important attributes of folk therapists: strong integration with the communities where they are active and identification of their own interests and values with group interests. A high degree of trust in a village midwife (old woman) delivering a baby and distrust of practitioners of paramedical professions is illustrated by quotations from physicians' memoirs of 1939, 'She [old woman-midwife-folk doctor, W. P.] bore six children, so knows all about it. She looks after women in labor as best as she can'. (*Pamiętniki lekarzy* 1939: 20). The overwhelming majority of folk therapists have a comparatively low level of education, this is evident especially among women, who do not have relevant medical knowledge (or very little of it). Woman folk doctors usually regard their proficiency as 'God given'; they guard it and keep it secret.

Describing typical examples of different specialties in the folk medical system, B. Seyda emphasizes the dominant role of women: witches, demons, old women called *wieszczyce* (seers, sorcerers), midwives, folk doctors and itinerant old women (Seyda 1962; Brzeziński 2000: 406-426). Several decades ago female folk (quack) doctors in the Polish countryside dealt with all functions related to the physiological conditions of the organism, because they knew them best from their own experience. They helped with menstruation disorders. They made both herbal contraceptives and aphrodisiacs, and performed abortions. They looked after pregnant women during labor and the postpartum period (puerperium), widely using plant products (chiefly herbs) and animal ones (urine, feces, and internal organs). Women regarded as 'wise' collected medicinal substances from plant flowers, fruits and leaves, which they prepared according to strictly specified rules to produce ointments, drinks, herb teas, plasters, etc. They also performed simple treatment procedures that required manual skills, precision and gentleness: cupping, giving enema, removing dirt from eyeballs using their tongues. While performing instrumental procedures, they used magical-mystical measures at the same time: shaking off illness, measuring, spitting, scaring off illness, tying it up, selling, burning, drowning, nailing up, locking, burying and roasting illness, or driving a stake through it (Czyż 1989: 161-164). Believing that the spirit of illness residing in the organism should be removed, they used bitter, burning, vomitive plant remedies, the purpose of which was to put the illness spirit off the patient's body. Old women-*wieszczyce* mainly specialized in mystical-magical rites. They indicated the persons one had to avoid, which objects were impure, which places, days and seasons of the year were unlucky for a person. They were attributed not only with magical healing powers but also, and of equal importance, with the ability to inflict or plant illness on someone, etc. They were suspected of having the power to inflict any ailment on a person with the sheer force of their look. The eyes of these women, like the eyes of some animals (wolf, viper, frog), were believed to be the source of their power. M. Zieleniewski writes that the conviction about the powers of the *wieszczyce* was directly influenced by their appearance, their terror-inspiring otherness, they were old, lean, with shrill voices. Their penetrating glances and joined eyebrows were frightening (Zieleniewski 1845).

The above-cited sociological studies conducted in the 1960s (I. Bejnarowicz) and 1970s (J. Szaro) and my own field studies (1990-1992) show that women still play an important role in folk healthcare and in self-treatment (Bejnarowicz 1969: 253-254). Therapeutic procedures they now perform contain fewer mystical-magical elements and more instrumental ones. The folk medical system and self-treatment are part of the cultural heritage of the past and cannot be disregarded in research studies.[32] I have records of current accounts (2007) concerning the 'social role' performed by a female village folk practitioner called *Serwinka*, who lives near Lubartów (Poland). She sees dozens of patients a day in a small summer kitchen, diagnosing and treating people, using traditional chiropractic methods. Patients maintain that she can 'read' X-rays and correctly interpret medical documentation that the patients bring with them. In the case of locomotor injuries that she deems very serious (the need to operate) she refuses to treat the patients. The therapist is a member of the family which has practiced chiropractic for generations.

2.4. Determinants of Illness Behaviors

It is generally assumed that there is a relationship between social determinants of life and the risk of occurrence of specific diseases. This connection is not easy to prove because we do not fully understand the causal relationship be-

32 My own field studies on the social effects of hemophilia (1990 and 1992) demonstrate that parents of hemophiliac children often utilize folk healthcare methods and services of modern healers (Piątkowski and Karski 1988, XIX, 3-4: 151-152). I obtained similar results in my pilot studies on the effects of ICP. (Piątkowski et al. 1994: 108-109; Szaro 1976: 467). The importance of folk therapists on the present-day health services market in the US was pointed out by W. C. Cockerham (2004: 175-176; see also Nettleton 2009; 35-36).

tween medical and sociological phenomena. Individual elements of social life do not act one by one but in a complex of other factors. Despite these doubts, sociology and its subdisciplines, ethnology, and medical sciences (hygiene, epidemiology) have repeatedly emphasized that the manner of being sick depends not only on the individual and his/her immediate environment, but also on other factors such as the State's economic policy, the form of social policy., access to medical institutions and professions, and cultural, psychological and demographic elements, etc. (Sokołowska 1986; Śliwińska 1974; Mackiewicz et al. 1970, 8: 695-705; Kawczyńska-Butrym 2002: 221-236; Skrzypek 2004: 76-77). Weiss and Lonnquist accentuate the macro-, meso- and microsocial behaviors in health and illness, and distinguish four categories of factors that 'structurally' influence health/illness: physical and environmental factors, historical factors and structural factors (2006: 332-333; and Kronenfeld 2011: 271-275).

The factors that occur on the largest social scale that shape the general living conditions of society, and that influence people's behavior towards health and illness, are political, economic and cultural phenomena.

2.4.1. Macrosocial Determinants

2.4.1.1. Social Policy and Ideology

In twenty-first century societies there is an increasingly widespread conviction that medical and health maintenance are one of the priorities of social policy. Factors that contribute to the growing commitment of modern States and political personalities to organized actions for public health include respect for the human right to develop and maintain maximum fitness, increased importance of human health in modern economy, the increasing influence of public opinion demanding affordable healthcare available to all, etc. (Elling 1981,2; Kościelak 2004: 181-202). This ideology took a long while to find its way into the public consciousness although some of its elements were espoused by enlightened social circles. It should be added that large pharmaceutical companies now promote self-treatment. The 2007 report on the subject reads '[…] self-treatment in the world has a positive effect on prevention, enhances the level of life and care of health, and makes it possible to save budget resources, and engagement of medical services' (*Rozważania o rynku OTC …* 2007, 7/8: 54-55).

From the historical perspective, the extremely adverse living conditions of the peasant class (poor nutrition, housing, hygiene) in the nineteenth century were well-known to the then Polish intelligentsia (Kosiński 1983). Gradually, social and administrative measures were taken aimed at improving the living, hygienic and working conditions of the rural population. These activities were supervised and coordinated, inter alai, by the Warsaw Hygienic Society. From the mid-nineteenth century onwards, parallel to the movement for hygienization of rural areas, steps were taken to organize a network of healthcare centers. An example of the social policies of the Tsarist authorities in the field of health was the establishment on Polish territory of the so-called 'zemskaya medicina' [local medicine, local-government-funded medicine in rural areas], which had already functioned in Russia. The local-medicine physicians were officials responsible for health in local communities. They recorded epidemics, morbility and mortality rates and prepared medical statistics. In some areas of the Russian partition regional, district and *gmina* (commune) physicians were allowed to practice. After WWI ended and Poland regained independence, the Ministry of Public Health was established in 1919 to coordinate health policies. It began legislative activities: a new sanitary law was passed, among others, and the organization of the rural health service was tied to the functioning of local governments. In 1934 the Ministry of Public Health was abolished, responsibility for healthcare having been vested in ten central government offices, including the Ministry of Internal Affairs. In the 1920s the local administrative authorities in Pomorze [Pomerania] and Wielkopolska provinces re-established Health-Insurance Funds, which were important only to a negligible number, of the 19.4 million citizens inhabiting rural areas (83% of Poland's population). The locally introduced social security funds, which provided an opportunity to access medical care, sick benefits, and sanatorium care, covered almost exclusively farm laborers. Memoirs of physicians of 1939 indicate that the insured village inhabitants eagerly used the services provided, and changed their attitudes and behavior in illness: they did not ignore symptoms, went to doctors in time, and did not stop treatment as soon as they felt better (*Pamiętniki lekarzy* 1939: 232). After the Health Insurance Fund closed down in the countryside, the behaviors of farm laborers in illness returned to 'normal'. Doctors wrote that hospital treatment was also reduced to the minimum. Only very serious, hopeless cases came to hospitals (Ibid). 'In the neighboring village the sexton provided medical help. Medical counsel was often sought in the pharmacy and from neighbors, because it did not cost anything' (Ibid: 990). '[...] most child deliveries were handled by old women-midwives or casual women neighbors. The effects of this help varied, but deaths and postpartum infections were a common occurrence' (Ibid: 821). The unsatisfactory state of health of the rural population in the interwar period totally collapsed after WWII: there was a drop in all health indicators. The first postwar health minister – peasant activist F. Litwin declared '[...] whether it is the peasant formerly deprived of medical care, or the worker or clerk, they all should have an equal opportunity to utilize medical care' (Litwin 1945,1: 4). Thus, an egalitarian healthcare system was promised; it was emphasized that the problem concerned 65% of the population. It soon became apparent that the State had failed to fulfill its declaration of providing the peasant population with medical care. In 1945 the Ministry of Health representatives blamed the failure to cover peasant families with the universal healthcare system on the lack of funds. Healthcare provision for this social stratum was limited during the first 25 years of Communist Poland to meeting basic hygienic and health needs and consisted in combating infectious diseases, care of mother and child, and assistance in emergency. Despite the limited character of State's healthcare, this was, however, noticeable progress compared with the interwar period. From the postwar memoirs of physicians (*Pamiętniki lekarzy*) and a book on the rural young generation in the People's Republic of Poland (*Młode pokolenie wsi Polski Ludowej*) we can learn about certain behavioral patterns in illness, which were doubtless the result of the new form of social policy. **Nevertheless, the most common health needs were still satisfied mainly as part of self-treatment and the folk medical system**. The lack of universal health insurance resulted in treatment being delayed as long as possible, 'Mother's illness progressed fast […] always no time, always loads of urgent work. You can't think of doctors and treatment because the doctor is far away and you are not dying yet […] Because you have to pay the doctor, and money is needed to patch a dozen budget holes: without doing so, it seems, things will not work any longer' (Chałasiński et al. 1968: 107).

Economizing on healthcare in rural areas was undoubtedly motivated by ideological concerns. Although the new Constitution of 1952 formally conferred the right to medical care on the peasant population, it was becoming clear that the authorities gave preferential treatment to workers (including farm laborers) at the expense of 'individual' owners, i.e. peasants (Kaja 1976, 1; 31-50). To implement their right to healthcare, peasants had to wait until the next political crisis. The extension of free medical care to peasant families on 1 January 1972 was clearly a political propaganda ploy instigated without having first prepared rural healthcare services for their increased responsibilities. This decision and its implementation revealed the great scale of health needs of the peasant population, which had not been identified before. There was a fourfold increase in the number of patients visiting doctors' offices, the number of house calls having risen by half (Świderska-Możdzan and Możdżan 1979, 2: 115-119; Kukiz 1974, 10: 889 et seq.). It turned out, however, that the medical care in the countryside, although still leaving much to be desired, resulted in a limited improvement in a number of standard health indicators. A deterioration in the state of health of the rural population occurred at the end of the 1970s and the beginning of the 1980s with the growing economic crisis and its diverse effects. This was manifested *inter alia* in lower life expectancy and in a distinct increase in excess mortality of men aged 40 (especially noticeable in the countryside). At the same time a positive phenomenon appeared in the mid-1980s: an extremely low infant mortality rate in Zamość province. These changes are difficult to interpret unequivocally but they do not seem to be directly related to the government's policy towards the rural areas.

In the last 17 years changes in attitudes and behaviors towards health and illness were determined *inter alia* by structural changes, such as the introduction of the KRUS social security system or Poland's entry in the EU (2004). Social transformations and integration processes rapidly accelerated the stratification, antagonization and anomie within the agricultural population. A small group of agricultural producers who control large farms earn very high incomes and use EU subsidies very well. However, studies show a generally pessimistic picture of the living and health conditions of the ageing rural population. Many village seniors rate their health condition as worse than the corresponding category of town population. Transformations, as L. Kocik stresses, are assessed as a 'social and cultural trauma". The number of people with health insurance in 1998 was only 1,417,000; after 1998 mortality rates worsened. A very low level of education (prevalence of only elementary or incomplete elementary education among the rural population aged over sixty) determines the traditional, passive way of reacting to innovation and structural changes (B. Fedyszak-Radziejowska 2000: 107). The crisis in the insurance system in the rural areas has also been pointed out (Skrętowicz 2000: 19; Kobielski 2003: 30; Kocik 2001; 9-10).

2.4.1.2. Economic Conditions

Sociomedical literature has adopted a thesis that the income level of a family has a direct effect on the behavior in illness (Twaddle and Hessler 1977: 282-283; Lahelma 2010: 71-84). The size of household budget and income per family member are highly significant as regards measures for the care of one's health, oriented towards the professional level of health needs, doctor-patient interaction, the period of playing the social role of the patient, and the commencement or termination of rehabilitation.

There is no doubt that over the last hundred years the income level of most peasant families has been lower than that of families in town. This fact was a major barrier cutting off the rural population from the achievements and benefits of urban civilization. This economic disadvantage not only resulted in inferior housing conditions, household equipment, diet, and educational opportunities, but also reinforced reactions to illness: ignoring symptoms, a tendency to 'walk through' the illness, treatment as a last resort when pain prevents one from working, premature termination of treatment with the first signs of improvement, etc. Interwar diaries and memoirs document the effects of peasant poverty and its impact on ways of treatment, 'The rural people are afraid of a doctor like a devil because his visit costs one cow, then how can you *not* be frightened' (*Pamiętniki chłopów*, 1936,2: 89). 'A doctor is a prohibitive luxury. You bring him in as a last resort, together with a priest' (*Pamiętniki lekarzy* 1939: 5). The high cost of medical services made people sell their only cow or last sack of grain, or take out a loan at usurious interest. When there was no money left, doctors were asked to provide treatment on credit, or people turned to a feldsher (paramedic), who was much less expensive, and could be paid with 'what one had, eggs or a chicken', alternatively, one could work off the fee. The economic situation of peasant families at that time was further aggravated by the worsening economic crisis and the falling demand for already inexpensive agricultural produce. Peasants did not have enough money to pay for a visit to a doctor's office or for medicines, even less so for a stay in hospital. An average appointment with the doctor cost 15-100 zloty, the delivery of baby – 100-150 zloty; at that time a family of several persons could live off 10 zloty for a week. In 1938 and 1939 the cost of hospitalization in a typical agricultural province such as the Lublin region, was from 3.5 to 9 zloty per day. Pharmacy drugs were also expensive. I. Solarz wrote, 'I know of cases where peasants came out of the pharmacy with a prescription alone without a drug – too expensive (Solarz 1937: 19).

After WWII health insurance covered only employees of agricultural cooperatives, state-owned farms, and peasants-workers, who were also employed outside of farming. Health policies in fact constituted one of the instruments of collectivization of agriculture. The fight against well-off farmers with larger farms (the kulaks) and strict enforcement of compulsory agricultural quotas reduced the incomes of peasant households, and thereby the possibility of covering medical expenses. The number of consultations increased rapidly when they were free; this was noticeable with tuberculosis and infectious diseases, and in medical care of mother and child. There is no doubt that lack of access of most peasant families to free medical care had an adverse effect on the state of health, especially of children in the rural areas (Rafalski 1961,11). The attitude to health in the early 1960s can be illustrated with a quotation from a peasant's diary, '[…] Time and first of all money must be for everything, and for saving life and health – in the last resort' (*Młode pokolenie wsi Polski Ludowej* 1968 :115). Of necessity, peasant families spent only a very small percentage of their income on healthcare; in 1963-1964 it was 1.9%. In the late 1960s those responsible for healthcare had to admit that despite high morbidity rates the peasants were reluctant to undergo medical treatment. The authorities were aware that the main reason was financial barriers (Dziadosz et al. 1970, 1/1: 11-12; Butrym 1976, 10: 37-43). Physicians - field correspondents of the Institute of Rural Health in Lublin - reported that monthly incomes of peasant families were 1900-2200 złoty, while a visit at a private practitioner cost 100-150 złoty.

A fundamental change in People's Poland's health policy was the introduction in 1972 of universal health insurance for individual farmers and members of their families. In the preceding period the number of uninsured farmers reporting to national health service centers was sixteen times lower than that of insured persons (Rudziński, Tokarski 1972, 4: 297 et seq.). Provision of free medical services for the peasant population did not entirely eliminate economic barriers. The treatment costs also included traveling to the doctor, the price of foreign medicines, often not available in state-owned pharmacies, specialist consultation fees, informal, often high payment for operations, cost of additional nursing care, and many others.

In the 1980s the stratification of the rural population continued with the growing poverty sphere, which covered first of all the aged, disabled, and living alone. Pensioners' families were those with the lowest incomes (Tryfan 1988; and 1992, IV: 90). This is how a village female pensioner describes her situation, '[…] I received a pension […] which is barely enough for me to buy bread, butter, and a newspaper once a week' (Matlęga 1989,1: 84). Old farmers were embarrassed by their situation. They would not go to hospital because they did not have adequate clothes; 93% of the aged did not use hospital treatment in recent years (Ibid: Piątkowski and Ostrowska 1994). Economic conditions changed after 1990. Some scholars maintain that a portion of the peasant population 'lost with the introduction of market reforms' (L. Kocik). The peasant farming economy changed slowly despite having absorbed technical improvements, and so did the structure of the peasant community. Economic analyses by K. Gutkowska and L. Goraj indicate that since the late 1990s farming conditions have deteriorated (Kocik 2001: 10). Technological impoverishment of farms and their poor economic condition are presented in J. Wroński's studies (Jastrzębska 2003: 17), and income differences to the disadvantage of the rural population are described in the analyses by J. Skrętowicz (Skrętowicz et al. 2005, 1: 37-52; Gutkowska et al. 1998, 26: 220).

2.4.1.3. Culture

Each human community produces its characteristic material objects, as well as values, beliefs, behavioral patterns, and lifestyles in the non-material sphere. The effect of cultural factors on behavior in illness has long been proved.

Hessler and Twaddle assert that the patient is not a mechanical whole reacting to stimuli from the outside environment ; rather, his decisions, choices and behaviors are influenced by such diverse elements as education, life experience, professed norms and preferred values. It is these elements that account for the fact that the value attributed to health varies in different societies (Twaddle and Hessler 1997: 282-283; Senior and Viveash 1998: 169-170). M. Sokołowska points to the role of culture and its effect on behaviors in illness, referring to M. Zborowski's classic discussion on reactions to pain and their association with cultural elements (Sokołowska 1986).The results of studies on non-biomedical healing systems show a significant influence by cultural elements on behaviors in health and illness, and the persistence of this influence (Tylkowa 1989).

An important cultural factor contributing to the formation of lifestyle elements associated with health and illness is education. It determines hygiene habits, diet, housing conditions, the manner of performing work, and, finally, the occurrence and range of preventive measures. Sociomedical and epidemiological studies have also demonstrated the relationship between the educational level of mothers and infant death rates, visits to doctors, knowledge of disease symptoms, and indicators of children's physical development. Most features of the peasant style of being sick are determined by the low level of education. During the interwar period almost one quarter of Poland's population could not read and write (illiterates and semi-literates), the overwhelming majority of these being peasants. A peasant diarist from the Vilna region wrote, 'Our fundamental trouble is ignorance […] this paralysis of reason prevents us from looking at the world in a realistic way, and traditional stupidity produces a lot of false beliefs that bring quite a few misfortunes on people. This fear of unknown natural phenomena causes a whole lot of superstitions in everyday peasant life' (*Pamiętniki chłopów…* 1936: 538).

Despite transformations in civilization, traditional attitudes and behaviors in illness persist in rural areas. The style of houses changes, household equipment and furnishings are greatly improved, the prevailing style of clothes is urban but the spread of biopositive health behaviors is very slow, e.g. hygienic neglect has occurred in the Polish countryside over the lifespan of two generations (Lewonowska et al. 1989, 2: 104-110). This is due to the fact that as recently as in the 1980s almost 20% of farmers had incomplete elementary education, while 52% had only elementary education. The level of education of the aged, who are exposed to diseases most often, is generally much lower. Studies show that the low educational level, especially among the rural older generations, persists. W. Pędich's investigations demonstrate that 'the level of education of Polish rural inhabitants is far lower than that of town population' (Pędich 2004: 16). Recent studies (2007) by R. Filip and R. Lenart point out that two categories of education are overrepresented in the country: elementary – 20.3% of the rural population and basic vocational- 33.2% (Filip and Lenart 2007, 1). We should add that in the typical rural province of Podlasie (Podlaskie) – as many as 7.3% of the rural population has only an incomplete elementary education (Wdowiak and Syczewska-Weber 2006, 3-4: 140-150).

A feature of folk culture, which influences behaviors in and attitudes towards illness among the peasant population is co-occurrence of mystical-magical elements. This applies as much to views on etiology, prevention and diagnosis as to therapeutic measures. In his discussions of folk culture, K. Dobrowolski emphasizes that one of its major features is 'a great role of magical beliefs and practices along with activities based on true empirical foundations, […] mystical powers that were personified in some cases in the form of numerous demons that controlled a broader or narrower section of reality [..] these powers could bring harm and disasters on man, or they could be brought under control and made to work to his advantage' (K. Dobrowolski 1966: 90). Mystical-magical acts influenced and still influence a number of behaviors in illness, which a peasant family exhibits. For example, illness was assumed to be caused by spells, charms and magic; and the use of holy relics, amulets or talismans was believed to prevent illness. People were convinced that revelation, inspiration or clairvoyance made it easier to diagnose an illness whereas casting spells, charms and the like would remove it effectively. Performance of magic acts was reserved for strictly defined persons who were believed to have contact with supernatural powers and who were thereby able to control them. The importance of magic can be related to the special 'mythology of illness' in folk culture. Illness was always treated as something hostile, alien, external, something that insidiously penetrates human life and destroys it. The less people knew about the real causes of illnesses, the more magical elements accumulated; this was the case with the alleged etiology of cancerous diseases. Folk knowledge, as part of folk culture, is a whole area of material and spiritual reality, the perception of phenomena in the connection of 'everything with everything' – cosmos, nature, and man (Libera 1989: 154-159). The expert on modern rural culture, M. Wieruszewska, says, '[…] let us look at the problem through the filter of culture. The rural culture has a wider range than folk, peasant, local, popular culture. From the viewpoint of long stability, we can discover in it the reserves of the legacy of the past […] equally dignified as those […] that we find in the tradition of peasant culture'. This quotation referring to the conception of J. Bartmiński shows the permanence and integrity of cultural transmission (Wieruszewska 2006, VI: 19). The same author points out that '[…] rural culture themes refer to the elements of former folk culture, usually without being aware and knowing of their own origins' (Ibid: 20). The permanence and strong presence of elements of culture and folk traditions in everyday life (especially of old people) are stressed by G. Orzechowska (2004: 46-52). In his study about transformation in peasant culture after 2000, L. Kocik writes, 'This retrospective system of references fulfilled a fundamental role in the reconstruction and continuation of the way of living. All kinds of changes were based first of all on the recomposition of previous cultural products and elements into new configurations without disturbing the fundamental features of the rural socio-cultural system' (Kocik 2001: 34).

2.4.1.4. Folk medical systems – the Perspective of Seeing the World

One of the founders of Polish post-WWII ethnology, Professor J. Burszta, drew attention in the mid-1990s to the broad cultural context in which the Polish traditional folk medical system functions. In this interpretation, healthcare is a fragment of a larger whole, which is folk knowledge, and this in turn constitutes an integral part of folk culture. Burszta stresses the distinct emergence of views related to health and illness out of this larger cultural whole, accentuating contradictions, diversities and inconsistencies that a student of this phenomenon will encounter (Burszta 1967, 3: 394-395). The crucial theme here is for example the character of etiological views. With the absence of knowledge about the true mechanisms through which diseases arise, the rural population created quasi-magical knowledge based on thaumaturgy and religious interpretations. Thus, illness 'entered' the human organism from outside, it embodied evil and misfortunes, and it was caused by evil spirits and demons. The consequence of adoption of a thaumaturgical etiology were the corresponding diagnostic methods (clairvoyance, revelation, etc.) and treatment techniques (casting spells and charms to cure or prevent an illness), undoing illness spells, etc. Of course, the mystical-magical elements overlapped with 'empirical' folk methods of fighting illness and eliminating it, which were based on centuries-old treatment techniques (herbal healing, setting broken or dislocated bones by the chiropractor, etc.) (Piątkowski 1990: 131 et seq.; Wieruszewska 1995, 78: 104-109). Burszta points out that the present-day interpretation of cultural facts around illness is greatly influenced by the past. He believes that identification of illness with evil (the devil, demons) from the Middle Ages until the present day is the accurate exemplification of this thesis (Burszta 1967: 295); hence the importance of religious elements supporting instrumental acts that we see when describing the social role of village folk practitioners today. An aspect of cultural interpretation of the development of illness, which could not be explained by real traumatic events (injury, catching cold, poisoning), were religious elements. Illness might have been an inevitable punishment for previous (consciously and unconsciously committed) grave and light sins and transgressions. The punisher was God as an 'impartial and just' judge. Conditions with such an etiology were mental diseases (Ibid: 403).

Another element taken from traditional peasant culture, which made its way to folk healthcare, is the belief that everything is related to everything in animate and inanimate nature. In this interpretation human life and illness depend for example on astral (cosmic) forces and stages of the moon, date of birth, solar eclipses, the appearance or non-appearance of a comet, etc. Similarly, other natural elements may have a direct or indirect effect on the state of health and illness, for example air and water. Diseases were said to arise from air, from water or from other constituents of man's natural environment (Ibid: 402).

Therapeutic procedures in the folk medical system stemmed as much from beliefs, habits, customs and practical measures as from folk empirical knowledge. All these elements were applied in full conviction that they were appropriate, suitable, purposeful and necessary to save that which was most precious in man: health. The cultural system of folk healthcare was self-sufficient, complex, integral and oriented towards specific therapeutic actions. Observe that prevention of illnesses (prophylaxis) when an individual had not experienced the clear adverse effect of a disease earlier was regarded as pointless and unnecessary (Tylkowa 1989: 13 et seq.). The many-years-long studies by D. Tylkowa, carried out in the Polish Carpathian Mountains, show that the aforementioned thaumaturgical-mystical and religious elements used in etiology, prevention diagnostics, and treatment, are **also present today** [*my emphasis*, W. P.] in the way of thinking and interpreting the world by the peasant population in southern Poland (Karpackie [Carpathian] province).

As demonstrated by the examples of field studies conducted in the 1960s (J. Burszta), and in the 1980s (J. Jeszke), the views and behaviors of some part of the rural population still show the traditional (close and real) connection between man and nature, cosmos and the whole of the surrounding world, this bond being indivisible and integral. Man is involved in and subjected to the influence of two conflicting and opposing forces: health and illness. The popularity of non-conventional treatment methods (bioenergy therapy, radiesthesia) present in the media, in which TV therapists (i.e. those most popular in the country, e.g. Zbyszek Nowak) appeal to extrasensory, non-material, intangible, miraculous elements, may strengthen the ordinary man's belief that the traditional folk approach to illness and to fighting it is accurate and effective. We can also ask whether the scenario, repeatedly predicted by doctors, will come true: that the folk ways of coping with illness will be gradually rationalized, and the elements regarded by science as mystical-magical will be eliminated. The answer is not unequivocal. both sides may retain their positions and convictions or some elements of the folk medical system will gradually penetrate into academic medicine (which may mean that orthopedic centers will recognize the manual proficiency of some chiropractors, or there will be studies by the Polish Academy of Sciences Institute of History of Science, Education and Technology, which will reveal the efficacy of products used as part of folk pharmacy). We may also witness faster adoption of modern health culture by rural communities. It should be remembered that this two-way process of a kind of osmosis, observable in field studies (Jeszke 1996), may intensify because we know that the same persons seek, in the complementary and parallel mode, both official and informal ways of help with illness (Stomma 1986: 192-196). There is much to indicate that this is the beginning of a process of change covering both parts of the medical system – official and informal. The folk medical system, an element of the traditional system of knowledge and peasant culture, will undoubtedly change and be enriched under the pressure of ubiquitous academic medicine: the question is to what extent and at what pace. At the same time, as a result of the effects of 'natural ways of treatment', medicine may become more tolerant towards 'non-biological elements', for example mystical-magical, especially religious, whose impact on the results of therapy is no longer challenged outright by clinical sciences. It is also possible that we will witness a better understanding of the folk medical system by physicians. Then the doctor's banal rationalization, when assessing incomprehensible effects obtained from time to time by some village folk therapists, will be more in-depth and go beyond the conventional saying 'faith can work miracles' (Kutrzeba-Pojnarowa 1977: 288 et seq.) This section of the book cannot be regarded as a complete reconstruction of the cultural system surrounding the Polish folk medical system. The issues have been presented here selectively. We have frequently referred to ethnological literature because there are practically no socio-medical studies to characterize the problems in question (the author has only a manuscript by medical sociologist Renata Tulli [1983]). Cultural changes in the folk medical system are also commented on by D. Penkala-Gawęcka [1995, 78: 185-186]). We have intentionally omitted certain elements of the cultural interpretation of reality, the discussion of which would require a more systematic analysis. A separate problem is *inter alia* the culturally determined significance of gender in the socialization for the social role of village therapist; especially interesting is the mechanism of preference for women as folk experts in the matters of illness (a separate section is devoted to this question in this part). Nor do we discuss the magic and symbolism of places defining the ecological framework of the folk medical system: fences, shrines, windows, balks, house corners; these specific sites determined the conventional boundaries between 'one's own' area and 'alien' area, and they protected against illness (compare Twaddle and Hessler 1977: 152-156; Cockerham 2004).

2.4.1.5. Religious Elements in the Polish Folk medical system

An important feature of folk culture, important for behavior in illness, is the presence of religious elements. They arose from the conviction about God's omnipotence, which creates and controls everything in an unchanging way. The will of God regulated the social order and individual fates, and all natural phenomena. Those who violated this order were liable to divine punishment while those who yielded to God's will could count on His favor. As the earlier, medieval influence of the Church established the conviction that illness was a punishment for sinning, it was necessary to win over the Divine Providence to avert the fate. This was the purpose of offerings, prayers, vows, and blessing of objects meant to protect against illness (figurines, crosses and pictures). Every disease had its patron saint, who was prayed to for recovery. Members of the patient's family walked to the places recognized as holy and offered votive gifts. In the 1960s the especially valued objects protecting people against illness included threads drawn out from the stole, blessed candles and holy water (Bejnarowicz 1969; Idler 2010: 133-158). In serious cases, the physician arrived together with the priest. Here is an example of behavior in illness with distinct religious elements, '[…] they told [parents] to carry me before the sunrise to the crossroads, there is usually a cross there, only they were not allowed to say a word so that theirs would the first words to the cross, to carry the baby to the cross to and fro, circle the cross twice with the baby and repeat: "Good Jesus dying on the Cross, take this suffering child with you or restore his/her health"' (Chałasiński and Znaniecki 1938, 3: 416). Studies by D. Tylkowa conducted in southern Poland demonstrate that even now religious elements are important in illness-related behaviors in the country (Tylkowa 1989; and later studies by Penkala-Gawęcka 1999, and Jeszke 1993).

The folk medical system and self-treatment is, as mentioned earlier, one of the major parts of Polish folk culture (Burszta 1967). Earlier investigations indicate that contrary to simplistic forecasts of the 1960s, the folk treatment methods have not only not disappeared in the rural areas but seem to be enjoying social acceptance (Penkala-Gawęcka 1991, 74; Tylkowa 1989: 97-98; Piątkowski 1995; 19-30), which is confirmed by ethnological, sociological and medical studies (bibliography can be found in Tylkowa 1989; Piątkowski 1990, Jeszke 1996). There also seems to be a large disparity between the broad scope of public popularity of the folk medical system and the comparatively negligible exploration of this field by individual disciplines; this is especially emphasized by D. Penkala-Gawęcka (1991, 2006). The delaying factor is the lack of coordination of such investigations at the stage of conceptualization and implementation, and their usually contributory character.

Behaviors and views associated with the biological elements defining the framework of human existence (illness, suffering, dying) had a special character in the rural areas and were, on a *pars pro toto* basis, an integral part of the whole peasant view of the world (Styk 1993; 17 et seq.; 1988, 20 (7): 101 et seq.). There were diverse manifestations of this specificity, for example death did not inspire the same amount fear that it did in urban communities because it did not disturb the rhythm of life and work in a local community. Illness, pain, and dying were the links in the logically consecutive stages of the continuing human fate, which could neither be challenged nor undermined: hence came the characteristic feature of the peasant psyche – fatalism. Highly internalized religious elements sometimes also permitted people to accept without resistance the successive stages of taking on the social role of the patient. They would say 'This was meant to be so', 'God so willed', 'death seeks no causes', 'God gave, God took away': in this way a passive and ambivalent attitude to illness developed. On the other hand, health (especially the farmer's) was a value in itself; it had its measurable price in the circumstances of continually doing hard physical work, which required efficiency and fitness. The peasant-farm owner could not afford to be ill for a long time, less so to undergo long treatment and convalescence, which is why he needed a quick and accurate diagnosis and therapy that would radically eliminate illness; with such expectations people sought help from non-professional and professional therapists (Borkowski 1980; 21 et seq.). Another characteristic feature of attitudes and behaviors towards illness was the low status of measures serving to preserve health, which was seen as a God-given, normal and stable state independent of one's 'biopositive or bionegative conduct. An important trait of the peasant's manner of coping with illness was and is the co-occurrence and intermingling of mystical-magical and religious elements (Burszta 1967, 3; Piątkowski 1990). In the past, religious elements determined the attitude of medical professions and institutions; distance and distrust were caused on the one hand by the faith in the efficacy of the folk medical system and self-treatment, and on the other hand by expectations of aid from the Divine Providence. The memoirs of the mid-1930s read, 'I won't go to hospital either [...] it would cost even more. God willing, the child will live, if not, s/he will die' (*Pamiętniki lekarzy* 1939). It is now difficult to find such shocking examples of such a defensive, passive attitude towards illness although, having conducted observations of behaviors and attitudes towards illness among the rural population in the Zamość region since 1987, I have repeatedly encountered manifestations of the absence of greater interest in the health of their own children by parents (Piątkowski et al. 1994: 107-109). More recently Lucjan Kocik, for example, asserts, 'bad fate is therefore an inherent element of rationalization and interpretation of the peasant's everyday experience' (2001: 32).

The foregoing description of certain attitudes and behaviors towards health and illness is the necessary background for determining the role of religious elements in traditional rural healthcare. Their significance stemmed *inter alia* from the belief in God's omnipotence, which created and controlled everything in a continuous and unchanging way. The Divine will regulated the social order and individual fates, and determined a person's health and illness. Those who violated this order deserved to be punished, while those who yielded to God's will could count on His favor.

In 1990 I presented my own conception of the internal structure of the Polish folk medical system and the manner of its functioning, distinguishing among others etiological, preventive, diagnostic and therapeutic elements. The modified form of this idea was presented in Part One. We will therefore look at this interpretation of the system and the position occupied in it by religious views and convictions.

A. Prevention of Illness (Prophylaxis)

As has been said earlier, the rural population did not pay particular attention to behaviors serving to prevent illness and increase one's own health 'reserve'. Nevertheless, village folk therapists often gave their patients preventive instructions. Of special importance were prayers to patron saints of particular diseases (Paluch: 1989: 7, 10). For example, prayers to St. Apollonia were belied to prevent toothache, to St. Otilia – eye diseases, to St. Valentine – nervous system diseases (e.g. epilepsy). Already, by the Middle Ages, every disease was assigned to its patron, who would answer the prayers of the faithful. Another type of behavior protecting against illness was pilgrimages to holy places. This is still observable today, not only in the case of pilgrimages to national sanctuaries such as Częstochowa but also to local places of worship, e.g. Wąwolnica, Krasnobród or Górecko Kościelne. To the sphere of the sacred belong places that are attributed with special religious-magical powers: crosses at the crossroads, and even fences, windows or doors of houses. These are conventional boundaries between good (health) and evil (illness); in this area prayers for health and well-being were believed to be answered especially often (Ibid: 10). Special objects also prevented illness; most often these were items of religious worship: holy medallions, small crosses, holy water bottles, and herbs blessed in May, which was regarded as the month devoted to the Heavenly Mother. The customary for the blessing of these objects were *inter alia* Palm Sunday and Corpus Christi. Sacred power also resided in threads drawn from the stole, pictures with images of individual saints, and recently even videocassettes with recordings of religious-therapeutic rituals (Bejnarowicz 1969: 251-255).

Significant elements increasing health reserves were strictly defined acts and behaviors performed during important church holidays such as Christmas or Easter. Recommendations included for example washing in running water after returning from the midnight Christmas Eve Mass, which would ensure good health all year round, and eating 'flawless apples' on Christmas Eve for protection against illness. In Beskid Żywiecki area members of peasant families sprinkled one other with holy water during Epiphany, while in Beskid Śląski people flogged one another's legs with willow twigs, as his was said to prevent rheumatoid ailments; in Podhale region holy water was drunk on Easter Sunday, and in Górecko Kościelne in Zamość district they still wash their bodies with water from the Holy Springlet on the day of the parish holiday devoted to St. Stanislaus (Stanisław) the Martyr of Szczepanów (Tylkowa 1989; and my field observations in 1987-2000 in Zwierzyniec district).

B. Etiology

In Polish folk medical lore, causes of illnesses had a material, (internal and external) and thaumaturgical character (I have presented the detailed structure of the folk healthcare system in Piątkowski 1990). Here we will be particularly interested in the latter factors. Christianity, J. Burszta emphasizes, was already exerting a growing impact on the folk medical system already by the early Middle Ages. Man realized that earthly life was only a short episode on the road to eternity, and the whole world was controlled by supernatural powers – God, saints, and angels on one side, and evil powers, devils and demons on the other. Illness was regarded as a condition decreed by God, as was health; sometimes, however, divine intentions might have been thwarted by evil powers. Burszta stresses that the theme of illness as a consequence of committed sins appeared very early in Church teachings. The Church taught that everything was in the hands of God, including health and illness, and that God wanted to try people by inflicting illnesses upon them (Burszta 1967). At the same time people are convinced that certain diseases are caused by infernal powers at work (mental diseases). These views continue to be reflected in sociomedical surveys of reactions to mental diseases or HIV/AIDS (Twaddle and Hessler 1977; 96-97; Jarvis 1989: 9-11; and my chapters in Barański and Piątkowski: 2002). We can say that the lower the knowledge of anatomical and physiological knowledge, the less that was known about specific, material causes of illness, and the less effective the treatment, the more frequently folk etiological views contained intermingled mystical-magical and religious elements.

C. Diagnostics

Various measures were taken and acts performed as part of the folk medical system and self-treatment in order to establish the nature of illness. For centuries the character and symptoms of diseases were a mystery to the rural inhabitants – they were not able to find relationships between certain states of the organism and the kind of disease; in the majority of serious cases the *morbus* (illness) developed in an unpredictable and incomprehensible way. The most frequent, prevalent belief was that illness was caused by supernatural factors: it was then that diagnostics based on thaumaturgical and religious elements were resorted to. Characteristically, while preventive measures as part of folk healthcare and self-treatment could be applied practically by any community member, diagnostic procedures were traditionally reserved for professionals with specialist knowledge, abilities and intuition. These phenomena were pointed out by J. S. Bystroń, emphasizing that folk therapists could sometimes be excellent intuitive diagnosticians (Bystroń 1947 and 1947a). The most frequent diagnostic techniques found in the folk medical system were the inspection of the iris (a distorted and simplified version of iridoscopy), examination of the tongue and human secretions and excretions (urine, feces, spit), examination of the objects belonging to the sick person (pieces of clothes, underwear), contemplation of the patient's pictures and his palm, and recently, bioenergotherapeutic and radiesthetic diagnosis. A separate kind of diagnostic method was to find the character of the illness through clairvoyance and revelation. By applying this manner of diagnosis, folk practitioners used *inter alia* the objects of religious worship: holy pictures, blessed candles, and those items that they termed holy relics. Very often there was a balance between the magic of words, signs, and acts. Trying to establish the character of illness, folk practitioners recited whole prayers or fragments thereof, making the sign of the cross over the patient, calling out the names of saints. With diseases of nose, ears or throat, St. Blasé was asked for help, St. Lucia was expected to help with eye conditions and with accurate diagnosis, while St. Catharine helped find causes and nature of gynecological conditions (Tylkowa 1989: 92). These mechanisms are permanent as shown by field studies (Bartoszek 2001: 76).

D. Therapy

The most developed segment of traditional folk healthcare is therapy/treatment. This is because the folk medical system is instrumental, based on ad hoc actions meant to remove illness quickly and entirely. Examples of utilization of religious elements at the treatment stage can be found both in the kinds of therapy (casting spells and charms to cure or prevent illness) and in therapeutic means (crosses, holy water, blessed chalk, blessed candles). An example of behaviors constituting the social role of the folk practitioner-therapist based on the magic of words and gestures is casting spells to cure or prevent an illness. Verbal formulas and therapeutic acts differed, depending on the kind and condition of illness, and the region, with mystical-magical and religious elements being often superimposed on material acts. For example, incantations were interspersed with fragments of prayers and invocations to angels, and driving off an illness concluded with the formula: 'I make the sign of the cross over you in the name of Holy Trinity', although care was taken to avoid saying the word 'Amen'. The most frequently used words were excerpts from such prayers as 'Our Father', 'Hail Mary' and 'Glory be to the Father and Son' repeated three or seven times. When saying prayers, the sign of the cross was made over individual parts of the patient, the sick areas of the body were incensed with blessed herbs and washed with holy water, while objects attributed with special powers had to be kissed, and geometrical figures and lines were drawn around the patient's body with a piece of blessed chalk.

The past and present theraupeutic knowledge is syncretic, combining material, thaumaturgical and religious elements; we find in it behaviors that reflect local healing traditions, e.g. in phytotherapy, modified and simplified fragments of the present and past views of academic medicine, and treatment techniques used by modern bioenergy therapists and radiesthetists. As a result of the wide access to the media promoting non-conventional treatment techniques (Z. Nowak's series of programs on the Polsat TV), growing costs of utilization of medical institutions, an increase in the percentage of chronic diseases resistant to conventional treatment, the progressive ageing of society and the occurrence of the wave of somatic dysfunctions accompanying old age, and finally, the growing criticism of the methods of academic medicine, the extent of acceptance of many methods in the 'natural' folk medical system and of their practitioners may continue to grow. Therefore it is necessary to investigate these phenomena in accordance with an interdisciplinary or team approach with such sciences as medicine, psychology, sociology, and anthropology. This is especially important because at issue are not only theoretical and sociotechnical advantages but a rational approach to the phenomena that are the basis of human existence. It is a paradox that the demand for such studies seems as much trivial as topical[33]. D. Penkala-Gawęcka's studies

33 Summing up the results of her field studies D. Tylkowa wrote, 'When observing the quick development of healthcare in the villages surveyed we might think that folk healthcare should not play any significant role there. By contrast, the rural population in this area preserved many superstitions and practices of the folk medical system (1989:103). See also the description of revival of folk healing methods using religious elements (Cockerham 2004: 171-175).

show for example permanent presence of religious elements in the therapies offered by present-day folk practitioners in Wielkopolska province. She describes for example the use of holy water of the Lichen sanctuary by the local village therapists. (!996: 153-156).

2.4.2. Mesosocial Determinants

2.4.2.1 Attitudes to Medical Institutions and Professions

A permanent feature of the peasant's attitude to illness and being ill is distrust of medical professions and institutions, stemming from the closed and local character of peasant culture - the division into 'friends and foes'. Distrust also provokes fear of the unknown, contacts of the rural population with doctors having always been limited and the possibilities of medicine disregarded and underrated.

On the one hand, people **believed in home self-treatment and in tried and tested folk healthcare** [*my emphasis*, W. P.], on the other hand, they sought Divine support, taking destiny into account. With this attitude, a doctor was not necessary – his visit was associated with the last stage of illness and death. If a doctor was called in, it was usually at the last moment. Even patients tried to evade calling one, being afraid that doctors would poison them (Witos 1978: 127). It was also generally believed that injections had to be particularly avoided as being dangerous for health. For the peasant, the meaning of injection covered all manipulations involving pinpricks and punctures with a needle (taking blood for examination, pleural fluid etc). The hospital diet was also highly feared as there was a commonly accepted opinion that hospitals starved patients (*Pamiętniki lekarzy* 1939). Doctors themselves pointed out that this distrust was often due to the low quality of treatments and the occurrence of iatrogenic errors. No less important was the fact that doctors thought and worked in the way that was different from folk medicine; therefore they could not meet the special expectations of the village people. When a peasant heard the doctor's words '[..] shattering his beliefs, he was deeply disappointed […] A common peasant does not expect learned diagnoses from a doctor. Basically, the peasant knows and recognizes only three types of diagnosis: a cold, overexertion, and becoming infected. If the doctor's explanations […] do not contain one of these diagnoses, the patient is dissatisfied' (Ibid: 626). What the peasant family required from a doctor was fast and effective measures to restore the ability to work, an explicit diagnosis, and painless treatment without operation. 'A doctor should know everything without X-rays. That's what a doctor is for. In the country we need a miraculous doctor. There is no time for X-ray and some blood examination. There is no time to go to the doctor's all the time so that he will identify the illness and treat it slowly. Work in the field won't wait' (Ibid: 605). The peasant's skepticism also applied to the representatives of other medical professions (certified nurses and midwives). When describing the rural attitude to medical institutions in the late 1930s, S. Kosiński emphasized that the rural populations shied away from hospital treatment for many reasons, and even expressed negative attitudes towards hospitalization (S. Kosiński: 1983).

Despite transformations in the Polish countryside, some skepticism and ambivalence towards doctors still persists. Epidemiological studies conducted at the end of the 1970s and the beginning of the 1980s show *inter alia* that only one fifth of peasant families responds to illness by going to the doctor, the respondents often wanted 'to walk an illness through' (always 14.4%, often 14.2%). Low health indicators in the rural areas go together with a comparatively still low level of hospitalization, especially among the aged who often fall ill. Critical opinions about the qualifications of doctors practicing in rural areas and confidence in medicine is not high (low – 16%, medium – 21%); about 10% of respondents admit that they utilize folk medical practices, 32% use doctor-prescribed drugs at their own discretion, 29% of those surveyed treat themselves (Wdowiak et al. 1980, 4: 239-246; Woźniak 1991; 203-204).

S. Lachowski's surveys (2001) point out that the most frequent reason why peasant families give up medical treatment of children is the lack of money. This accounts for 29.45 of those surveyed. 18.2 % of mothers used self-treatment in illness almost always, and 59.7% used it from time to time (2001: 280:297).

2.4.3. Microsocial Determinants

2.4.3.1. Nutritional Patterns

Medical sociology generally assumes that the character and quality of environmental conditions have an effect on the rise of many illnesses. S. Graham presented the concept of the etiological chain, which places emphasis on such elements as nutrition, housing conditions, stress level, etc. (Graham 1974, 64, 11: 1046-1047).

A characteristic manifestation of folk culture and customs related to the rise of illnesses is nutritional habits. Despite general diffusion of cultural patterns and the influence of the media, these customs exhibit amazing persistence (Kosiński 1983). On the basis of personal documents and medical reports the following characteristic features of the nutritional patterns of an average peasant family (which were still present 70 years ago) can be distinguished: periodical stages of hunger (especially during the preharvest period) which caused lower resistance; susceptibility to and more serious course of illnesses; better food on holidays and inferior food on other days, regionalization of nutritional patterns; elimination of components with a market value (poultry, butter, eggs); monotonous diet; irregularity; careless preparation of food; rationing of portions depending on the position in the family hierarchy; skipping or not finishing meals; deficit of high-calorie products, fruit and vegetables. A peasant diarist recalls the 1930s, 'Many a time […] I was ill. Partly because of cold, partly because of not eating right. As I remember, in winter the only food was potatoes and beetroot soup, sometimes brown bread' (Chałasiński 1938: 122). J. S. Bystroń observes, 'Our people cook awfully; the best meals are so sloppily prepared, undercooked (potatoes, cabbage) and tough that they cause grave stomach suffering' (Bystroń 1947: 157-159).

Postwar studies on the peasant diet report people eating meals irregularly and consuming them too quickly, eating cold and not fresh dishes, drinking cold water after meals, a monotonous diet, and not enough fruit and vegetables. Dieticians maintain that bad nutritional habits cause insufficient growth, low body weight, rickets and dental caries. They point out that improper nutrition produces lower resistance to and more serious course of illness (Sikorski et al. 1964; Tokarski 1992: 44-47). Field studies on the nutrition of rural children by A. Dyjak demonstrate that children and teenagers in the country eat worse than their peers in towns (2005: 92-95). In her analysis of the satisfaction of nutritional needs, K. Gutkowska (2003: 150 et seq.) observes that when the income of a farm deteriorates, 'people save on food'. The rural diet means *inter alia* the low consumption level of eggs and dairy produce. In 12% of farms (especially in the elderly rural population) the level of nutrition is insufficient .

2.4.3.2. Housing Conditions

J. Szczepański writes in his study that 'The house organizes (or disorganizes) the coexistence of the family [..] it determines how children are brought up and their health' (1971:435).

Housing conditions were and to some extent still are visible proof of the disadvantage of peasantry. Until recently some peasant families lived in cramped, small, dirty, dark rooms, sometimes even without a floor. They usually lived in one or two rooms, even two families living in one room in extreme cases. Often several persons, usually children, slept in one room. Because there was not enough coal or firewood, the rooms were cold: this did not encourage hygienic practices and did allow isolation during sleep or at rest. One-room housing had, of necessity, to perform the universal role of workplace, storeroom, playground etc. As late as the 1940s and early 1950s rural housing conditions did not change considerably, modernization processes were slow but summer kitchens were already built, roofs were covered with non-flammable materials, etc. The crucial changes in rural housing construction took place in the 1960s and 1970s: in the new house the living premises were separated from the agricultural part, bathrooms were fitted, and the number and size of living rooms began to increase. By contrast, the elderly persons in the countryside lived in far worse conditions. It is emphasized that 7.4% of houses where elderly people lived were built in the nineteenth century. 17.3% of flats are over sixty years old. Furthermore, one out of four flats occupied by the aged has no gas, and in 28% of them water is drawn from the well. Health standards are met in the houses built during the last thirty years. It should be suspected, though, that in many peasant families the habits established in childhood and young years are passed on to the new house and do not change significantly. In some cases sick person are still not isolated and the patient's bed is occasionally used by another person (Kosiński 1983).

longitudinal studies by K. Gutkowska on the housing conditions of the rural population show that, even today, some proportion of peasant families (about two million people) also live in houses in bad technical condition: one out of four rural houses was built before 1946; 40% of them having no central heating, 30% have no toilet. On the whole, 18.4% of the rural inhabitants live in very bad conditions (against only 8.4% in town). It is stressed that bad living conditions are an etiological factor in many diseases. W. Pędich believes that, in typical 'eastern wall' provinces [i.e. in eastern Poland], the percentage of housing with bad standards amounts to 19% (Gutkowska 2003).

2.4.3.3. Hygienic Habits

The type and manner of the farmer's work was not conducive to the popularization of hygienic behaviors. Peasants did not see the virtues of personal hygiene and cleanliness. Even though people washed quite often, it was to refresh themselves rather than perform a hygienic function. Peasant farmsteads were dirty, waste was poured out into the yard, and toilets were often situated quite close to from wells. Water was also taken from pools, ditches, and shallow wells, and was drunk without being boiled. Special nightwear was not used, sometimes people worked and slept in the same clothes, and farmhands slept without undressing with the horses in the stable. It was only in the last few decades that important changes have occurred in hygienic patterns, especially among young women: readers of the press, radio listeners, and TV-viewers, (and recently internet users) are interested in developing new hygienic patterns. It is women who are most concerned with cleanliness (their own and that of their environment), rational eating, and optimum conditions for rest (Ibid). Generally speaking, hygienic patterns in the country are quickly becoming similar to those observed by the urban population.

When assessing the sanitary conditions in recent years, we should say that they are influenced not only by substantially lower incomes (as compared with town dwellers) of an average farm, but also the hard physical work conditions of most farmers. Lower income cause farmers to economize on expensive toiletries and household detergents, and buy the least expensive ones (of poor quality) or give them up altogether. F. Bujak's research report demonstrate that working conditions often cause farmers to be overworked, 'My observations and contacts with farmers […] every day show that many suffer from being workaholic: they get up at 3 or 4 o'clock in the morning, all day in a hurry […] After so exhausting a day they just lie down in bed without taking their shoes off, without having the strength (or will) to wash properly, sleeping lightly and thinking what they yet have to do, looking at the window with one eye to see if the morning is dawning so that they will not oversleep' (Bujak 2001: 200).

2.4.3.4. Psychosocial Factors

In traditional folk culture, feelings play a specific role and are shown to family members depending on their usefulness on the farm (Chałasiński 1938). This situation undoubtedly influences behaviors in illness. Of greatest value for the functioning of the farm was its manager – the farmer and head of the family - followed other men and, finally, women and children. Peasant diarists wrote 'if the one who earns a living for the whole family – the main force in the farmstead – is ill, and illness is prolonged, then they take last stores of grain […] and take the patient to the doctor's' (*Pamiętniki chłopów* 1939: 13). 'The year 1934 was very hard for me […] because it was then that my husband fell ill. For a year he stayed in bed, and we had to have money, whatever there was to sell, we did sell' (Jakubczak 1976, 3: 130). Reactions to illness among those who were not valuable labor on the farm were entirely different. Children and the aged were hardly ever provided with expensive medical care, or not even ordinary care (Kosiński 1983). Peasant memoirs read, 'I won't go to hospital either […]. It would cost even more. God willing, the child will live, if not, he will die' (*Pamiętniki lekarzy* 1939: 7). From the standpoint of the dominant economic interest and the importance of farming, farm animals were of higher value than any of many children: 'A cow feeds the whole family, it is easy to make a child'(Ibid: 45).

In peasant culture, illness, especially serious illness, was treated as something embarrassing which degraded man before his family and the immediate environment. People were especially ashamed of diseases regarded as the results of sin and indecency, and of diseases whose symptoms were located in the 'embarrassing' parts of the body. Then patients hid their illness even from household members, were ashamed to go the doctor, or demanded that examination be made 'through the clothes'; they were also afraid to go to hospital. Obviously, in the case of dangerous infectious diseases, women's diseases and tumors, the result of this embarrassment was the exacerbation of illness or premature death. Here are doctor's accounts: '[…] the woman's crotch burst during the first labor […] A country woman will not call a doctor to stitch the crotch […] She will not die because the opening will be larger […] between her legs there is a hanging sack the size of baby's head, covered with festering wounds […] she has never been to the doctor's (Ibid: 22). 'A father brings a twelve-year-old girl to me […] I take her blood for typhoid and tell them to come after three days […] But the father did not come. He was offended that I dared to suspect his daughter of having an infectious disease' (Ibid: 28). People were especially embarrassed about having venereal diseases regarded as sinful and impure. The absence of prevention caused frequent cases of congenital syphilis, '[…] a married couple come with a baby […] The several-days-old child covered in rash […] how many children have you had, I ask. This one is the thirteenth, says the peasant, all the others died when they were very little' (Ibid: 28). The parents never showed up again, they were ashamed of the disease and lack of money for treatment; the child died.

An especially characteristic feature of attitude towards illnesses in the peasant family was fatalism, generally associated with religious elements but also with peasant mentality marked by passivity, submission, and a sense of inferiority. Fatalism stemmed from the belief that everything depended on God, that God's will must not be opposed, and from the peasant's feeing of helplessness and powerlessness in the face of serious illness. Cut off from professional medical care, left to himself, he could only hope that the disease would pass or try to cast spells and charms on it, 'kill it', transfer it to another person or object, bury it or frighten it away. Being usually convinced that he could control neither his fate nor his family's, the peasant waited for 'what God will dispose'. Apart from passivity and apathy, this led to the acceptance of fate even if punishment in the form of illness was considered undeserved. The peasant mentality did not take into account the possibility of actively opposing evil. Illness was evil, but it was also part of the supernatural world, remained impenetrable and mysterious. In this way fatalism – both a part of culture and an element of the individual mind – impacted on behaviors and attitudes towards illness. Peasants would say 'It's the will of God, so be it. God will not harm the poor man, you have to believe in God's grace'. The father of a family with many children wrote, " I had six children, and buried three [...] what God wants to take away, he will, everything is in God's hands' (Ibid: 13). A popular saying in the country said that doctors would not help if you were ill with death'.

The well-known community-committed doctor A. Bałasz characterized his patients in this way: 'The patience of rural patients is amazing. The sick waiting in the hospital corridor, who often had to spend a long time waiting until I returned never reproached me or complained. On the contrary, they were glad although they spent all night cramped in the small room unsuitable for a waiting room' (*Pamiętniki lekarzy* 1964: 817). In the early 1950s the peasant patients treated medical care as a privilege rather than a right. The peasant coping with everyday adversities, with no possibility of influencing his life, and living in the manner determined by the natural calendar, was patient. He suffered pain in patience, he waited for months for his health to improve, and that is why he was able and wanted to wait for the doctor, whom he called 'our doctor'. Did this kind of 'peasant mentality' change at the turn of the twentieth century? Not entirely. M. Halamska points out that 'the mentality of agricultural peasant groups' is still traditional (2000: 32-33). B. Fedyszak-Radziejowska (2000: 107) emphasizes in conclusion of her studies that farmers (especially of older age) are characterized by 'the traditional, passive way of reacting to innovation and hazards'.

The foregoing remarks do not exhaust all the problems related to the peasant style of being ill and to its social, cultural and economic determinants. The role of work in shaping behaviors in illness and the importance of demographic factors have been marginally treated here. The main objective of this chapter was to draw attention to **considerable gaps in the sociology of illness in the peasant family and to show the social background of the folk medical system and self-treatment practiced in the past and partly in the present**. The fact that Poland has one of the highest percentages of peasant population in Europe and that this population was disadvantaged for years, including in terms of conditions determining their state of health, should provide a strong impetus for continuing research into these issues.[34]

34 The theoretical framework on the borderline between family sociology and medical sociology is defined by A. Ostrowska's study (1990,2; 83-97); the complementary character of the two subdisciplines is emphasized by Z. Kawczyńska-Butrym (Ibid: 65-81). The role of family as a significant link in the care of the sick and disabled is stressed by Z. Woźniak (1991, 2: 217). Studies by L. Solecki show that the percentage of the aged of both genders is higher in the country than in town. It is estimated that 17.5% of people aged over 60 live in the country, and rapid 'feminization of old age' is noticeable. The economic and health condition of this population category is actually worse than that of their town peers (Solecki 2004: 16 et seq.).

PART THREE

THERAPIES OF MODERN HEALERS. SPECIFICITY, CONTEXTS AND INTERPRETATIONS

1. Sociological Description of Non-Professional Ways of Meeting Health Needs in a Pluralistic Society

We will start from 'a brief history of Lublin themes' in sociological studies on the non-medical healing systems discussed at successive All-Polish Sociological Congresses in Poland. The results of research work on the traditional medical system conducted in Lublin's sociological center (UMCS) were first presented by this author and by S. Kosiński at the 7th All-Polish Sociological Congress in Wrocław (1985) during the session held by Professor Magdalena Sokołowska. Discussions on the revival (or persistence) of traditional forms of diagnosing, treating and preventing illnesses sparked considerable controversies at that time. There were disputes over the causes of the increase in the social popularity of methods regarded not long ago as anachronistic, backward, irrational or superstitious. When summing up this theme of the Wrocław proceedings, Magdalena Sokołowska emphasized diverse contexts (cultural, social and religious) and the relative character of the term 'rationality'. She emphasized the fact that the plurality of kinds of suffering may prompt patients to seek pluralistic forms of help in illness. Finally, she stated that the study of non-professional methods may be facilitated by the familiarity with such sociological materials as diaries and memoirs; in this context attention was drawn to the wealth of information contained in the interwar *Pamiętniki lekarzy* [Memoirs of Doctors] (1939), *Pamiętniki chłopów* [Memoirs of Peasants] (1936) or *Młode pokolenie chłopów* [Young Peasant Generation] (1938).

During the 9th All-Polish Sociological Congress in Lublin (1994) the issues in question were discussed twice during the session of the thematic group *Towards the New Paradigm of Medical Sociology* organized by A. Titkow. The presentation covered *inter alia* selected results of studies conducted at the UMCS Institute of Philosophy and Sociology (Department of Medical Sociology and Family). These analyses (to be referred to throughout this section) allowed us to indicate the main dilemmas and methodological difficulties related to the implementation of the contemporary research subjects (it was agreed that the optimal condition is balance and complementary treatment of quantitative and qualitative methods). The exploration of the problems covered the following: social determinants of the choice of 'other medicine' as alternative or complementary methods of treatment utilized by modern Poles; temporal variability and cultural determinants of terms associated with this way of meeting health needs, for example 'drug', 'health', 'illness' and 'improvement/deterioration of health'; finally, the prospect for further studies was outlined (Sułek and Styk 1995, 2: 288, 303 – Session Program no. 13).

Sociomedical studies presented at the 10th All-Polish Sociological Congress in Katowice (1997) was the third attempt to discuss the issues which some medical sociologists recognized as crucial to an understanding of changes in health behaviors in Polish society during transformation, a society increasingly pluralistic both in the sphere of social consciousness and in the kinds of social activities. I do not attribute subjective importance to the problems discussed here only because I am personally involved in the research projects. They are also objectively essential as this social area concerns the matters of utmost significance in every person's life: health and getting better, illness and being ill, and utilization of increasingly diversified methods of aid (treatment) that are intentionally offered to the Poles more and more often by lay practitioners without formal medical qualifications (Piątkowski 1998: 314-332).

A survey of the results of European sociomedical studies of 1990-2007 shows that systematic investigations of non-medical healing systems were practically not conducted except in Poland. At the 5th European Conference of Medical Sociology in Vienna (Piątkowski 1994) I presented a paper on the subject, and at the 6th Conference in Budapest (1996) four reports, including mine, were devoted to these problems Bajka and Bajka 1996: 115; L. Budak et al. Ibid: 112; Sciupokas Ibid: 113; Piątkowski Ibid.). At the 11th European ESHMS Biennal Conference (2006) held at the Jagiellonian University, Krakow, the problems in question were the subject of the whole plenary report by Judith Shuval, who summed up her longitudinal research into complementary medicine in Israel. The main thesis of her studies was to show actual examples of the areas of cooperation between academic medicine and CAM (complementary and alternative medicine). She also defined the spheres excluded from the growing rather than decreasing possibilities of healers' activities (Shuval 2006: 9). It is therefore necessary to conduct intensive, interdisciplinary (sociological, anthropological, psychological) investigations of the social context of 'other medicine' because this phenomenon is permanent and on a mass scale while the degree of its exploration is still unsatisfactory. The results of these studies should be regularly published and thoroughly discussed. It also appears that the reasons why such important research topics are not fully present in the current 'market of sociological ideas' are diverse and complex. Therefore they need to be provisionally described. Interdisciplinary studies on the subject were reported in the recent joint publication *Socjologia i antropologia medycyny w działaniu* [Medical Sociology and Anthropology in Action] (Piątkowski and Płonka-Syroka 2008).

1.1. On Methodological Disputes Once Again

I have already written about the question of taxonomy in part I (1.1.1. and 1.1.2) but this is a multifaceted issue and needs to be revisited. A formidable obstacle, which I have repeatedly mentioned in this book, is the problem with final standardization or uniformization of terminology concerning treatment methods and techniques not accepted in the past or at present by academic medicine although in medical sociology, ethnology and medical history many students of the problem use the term, which I have introduced: non-medical healing system divided into its three constituents of self-treatment, traditional folk medical systems, and therapeutic practices of modern-day healers.[35]

Another problem, which may obstruct investigations, is that representatives of natural sciences challenge the existence of phenomena and concepts applied by ethnologists, medical historians, sociologists, and even healers when trying to explain the phenomenon of 'the non-conventional therapist's influence on the patient's body' (Nardelli 1986). Since the question of difficulties in starting research work appears crucial in our discussion, we will devote more room to it. A typical representative of students of supernatural phenomena is English physicist and mathematician J. Taylor. The results of his longitudinal, interdisciplinary team studies can be reduced to several major conclusions, which we will try to describe. As early as the seventeenth century physics endeavored to investigate esoteric phenomena (Glanvill 1650-1680). Adopting the principle of objectivity and criticism, Glanvill assumed that some of the paranormal phenomena investigated were empirical. Looking at the results of his investigations from later perspectives, we can notice some credulity in Glanvill, who lacked proper instruments to precisely verify or disprove his adopted hypotheses. J. Taylor points out that current systematic studies on paranormal phenomena in non-medical healthcare conducted by various centers (mainly in the USA and Japan) are based chiefly on medical statistics and probability calculus. Physicist A. K. Wróblewski asserts that without the knowledge and application of statistical laws and rules we cannot settle any problems concerning for example distance healing and radiesthesia, etc (Wróblewski 1990). It is believed that any objective assessment of phenomena related, for example, to spiritual healing has to take into account a high probability of accidental coincidence of events in the causal chain. The use of a statistical approach, Wróblewski maintains, entirely disquali-

35 I presented the first complex suggestion of taxonomic terminology in 1990. It was discussed or adopted *inter alia* by J. Jeszke, D. Penkala-Gawęcka, S. Sterkowicz, B. Tobiasz-Adamczyk, M. Libiszowska-Żółtowska, I. Jaguś, A. Kubiak, E. Więckowska, K. Imieliński, A. Firkowska-Mankiewicz.

fies diagnostic effects obtained by radiesthetists. Interestingly enough, physicists and mathematicians enter, in a sense, the sociological methodological field when they warn against the doubtful evidentiary value of accounts of eyewitnesses to miraculous recoveries, as they are easily manipulated, suggestible, and likely to fall victim to their own emotions.

From the standpoint of logic of natural sciences, the interpretation of faith healing (healing with psychic powers) should, apart from using a uniform taxonomy, be connected with objective quantitative description. In order to achieve that, different features of the investigated phenomena need to be related to exact classes of statistical quantities. Also the features of the object studied should be described in an exact way because even in descriptions of such obvious and unambiguous properties as for example the human body temperature, there are differing accounts by therapy session participants. J. Taylor also proposes that paranormal phenomena be systematically measured although he admits that it is difficult to implement this postulate because they (phenomena) tend to be unique and difficult to record with standard research instruments. Generally speaking, skepticism and criticism cannot lead, Taylor asserts, to a denial that healing (or self-treatment of) others with one's own psychic powers can be a genuine fact (Taylor 1990: 55). Consequently, we should recognize as actual, for example, spontaneous remissions that happen in the course of cancerous diseases. Several hundred such incidences have been objectively confirmed by academic medicine.

A separate problem is the effect on the recovery process of other factors outside the influence of the faith healing methods, for example, the healing effect of parallel administration of measures of technochemical medicine (pharmacotherapy, operation results, etc.). It should be pointed out that it is difficult to assess whether and to what extent psychosociological factors impact the course and effects of the treatment process. The results of Taylor's studies and similar analyses strongly reject for example the possibility of psyche breaking the continuity of tissues in the human body. From the standpoint of natural sciences, this portion of modern healing methods practiced, for example, in the Philippines is based on suggestion, delusion, hypnosis, and on clever deception and mystification. It is emphasized that none of the operations of this type has ever been performed under satisfactory conditions permitting sufficient control of all variables and fully legitimate conclusions.

Science can also offer a partial explanation for another phenomenon of interest to students of non-medical healing systems: biofeedback. This consists in the ability of the patient o exert controlled influence (*inter alia* under hypnosis or suggestion) on such processes and phenomena as drug action, pain, blood pressure level, activity of endocrine glands, etc.

A different factor associated with faith healing that should be recognized as one capable of objectively influencing health and illness is *élan vital* (vital force, vital impetus), a strong subjective conviction that 'you have to live' or, in the absence of it, 'you have to die'. Empirical results thus confirm the fact that we cannot deny the cause-and-effect relationship between health and a strong faith (for example religion-motivated) in being cured. Similarly, the placebo effect on psychosomatic phenomena is recognized and undisputed. Taylor et al. report that the efficacy of a placebo in reducing some pain symptoms can amount to as much as 40% (Ibid).

All these may prompt us to say that, from the standpoint of natural science, the phenomenon of healing with spiritual powers can be reduced to a sociopsychological (rather than physico-biological) impact on the patient's mind and emotions, and her/his state of health. Many other hypotheses proposed by healers and concerning all kinds of 'energy', 'healing power', 'waves', 'radiation', should be regarded as false in light of the methods and concepts utilized by modern natural sciences (we are speaking of evidence-based medicine; Ibid: 71). The results of experiments obtained by Taylor, Balanovski et al. and the results of those of other similar reliable studies conducted in the 1990s are of essential significance to social science scholars. On the one hand they disprove all manner of even the most fantastic views of healers about a strong impact of 'bioenergy', 'bioplasm', or 'biofield' on the physical state of health and illness of their (the healers') patients; on the other hand, they emphasize that the source of many spontaneous recoveries are sociopsychological factors of varying strength in different configurations, which underlie such mechanisms as biofeedback, *élan vital*, or the placebo effect.

The results of similar analyses are continually challenged by influential representatives of medical science, who are critical of any studies whatsoever on non-medical healing systems. Public interest in non-conventional methods tends to be explained here by demands of the 'intellectual proletariat', difficulties associated with distinguishing science from pseudoscience, educational deficiencies in modern societies, or by tolerance of diverse pseudoscientific hoaxers. In this context it can be is asked whether the growing democratization of science is not its misfortune consisting in the failure to assess and classify the results of studies quickly and exactly, and to the spot pseudo-achievements of false science.

Among the representatives of academic medicine there is growing criticism of fraud and pseudomedical abuse allegedly committed by healers. For example, M. Chorąży emphasizes that non-conventional medicine misrepresents the knowledge of the structure and operation of the human organism and duplicates erroneous views. The author (professor of clinical oncology) concludes, 'I do not want to recite the endless list of all the nonsense, superstitions, and rubbish [...] I cannot stand by indifferent to the spread of pseudoscience, ignorance, superstition, or tolerate manipulation [...] (Chorąży 1998, 3: 69-70). Another representative of clinical medicine who assesses 'paramedicine' is M. Pawlicki, frequently quoted in Part One. In his recapitulation of clinical studies he writes that practicing healers are one of the three main reasons why oncological treatment is delayed in Poland. Three to five thousand patients die every year because of delayed visits to the doctor, for which healers are to blame.

Can we, however, account for the growing public interest in and increased tolerance of most non-conventional methods only with reference to commercialization of science and its endeavors to woo the 'ordinary patient' or does the popularity of healers merely create the myth of their alleged persecution by physicians? Even if manipulations around homeopathic theories have been exposed, should we conclude from this fact that we must throw the homeopathic baby out with the bathwater? (Gryglewski 1995: 34, 36). The homeopathic conception also shows good models of doctor-patient interaction, effective use of the placebo effect, etc. We may ask whether it does not follow from the foregoing studies by Taylor and Balanovski that the core of the healing effect is not mysterious, unexplored and unreal phenomena such as 'bioenergy' or 'healing radiation' but measurable social acceptance, faith and hope invested by some patients in the healers who treat them. We should also remember that in social sciences we are not moving in the circle of unverifiable hypotheses, but that the explanation of social popularity of healing can be found in the results of sociological, psychological and ethnological studies on non-medical healthcare (Sokołowska 1980; 1986; Piątkowski 1990: 111-115; Piątkowski et al. 1998: 133-135; 1999: 99-105; Penkala-Gawęcka 1998; furthermore orthopedics professor Gregosiewicz (2002, 5: 26 et seq.), who demonstrates that, from the natural science perspective, bioenergy therapy, acupuncture, iridology and homeopathy are evident 'medical hoaxes'. We should also remember that surprising effects of 'spontaneous healings' obtained by some lay healers in sociopsychosomatic diseases are achieved by trial and error, most often without any scientific competence in socio- and psychotherapy. These examples allow us to see a possibility, in the treatment process, of combining the therapist's charismatic personality with scientific knowledge of behavioral sciences, at the same time respecting ethics and deontology.

The confirmation of the fact that the essence of a large portion of good results obtained by healers is not the presumed material factors but **the actual direct or indirect influence of specific, identified sociopsychological elements upon the patient's emotions and mental states, which, as a result, help achieve 'the subjective state of health' or produce a placebo effect**, opens the door to the therapeutic use of behavioral sciences 'at the patient's bed'. This in turn can lead to a legitimate conclusion that in the market of the previously non-professional health service provision there should finally appear professionals equipped with socio- and psychotherapeutic knowledge, e.g. general practitioners or psychology and sociology graduates specializing in helping patients with psychosomatic problems (chronically ill, disabled, the aged, those with mental disorders, etc.).

Summing up this discussion we should say that on the basis of concepts and research tools of natural sciences we cannot arbitrarily classify problems investigated by sociologists or psychologists practicing non-medical healing as pseudoproblems and regard them as ostensible, non-scientific, or marginal. Phenomena which it is now impossible to explore from the perspective of physics, chemistry or medical sciences can be investigated using qualitative or quantitative sociological methods, and the results of these studies can be valuable (Piątkowski 2002: 219 et seq.).

In short, the criticism and skepticism of natural sciences (especially medicine) stemming from efforts to disprove many 'healing theories' that attempt to explain the influence of the therapist's organism on the patient's body, and the dynamics of processes of recovering and being ill, cannot be translated into the field of humanities and cannot challenge the values of the research conducted here. The sociology, psychology or anthropology of non-medical healthcare describe actual social facts using tried and tested research procedures, and as a result they can accumulate and interpret information having substantial cognitive and practical qualities.

1.2. Social Causes of the Phenomenon

A systematic presentation of many scattered results of studies on the popularity of non-medical healing systems has already been partly discussed in the Introduction and Part One. We should therefore select the existing sources and reinterpret the research results. This procedure seems necessary because earlier empirical analyses of non-medical healing systems did not start in Western countries until the 1970s and 1980s (Grossinger 1980: 27-35; Stanway 1982: 31-33. The core feature, however, of the research approach to these problems is interdisciplinarity; consequently, the resulting studies are situated not only in diverse research fields and within different disciplines, but also within individual, comparatively autonomous groups of sciences. The results of studies on non-medical healing systems obtained through methodologies characteristic of a particular science are thus produced in medical sciences (from medical history to clinical medicine to ethnopharmacy), in the humanities (from medical sociology to anthropology to psychology), and in exact sciences (physics, chemistry), etc. This characteristic heterogeneity (methodological, taxonomic, and theoretical) in the approach to the same field of inquiry creates the state of a peculiar *embarras de richesse*. (Libiszowska-Żółtkowska et al., 1998). An attempt to avoid these dilemmas here is through selection i.e. omission of the results of investigations conducted by disciplines other than sociological ones (selected results have been presented in the state of research section).

In conclusion, in this section we will only present and briefly interpret the selected results of sociological investigations conducted by the CBOS [Public Opinion Research Center] and OBOP [Public Opinion Polling Center], which cover the problems in question and are not widely known, and we will discuss selected results of my studies conducted in the UMCS Department of Medical and Family Sociology. The results will be compared with the most recent research into non-conventional healthcare in the Netherlands and the United Kingdom because they are representative, being an effect of longitudinal scientific observations (Trevelyan and Booth 1998: 1-17; Corin 1995).

To begin with we should emphasize that, when interpreting the extent of social acceptance of non-conventional treatment methods, we touch upon the whole complex of transformations in modern culture and changes in the social consciousness of the people at the turn of the twentieth century. These changes arose owing to Poland being wide open to foreign and previously unknown ideological, religious and political ideas flowing freely from Europe and the rest of the world. This will be dealt with in the subsequent chapters. We may only mention the penetration, via the media, of postmodernist issues, the New Age ideology, Age of Aquarius consciousness etc. into this country. Representative public opinion surveys show that more and more Poles are convinced about the parapsychological capabilities of the human mind (telekinesis, telepathy, clairvoyance). Those polled accept the view that 'we are not alone in the Universe' and believe in psychic contact with the deceased. Moreover, people not only seem to believe in paranormal phenomena but also apparently experience them to a varying extent (*O niektórych aspektach... Komunikat z badań CBOS* 1997: 13-15; *Czy Polacy... Komunikat z badań CBOS* 2006).

Convinced of the broader context of the results obtained, the author of this study examined the background of the views in question, dividing the causative factors triggering the expansion of 'other medicine' into two principal groups: socio-cultural and those associated with transformations in the medical system. The former include *inter alia* the following: the role of the commercial media which promote the attractive topic of alternative medicine; changes in lifestyle consequent upon the emergence of a new ecological awareness and the rise of the consumer movement; a fashion for an alternative, 'natural' lifestyle, which covers not only the kind of clothes we wear, choice of ecological means of transport, and healthy diet, but also preference for natural ways of treatment comprising both methods and therapeutic agents. The next factor is the widespread cult of the healthy and beautiful body and at the same time the popularization of the 'natural ways' of achieving these goals, subjectively important to modern man, also through 'alternative medicine'. The way to the healthy body is by means of natural ways of treatment, avoiding 'toxic medicine', towards healthism which is growing popular in Western countries (Nettleton 1996: 209-214); Piątkowski and Brodniak 2005).

Another factor accelerating the move away from 'technochemical medicine' is the growing realization by healthy people of the iatrogenic effects of commercial medicine. Examples of such criticism of academic medicine (possessive, maximum-income oriented, and treating the patient instrumentally) are, respondents report, the reason why people lose trust in many health services and are increasingly convinced that although alternative treatments may prove ineffective they do not carry the risk of health deterioration (Nettleton 1996; Cockerham 2004: 171-175). We should also mention the slowly but steady decline in the prestige of the doctor's profession; with the growing increase in patients' general health culture, doctor-patient interactions are becoming highly democratized, while medical recommendations warning people against the adverse effects of utilization of lay healing services are usually ignored and do not affect decisions to choose a healer as a partner in fighting illness.

Another element determining the growing public interest in non-medical healing systems is liberal administrative law regulations, which permit one to provide treatment services without recognized medical qualifications. This mode of earning a living can be legally registered as a craftsman's business. It should added that the negligible legal consciousness of the Poles and the habit of circumventing the law contribute to the fact that healers' patients are unaware that pursuant to the Law of the Physician's Profession (1997) and the Code of Medical Ethics, provision of treatment and rehabilitation is reserved exclusively for medical doctors qualified to practice whereas their possible cooperation with lay healers is considered reprehensible and liable to prosecution.

Apart from socio-cultural changes the factor that enhances social acceptance of and interest in non-conventional treatment methods is transformations noticeable within the medical system. Previous studies have defined some of them. The extent of tolerance towards methods not accepted by academic medicine undoubtedly increased with the appearance of ideologies of holistic medicine in the West and then in Poland. These conceptions, drawing *inter alia* upon oriental philosophical and healing traditions, permit the coexistence of different and equal medical systems in 'healing the body and the soul' of the whole man (Klamut 1996, 4). Holism attempts to define the framework of humanistic medicine, thereby opening the door to methods used by non-physicians as part of various non-medical treatment techniques (both non-conventional psychotherapists and Filippino healers applying psychic forces refer to the holistic ideology). An issue of no small consequence, which makes non-medical healing systems tolerated (even if they do not meet scientific standards) by some part of the medical community, is financial matters. A comparison of technochemical treatment expenses with the money spent for example on homeopathic therapies (placebo!) in fighting rheumatoid diseases showed that the sums spent on homeopathy are several times lower. These results confirm doctors in their permissive attitudes (Boisset 1944, 21).

Clinical analyses conducted in the 1990s on the efficacy of several dozen methods practiced outside of academic medicine and the analysis of possible dangers resulting from their use led to the conclusion that the vast majority of these methods cannot cause deterioration of the patient's state of health (if we disregard the healer-imposed abandonment of traditional hospital treatment when the prognosis for an illness is good). It was also found that the therapeutic success that can be achieved as a result of non-medical therapies can be explained in terms of behavioral sciences (the placebo effect, 'subjective state of health') rather than within the natural science paradigm. Reports usually end with a conclusion that these are inexpensive and 'comparatively harmless' natural methods that can be used in medicine as 'supportive means' (Walsh 1993, 37; Boström and Rosner 1992, 2; Jonas and Levin 2000: 59-73).[36] The fairly popular opinion that these methods are harmless and 'sociopsychologically' effective is also important, as expressed by most patients (especially those better educated) who utilize them. At the same time the medical community realizes that the efficacy of some conventional therapies used in the treatment of chronic, painful, old-age-related, socio- and psychosomatic diseases is highly limited. It is in cases of these diseases with hopeless prognosis, when pharmacological treatment or surgery cannot be used, that all kinds of healers try their hand. Therefore, classic medicine, when faced with diseases with increasingly notice-

36 Recent clinical studies taking the sociological and medical standpoint into account show that with cardiological and oncological diseases the services of paramedicine are utilized by a large percentage of patients. The authors say that these therapies have no healing value in the biomedical sense. In conclusion they write that 'to eradicate this extremely widespread superstition requires […] expenditure not only on progress but also on the art of treatment' (Świątoniowski, Łaniewski et al. 2002, 5: 81-86).

able non-biological components, hands the initiative to non-professional non-physicians instead of to specialists in medical sociology and psychology. In these circumstances the urgent task of behavioral sciences is apparently to continually show their efficacy and usefulness, which in the long run, will partly prevent lay practitioners from providing services to patients, especially in treating socio-psychosomatic conditions with which specialized clinical medicine cannot quite cope.

Two more factors within the medical system that, apparently, accelerate the expansion of healers into the free healthcare provision market, are the growing importance of nursing sciences and the ideologies of friendliness towards non-conventional healing methods, prevailing in this increasingly influential community. Nurses have always been closer not only to the patient's body but also to his/her mental conditions, emotions, moods and social situation. They were also traditionally sensitive to the views and opinions of supporters of 'other medicine'. It is also not without significance that the nurse's professional training enables him/her to better understand non-biological, including sociopsychological, aspects of the treatment process. It is therefore not surprising that, for example, in the UK, at their 1972 National Congress the nurses passed a resolution demanding that research be undertaken on treatment methods that are outside of academic medicine. Representatives of this profession repeatedly voiced their willingness to include such therapies in nursing education but also supported patients demanding that the National Health Service refund treatments by healers. Members of nursing occupations, being aware of the growing emancipation of their profession, are valuable allies of healers who demand that any discrimination against non-conventional methods be abolished and that such methods be termed complementary to the offer of academic medicine (Pfeil 1994, 3).

1.3. The Extent of Use of Non-Conventional Therapies

We will now look closely at the social popularity of non-medical healthcare, which we first mentioned in the Introduction. We will present only selected results of nationwide sociological representative surveys conducted by the CBOS and OBOP since 1990, i.e. showing the changing attitude to non-medical healing systems in the context of great social transformations occurring in Poland.

We will begin with the CBOS survey of 1991. This analysis allows us to determine the

scope and framework of the social phenomenon, which is the utilization of non-professional treatment methods at the beginning of the systemic transformation. As many as 53% of adult Poles were 'very' or 'a little' interested in the activities of various healers. This is a far greater range of interest than we were able to observe in Western societies: for example only 4% of the Dutch population were more interested in such methods and knew of at least one 'alternative medicine' technique (Oojendijk and Mackenbach 1981, 4; U. Sharma 1996). The CBOS survey demonstrates that the Poles regard non-scientific methods as a good complement to medicine; this opinion was shared by as many as 78% of those surveyed, while 13% were opponents of non-conventional treatment methods. At the same time, in my own studies (Piątkowski 1990: 11-115) as many as 98.4% of patients of the well-known healer C. Harris were convinced of the need for cooperation between academic medicine and non-conventional healing systems. Conversely, the following figures for Dutch respondents show the types of patient behavior in the case of illness. Most of them used services offered by official medical institutions (83%) while 18% of those surveyed utilized non-conventional methods, treating them most often as complementary to methods offered under the medical system. The Polish 1991 CBOS study also permitted the listing of individual non-medical techniques by the criterion of their popularity. Of the 53% of respondents who were 'very (12%) and 'a little'(41%) interested in such methods, 15% had contact with herbal medicine, 14% took part in televised therapy sessions (chiefly teletherapy by A. M. Kashpirovsky), and 7% practiced various osteopathy methods. The CBOS survey also revealed the opinion of those polled about the efficacy and methods/techniques of non-conventional treatment. The respondents who used them rated the efficacy of chiropractic the highest (52% reported that illness symptoms entirely disappeared, while 27% reported that troubles lessened). Following the use of phytotherapy, illness symptoms entirely disappeared in 18% of patients, while ailments were reduced in 42%).

A comparison with the Dutch survey shows distinct similarities: in the Netherlands herbal medicine and chiropractic also enjoyed the highest popularity, and, at the same time, the two were rated the most effective. The difference was that the Dutch rated homeopathy - comparatively less known in Poland (although increasingly popular) - among the most effective methods. The analysis of personal particulars in the CBOS survey showed that at the beginning of the transformation period an interest in the best-known non-conventional methods (herbal medicine and chiropractic) was taken significantly more often by persons of higher socioeconomic status (the intelligentsia, executive personnel, office workers). The Dutch survey displayed an identical tendency – the majority of patients utilizing non-conventional methods as complementary ones had a comparatively high social status and large incomes. To sum up we should again emphasize the widespread belief of respondents that methods of 'other medicine' can be used as complementary treatments and, even if their positive effects cannot be seen at once, they will certainly do no harm to our health *(Opinia publiczna... Komunikat z badań CBOS* 1991).

In the early 1990s, TV programs featuring non-conventional therapists enjoyed immense popularity. For almost three years Polish TV Channel II broadcast regular programs with A. M. Kashpirovsky. The programs were surveyed by the OBOP on a representative sample of the Polish adult population (*Telewizyjne... Komunikat z badań OBOP* 1990). Here are some characteristic results. As many as 59% of Poles watched the programs in which this therapist appeared, one fifth had not heard about the program, while 3% of those surveyed reported that teletherapy had a positive effect on their state of health (in absolute figures - 840 thousand people). Although most TV-viewers did not feel any positive somatic changes in their health, as many as 73% of them wanted the program to continue. They did not necessarily expect instant somatic improvement, but some of them hoped for later improvement in their physical or mental state of health, or assumed that they simply did not notice any improvement. Still others were convinced that Kashpirovsky's programs increased 'health reserves', and were thus of preventive importance; almost all those polled believed that 'there was something to it' and identified with the view that 'if it does not help, it will certainly do no harm.' Only 5% of those surveyed shared the opinion already known from other studies that healers in Poland should be allowed to practice on a wider scale but would have to treat people under medical supervision. Only 6% of respondents asserted that non-professional healing practice should be banned. The Kashpirovsky phenomenon will be discussed in section 3.

The next OBOP survey concerning the problem of non-medical healthcare was conducted in February 1996 (*Co robi... Raport z badań OBOP* 1996: 1-3). Here are the most important results related to the problem of social reception of these kinds of healing practices.[37] When they felt illness symptoms, almost half of adult Poles (48%) used home methods as part of self-treatment, i.e. the most popular way of coping with illness and at the same time the oldest form of non-medical treatment according to the division presented in Part One. It should be emphasized that when treating their own illnesses, respondents used natural substances (e.g. milk with honey, herbs, garlic) (*Co robi... Raport z badań OBOP* 1996). Even if those surveyed used pharmacy drugs, they took them at their own discretion, buying them prescription-free. Only 31% of informants consulted

37 In 1990 we divided non-medical healthcare (healing systems) into three distinct, historically developing traditions: help in illness, or self-treatment, folk medical systems (folk practitioners), and modern-day healers (bioenergy therapy, mesmerism, homeopathy etc.).

a doctor after having noticed illness symptoms. Characteristically, non-professional healing methods were preferred by people of low educational and economic status, for example housewives (64%); however, for entirely different reasons, they were also preferred by professionally active, educated thirty-year olds (57% in this group).

Finally, we will look at two CBOS surveys: of December 1997 and April 1998. We will compare them with the above-mentioned British analyses by J. Trevelyan and B. Booth (1998). The first survey was conducted on a 1168-person representative sample of adult Poles (*O niektórych... Komunikat z badań CBOS* 1997). We will start with the social extent of the phenomenon. One in three respondents (35%), when asked 'a very broad question,' answered that s/he or her/his family were currently utilizing some form of non-medical healthcare or had done so in the past. This is a far greater percentage of persons not only interested in but also practicing such methods than, for example, in the Netherlands or in the UK. A comparison of the above-quoted sociological studies of 1990 and 1991 with these CBOS analyses shows that the level of interest in non-conventional healthcare methods is not only *not* declining, as doctors repeatedly predicted, but is steadily growing. We should emphasize that apart from complementary healing methods and techniques described earlier in this text, new therapeutic modes, related to oriental traditions, appeared in the late 1990s. This may be an element of expansion of the New Age consciousness as we wrote in the earlier sections. One in five respondents (or their families) had utilized non-medical healthcare many times (20%), with 4% of adult Poles using these methods very often. We should emphasize once again that, as in my earlier analyses (1990), this survey shows that an increasingly greater percentage of persons preferring these healing methods and treating them as a complementary therapy alongside official medicine are rational, well-educated middleclass people with comparatively high incomes. The December 1997 CBOS survey reports that these respondents defined their status as executive personnel, the intelligentsia, and private businessmen from the largest cities. On the other hand, such methods were also utilized by impoverished people, who were counted in the category of housewives (Ibid). As in the previous surveys, respondents were rather satisfied with the results obtained by non-physicians (25% definitely, 36% rather satisfied), only 13% were very disappointed with therapy results. Like the Lublin study (1990), this survey showed that there was a numerical predominance of women over men (66% vs. 61%) among patients utilizing methods not accepted by medicine. The 1998 CBOS survey (*Leczenie się.... Komunikta z badań CBOS*: 2-3) confirmed the stable tendency in the Polish medical services market: different forms of non-medical healthcare (including self-treatment) were utilized in the past or are utilized now by over a half of adult Poles (57%), of which healers' services were used by 5%, while 52% use self-treatment on their own (Ibid). We should stress that as many as 40% of those surveyed rely on their own home medicinal agents, without using pharmacy drugs, but most of them combine the use of pharmacotherapy with natural substances. In the case of illness (usually with a mild course) only 9% of respondents seek only medical advice. The most frequent reason for avoidance of contacts with medical institutions and professions is the prevailing conviction that an illness is not serious or will pass of itself; people may also distrust a doctor, believing that he will not contribute anything to their own diagnosis or therapy. Finally, they may not have enough time or money for lengthy and ineffective treatment.

Apart from the Dutch survey, our point of reference was the results of sociological analyses conducted in the UK in the 1980s and the 1990s. Recent results of studies on the subject were discussed in Part One. These surveys showed that the number of consultations provided by healers rose five times as fast as the number of instances of medical advice in the last decade. Other results are also interesting. It turned out that, in 1992, one percent of British adults used acupuncture, while two percent used homeopathy. Since the early 1990s complementary therapies in the UK, for example osteopathy, chiropractic and homeopathy have been available under the National Health Service. The authors state, as we have already indicated, that the fast development of non-medical services is conditioned *inter alia* by the favorable attitude of nurses to these kinds of offers. The cited English authors believe that the role of this type of aid in illness and in health promotion activities may increase in the EU countries (Trevelyan and Booth 1998; Baer 2010: 379-381).[38]

Apart from the foregoing studies, we should refer to the figures published by the Main Statistical Office (GUS) in 1997, which show that at the end of the twentieth century, healers' services were sought by 4% of the Polish population, i.e. ca. 1.3 million people. Among those, the patients were largely women and the rural population, with a predominance of middle-aged and elderly persons (*Stan zdrowia...* GUS 1997: 100).

According to the figures quoted by the media (20002) it is estimated that over 70 thousand non-medical therapists earn their living from practicing non-medical healing methods (the "Polityka" magazine reports that in Poland there are 50 thousand registered healers, Walewski 2001, 18: 4; Konarska 2002,18: 14-18).

38 Figures obtained in the European Social Survey (Round 2, 2004) show that in the case of back pains respondents would seek help from non-physicians: in the UK – 8.3% answers, in Germany – 4.6%, in Poland 2.4%; when asked about specific therapists the Poles usually indicate bioenergy therapists (3%), the British – chiropractors/osteopaths (5.6%), and Germans – acupuncturists/ acupressurists (6%).

The main conclusions from the foregoing surveys are the following:

- The use of non-conventional, non-medical treatment methods is a permanent, important element of the changing health culture of Polish society. This phenomenon is slowly but steadily growing.
- The most popular methods of non-medical healing are self-treatment techniques (home ways of treatment).
- The above-discussed factors that make up the syndrome of causes determining the quick expansion of 'other' medicine are located both in the socio-civilizational supersystem and within the medical system.
- All the studies quoted show that non-physicians are most effective in treating socio- and psychosomatic diseases (heart conditions, pains, neuroses, depressions, etc). Improvement symptoms last for a least several weeks.
- The main recipients of non-conventional health services in Poland are, for different reasons, two distinct client groups. One comprises people with low education and low income: they most probably find it difficult to access medical services, especially if we take into account the grey market of paid medical practice. On the other hand, yuppies choose these methods deliberately as a fashionable, 'non-toxic' path to health, without running the risk of iatrogenic errors and side effects of biotechnical medicine. This group seems to be growing.
- My own studies (1990, 1993) showed that the element that enhances the prestige of non-medical methods and therapists who use them is the support provided by some priests and church institutions.
- A social phenomenon of such importance and reach (matters of health and illness) requires systematic, full-scale, interdisciplinary and comparative studies, involving joint cooperation of specialists in medical, behavioral, ethnological, historical etc. sciences.

1.4. Healing – Methods of Treatment, Culture, and Ideology

I have returned to methodological issues several times (Introduction, Part Three): because of their significance we have to examine them once again from different points of view. When conducting studies on non-medical healing systems in the early 1990s we faced challenges brought by the new social reality, including the scope and pace of social transformations. This was accompanied by the conviction that the character of macrosocial transformations occurring in Poland in the spheres of culture, consciousness and structures of community life would certainly accelerate and expand the extent of utilization of non-conventional healing methods by the Poles. The hypothesis put forward when commencing the sociological analysis of the so-called Kashpirovsky phenomenon was fully confirmed (Piątkowski et al. 1993). At the 9th All-Polish Sociological Congress in Lublin, during the proceedings of the sociomedical session, a thesis was put forward that the best way of getting to know this new social reality was to conduct investigations combing quantitative and qualitative approaches. Analysis of personal documents was suggested as a major method of studying this area (Piątkowski and Latoszek 1995, 2: 288, 303). Emphasis placed on the need to appreciate qualitative methods in sociomedical inquiries (especially into non-conventional treatment methods and sociology of illness) followed from the experience of analyzing over three thousand personal documents (letters) sent to the Polish TV Channel II by people who took part in the sessions with the non-conventional psychotherapist Kashpirovsky (I have discussed this in greater detail in the Introduction). The partial move away from application of quantitative methods in medical sociology may have resulted from a wider range of causes including the intensifying anti-positivist (anti-scientistic) movement and growing popularity of the interpretive paradigm. It is not clear whether this is the emergent rise of the conception of post-positivist sociology or a passing fashion drawing upon strong traditions of Polish humanistic sociology.

I omit here the broader, historical context of discussion on the usefulness of quantitative methods present 'for ages' in the Polish mainstream sociology. Observe only that, as early as 1937 Stefania Skwarczyńska wrote that the letter characterized the social world, 'it belongs to life, strives for life, and describes life'. She was one of the first scholars who emphasized already in the early 1930s that the letter was a document, which should by also studied by sociology (Skwarczyńska 1937: 1-8).

We can also assume, as I have written in the Introduction, that sociologists' positive attitude to biographical methods (methods of personal documents analysis) goes back to the 1920s and 1930s, when the first volume of the work by W. I. Thomas and F. Znaniecki *The Polish Peasant in Europe and America* appeared. The materials gathered by the two scholars allowed them to reconstruct subjective features of social groups, customs, religiousness, kinds of social bonds, experiences of members in the communities studied, and social factors producing psychic states. In Piątkowski et al. (1993) we used letter analysis as the fundamental sociological method, this material serving both to prepare a statistical study and to present large excerpts from the collected written accounts, which exemplified the author's conclusions. It was thus an attempt to present direct accounts of events, which those surveyed participated in and directly commented on. The material obtained was selectively examined and, following the earlier criteria of information significance, this permitted reconstruction of facts serving to describe and interpret broader phenomena related to the sociology of health and illness (Szczepański 1973:615-648).

I indicate a methodological issue here, being convinced that this type of 'soft' research approach shows its special virtues in investigating cultural phenomena surrounding non-medical healing systems (especially in the context of illness): it does not impose the researcher's conceptual framework on the respondent; it ensures the researcher's openness to the reality analyzed; and it permits the recording of intimate, sensitive, traumatic and dramatic phenomena, and ensures the subject's autonomy, the researcher and the subject (respondent) being equal partners. The sociologist can be not only a witness to but also a participant in the events studied (which was the case in analyses of the Kashpirovsky phenomenon). Having accepted this approach, those planning and implementing research projects obviously need ethical qualifications, and more responsibility should be taken for project execution and interpretation of results (Piątkowski et al.1993; Wyka 1993; Kempny 1993: 291-303). Therefore, accepting a methodological approach close to humanistic sociology, we can apply it to relevant countercultural and subcultural ways of thinking that justify the value of non-conventional therapy methods and encourage patients to use these modes of coping with matters of health and illness.[39] Generally, a broader research question arises: during the system transformation, is a mature 'alternative culture' developing in Poland?, and if so, apart from ecologism, the struggle for animal rights, or healthism, is the revival of interest in, acceptance of and practicing of 'natural ways of healing' as part of non-medical healthcare a fragment of this culture? In my own studies I was able to determine and characterize the main sociocultural phenomena surrounding non-medical healing systems in the postmodern age. I support the view that the causes of the phenomenon of alternative medicine can be divided into two principal groups: those relating to the socio-civilizational supersystem and those to the medical system. The first group, which defines the cultural background, would include, *inter alia*, changes

39 It appears that having studied and analyzed thousands of letters sent to the TV Channel II after the A. M. Kashpirovsky sessions, we managed to get to know changes in health awareness at the beginning of transformation processes, to describe mechanisms of changes in attitudes to health and illness which appeared in Polish social reality, to get to know the motivations of the sick and the healthy, who realized their health needs partly without contact with medical doctors and medicine. In this sense this material can be counted as sociological because, as F. Znaniecki observed, the object of study of the discipline is a social group (although here without physical contact) strongly identifying with the person- an important point of reference (in this case with the charismatic healer) (Znaniecki 1988: 204-205 et seq.)

in consciousness brought about by the popularity of postmodernist ideology appealing not only to the cult of health and the human body (corporality) but also to focusing on one's own emotions and psychic states (Kubiak 1998, 14: 40-53; and 2005: 42-54).[40] The idea preferred by healers is equilibrium, which should be between the somatic, psychological and social spheres determining an individual's health. Equilibrium is needed to avoid dangers of illness, build up wellness reserves and enhance life quality. Proponents of non-medical healthcare (who call themselves 'makers of alternative medicine', e.g. A. Stanway) urge people to learn pro-health skills, especially by self-treatment methods, through which self-recoveries can be achieved. Post-modern man is thus both the maker of his health and the cause of his illnesses. There is a similarity here to the health promotion ideology, hence its rules have been quickly learned by healers (Stanway 1982: 21-22). The concepts defined in college handbooks such as positive health, self-checking, self-care, and prohealth choice function in parallel although they are often interpreted selectively and tend to be distorted in many publications on healing (Słońska and Misiuna 1993). Terms borrowed from the field of sociology or psychology of health are used in the healers' subculture to make a theoretical framework from frequently chaotic and inconsistent arguments meant to create intellectual foundations for the alternative art of healing, 'sensory medicine', etc. There are suggestions that this global system of alternative medicine will radically change or eliminate orthodox (scientistic-empirical) medicine from the market, since it is expensive, ineffective and inhuman (Stanway 1982: 36-42).

The cultural phenomenon accompanying post-modernity and referring to the non-conventional approach to the sphere of health and illness is the New Age philosophy. We will omit a general sociological description of the phenomenon, which can be treated both as an ideology and as a type of dynamic social movement. The New Age's 'new thinking' also contributes to views on health, illness and the human body. According to this philosophy, the etiology of most diseases is caused by the capitalist economy's devastation of nature, which disturbs ecological equilibrium, thereby giving rise to social diseases. The cult of economic growth is a real health-threatening factor at the social and individual level. Capi-

40 Present-day studies on cultural changes in Poland from the perspective of Poles' everyday lives show the significance of health issues, which are the main elements of ordinary people's interest. Analysis of letters sent to the "Poradnik Domowy" monthly (2002) by S. Siekierski shows a growing sense of importance of health and of prevention and self-treatment. Siekierski points out the growing criticism of medicine by female authors of the letters; on the other hand, under the influence of the media, women readers of the magazine increasingly believe in 'non-convnetional medicine starting with honey and chamomile to all kinds of wonder-working frauds' (Siekierski 2003).

talism is bad, *inter alia* in the sense that it disregards standards of life quality. That is why, as healers who invoke New Age values emphasize, we have to build not only alternative economics but also human-friendly alternative (natural, ecological) medicine (Gottschalk-Olsen 1990: 3 et seq.).

The interest in seeking a general theory of treatment that would take cultural elements into account and explain the phenomenon of effects obtained by non-conventional therapists is also seen in American cultural and medical anthropologies. In the encyclopedia on alternative medicine by K. Gottschalk-Olsen (1990: 3-8.) there are six fundamental questions which, the author believes, help in the general discussion on the essence of healing: whether a therapy is safe, whether it is theoretically reliable, whether it is comparatively inexpensive, whether it is effective, whether it has been practiced for at least five years, and whether there is no other therapy that would meet these criteria (Ibid). In K. Gottschalk-Olsen's approach the main argument for choosing 'other medicine' is that it is safer and less expensive than conventional therapies.

Another example of the search for the theoretical framework of the problems in question is the chapter *Toward a General Theory of Healing* in the book by the American anthropologist G. W. Meek *Healers and the Healing Process* (Meek 1979: 193-200). Its author believes that he was able to create a theoretical construction that explains paranormal healings (Ibid: 153; Stanway 1982: 21 et seq.). The foundations of this conception are the views of Bohm and Watson concerning Puharich's 'ethereal theory' and relating to the new 'mass theory'. Meek distinguishes eight areas crucial to the creation of the theory of paranormal healing. These are:

1. The conception of self-treatment mechanisms.
2. Theory of intercellular communication
3. Theories of mechanisms of cell atrophy and formation.
4. The role of water (fluids) in human physiology and its susceptibility to therapeutic radiation
5. The molecular conception of the human body.
6. Theories of body-mind relations
7. The brain as the programmer of psychosomatic processes.
8. The role of magnetic fields in the electrodynamic theory of life.

G. W. Meek argued that his research model could be the basis for explaining *inter alia* the phenomenon of healing with faith. The presented conceptions are not the only ones that function in medical anthropology. For example, Morrey Last treats 'paramedicine' as an integral part of the overall system of healthcare. Last discusses three basic models of relations between CAM and academic medicine: tolerant, integrative and exclusive. The closest to Polish solutions seems the exclusive model (France, Belgium), in which medicine as a system is controlled by the State and 'paramedical' practices are illegal. The American model is a hybrid one because legal provisions defining the possibilities of non-physicians offering services are partly regulated at the state level (licenses) and partly by the federal authorities and agencies. American cultural anthropology and medical anthropology also describe healers' therapeutic practices from the perspective of the intensifying civilizational transformations (globalization) and the revision of such concepts as tradition by applying them to 'other medicine' (Goldstein 2000: 292-294, 383-385 et seq.).

The ideologist of alternative medicine - Gothschalk-Olsen writes that we must create a system of holistic healthcare based on safe non-operative and non-pharmaceutical methods (Ibid:5 et seq.). In this type of medicine the patient should be treated as the subject; s/he should also be active and independent, expecting not only 'the removal of illness in the biological sense' but also the achievement of 'the subjective state of health (wellness, wellbeing) etc. P. Macura emphasizes that anthroposophy, holistic medicine, non-conventional medicine, traditional medicine and shamanism should bring about the transition of individuals and then societies to **the higher level of consciousness** [*my emphasis* W. P.] (Ibid; 11). A similar way of reasoning can be observed in other alternative medicine theories, which emphasize the values of spirituality in the broad sense, and the need to build a new type of global (cosmic) self-awareness in patients. The path to understanding this ideology is 'mystical illumination' and unification with one's own self (Ibid: 11). A significant role in the 'New World Medicine' (as in the Polish traditional folk medical system) will be played by women, whose spirituality, sensitivity, ease of reacting and 'understanding with their heart' makes them especially desirable healers. The connection of this healing ideology with its theoretical background i.e. ecologism seems to be noticeable here. M. Ferguson, a Californian Age of the Aquarius ideologist, maintains that the criteria determining whether a person is part of the 'new consciousness' include an element currently present in the non-medical healing systems, utilization of biofeedback, which permits one to control and use the unity of one's body and mind, assess the state of one's mind (life actualization and regeneration), study susceptibility to hypnosis and self-hypnosis, and participate in social movements (self-help) that form the new consciousness, etc. (Ferguson 1993: 21). Ferguson believes that present-day post-modern man also has to be able to use Hatha Yoga, Reichian therapy, the Alexander Technique and other alternative medicine techniques. Curing ourselves and then and then the people around us, our friends and acquaintances, should be the beginning of healing the whole of society. She asks, 'if the mind can heal and transform, why can't minds join to heal and transform society?' (Ibid: 29). Ferguson's views have consequences for studies conducted within the sociology of non-medical healthcare (Libiszowska-Żółtkowska 1998: 39-51). Discussions in social sciences on diverse consequences of post-modernity, ongoing since the end of the 1980s and beginning of the 1990s, also concern medical sociology, which is clearly transforming into the sociology of health, within which studies are conducted on building foundations for 'the sociology of non-medical healthcare'.

Within the sociology of healthy man, and not without some influence of supporters of alternative medicine, the concepts of health and illness were also redefined. As in modern healing, health extended its scope, and was treated *inter alia* as a way of achieving a better life, the key to its new quality, the path to fully understanding oneself, the means leading to new consciousness, etc. The concept of illness was also broadened with new interpretations emphasizing its subjective character (subjective state of illness) and specific etiology placing emphasis on the pathogenic role of technochemical medicine, one's incompetent, pathogenic lifestyle or lack of acceptance of positive thinking. Healers stress that the foregoing factors may disturb the energy flow, impede its free circulation, cause disorders in the organism's self-regulation and, as a result, cause pathological changes (Nettleton1996: 209 et seq.). The discovery of 'vitalism', 'sociopsychosomatic equilibrium', 'the ability to clean the organism of 'bad energy' and to accumulate 'good energy', acceptance of nature and the natural, the turn towards new (alternative) mental and religious experiences, learning to think positively, and gaining 'positive health' are some of the values built by healers around the healthcare that is in opposition to 'capitalist, toxic, profit-seeking, reductionist medicine which reifies the patient and treats health and illness as one dimension (Piątkowski 1995; 2005; Pilkiewicz 1994: 395-413).

The classic sociology of health, illness and medicine perceives the role of cultural factors as fundamental elements determining behaviors in illness and answering the question why people living in different cultures use different strategies of coping with the same illnesses (e.g. within self-treatment). The cultural determinants of what is 'good' or 'bad' for our health, Hessler and Twaddle write, define the framework of our activities in this area. The world of social values - norms, behavioral patterns, hierarchies, and adopted values - are the context of specific behaviors related to health and illness. Nettleton in turn emphasizes the role of culture as a factor determining lifestyles and the mechanism of taking or not taking care of one's health or the health of family and friends. Culture determines the indicators and scope of one's own responsibility and initiative in this field, or whether one has a passive attitude, counting on luck, Divine providence, or hoping that a disease will pass of itself without anyone's intervention. (The role of factors impacting health and illness has been dealt with at length by Hessler and Twaddle 1997: 41-42; and Nettleton 1996: 186-189). Can this system of values underlying 'miracle medicine' really produce a genuine (including cultural) alternative to academic medicine? Can the norms, preferences and ways of thinking of 'other medicine' create elements of a stable and universal 'alternative culture'? Much depends on the medical system, especially on its ability to adapt and on the depth of reactions to changes. There is no doubt that medicine, also influenced by the presence of healers' counterculture, is changing to some extent, accepting for example holism to a greater degree, appreciating the importance of sociopsychological elements, and becoming more anthropocentric. At the same time non-medical healing systems may also evolve, ad healers should look at their achievements with self-criticism, eliminating chaos, pseudovalues and dishonesty toward patients, because this is the area where fraud and deception may easily have tragic results. Apparently, the future strategy for restoring health will have to combine the competence of modern clinical medicine with the competence of behavioral sciences (sociology and psychology of health and illness). Only this offer is honest and reliable to the patients. Some conceptions of non-medical healthcare will probably be absorbed by modern socio- and psychotherapy (variants of use of the placebo effect), which will make them more legitimate. Some others (osteopathy, chiropractic, acupuncture) will be used selectively by physicians; the remainder, when they prove ineffective and fraudulent, will be forgotten (Piątkowski 2000: 62).

2. Lay Healing Practices – A Theoretical Approach. Symbolic Interactionism, Phenomenology and Ethnomethodology as the Sources of Research Conceptions Used in the Sociology of Non-Medical Healing Systems

The author's goal is to draw attention to the fact that areas of daily life, *inter alia* everyday ideas of health and illness, value hierarchies, patterns of health behaviors, and health awareness have a stronger effect on mortality and incidence rates of most diseases than the influence of institutional medicine (Piątkowski et al. 1998: 24; Nettleton 1996: 38-39; Puchalski and Korzeniowska 2004: 116-125; see also Fox 1989: 23-24). Paradoxically, this domain comprising social attitudes and behaviors has not been systematically studied to date in Poland by significant representatives of medical sociology. It is therefore necessary to attempt to describe and interpret facts, phenomena and processes that constitute this special 'non-presented world' (I inspired one such effort – Kaliszuk 1999, 17: 109 et seq.). Inquiries into the daily lives of ordinary people are of paramount importance for studies on non-medical healthcare since it is common knowledge that most behaviors in illness in Poland have the form of self-treatment, a considerable portion of such needs being realized outside of medical institutions in contact with diverse healers. As has been said earlier, this theme has both theoretical and methodological aspect. Subjective human needs, irrational attitudes, prejudices and superstitions are not easy to investigate by means of standard quantitative methods. What is needed here is an analysis using more subtle instruments of humanistic sociology and qualitative techniques of data accumulation (free interview, participant observation, analysis of personal documents etc.) (Csorba 1993; Silverman 2008: 27-39). In studies of this kind the role of the human factor or humanistic coefficient are taken into account, which permits us to look, without the empirical scholar's paternalistic superiority, at the world of emotions, views and beliefs, which until recently used to be regarded as banal, unimportant and unworthy of scientific cognition (Kaliszuk 1999).

The so-called ordinary man's views about etiology, diagnostics, prevention and therapy, and about criteria for health restoration and deterioration of health were usually ignored or even discredited by medical experts defending their professional competence, prestige and exclusiveness (Nettleton 1996: 38). Disregard for this sphere of consciousness and everyday behaviors was puzzling, the more so that in Poland (in the West from the late 1960s) emphasis was placed on the fundamental importance of self-treatment as elementary behavior, commonly used in illness. We should remember that when they feel ill, 59% of the Poles surveyed use their own tried and tested **home methods of treatment** [*my emphasis*, W. P.]. At the same time, when their health is threatened, only 31% (!) of respondents go to the doctor's at once (*Co robi... Raport z badań OBOP* 1996; cf. Thomas 2003: 26-27). Apart from self-treatment, the sphere of everyday commonsense views and actions concerning illness are practices of healers popular in Poland, whose services are utilized systematically or occasionally according to GUS by 4% of adults or over a million people (Statistical Yearbook 1997: 100). In the late 1970s and the early 1980s there was a steadily growing conviction that the previously unnoticed or ignored area of everyday knowledge on health and illness could no longer be disregarded in the conceptualization of scientific research.

In sociomedical analyses of everyday views, attitudes and behaviors around health and illness three theoretical conceptions appear to be especially useful: **symbolic interactionism, phenomenology and ethnomethodology** (Piątkowski 1998; Uramowska-Żyto 1992: 97 et seq.) We will start with some introductory remarks. For at least two decades in medical sociology the dominant functional approach to illness and being ill was that presented by T. Parsons in his books *The Social System* (1951) and *Social Structure and Personality* (Polish edition in 1969). We should remember that the author distinguished *inter alia* the feature of the social sick role i.e. the patient's role, emphasizing that s/he only has to yield to professional (medical) domination when s/he wants to recuperate. In Parsons's approach, illness was treated as a social deviation because it was associated with failure to utilize basic rights, responsibilities and duties, which prevented one's career and advancement, etc. In contrast, health was the only mode guaranteeing tan effective way of realizing the roles and tasks assigned to an individual by a community (Parsons 1969: 405; 1951). Parsons's classic functional-structural conception is, however, complemented more and more often with the study of commonsense knowledge about health and illness and about non-professional ways of help in illness that constitute the three forms of non-medical healthcare. From this standpoint we find two theoretical orientations to be the closest: phenomenology and symbolic interactionism (Uramowska-Żyto 1992; 9, 97-122, 131-149; Cockerham and Scambler 2010: 7-9). In these conceptions special importance is attached to investigating the subjective social reality specific to a particular patient and defined by the concepts of health and illness, and commonsense knowledge different from and even contradictory to the fundamentals of the medical paradigm is analyzed. An incentive to study non-professional forms of treatment is the gradual evolution of sociology in medicine (in R. Straus's terminology) towards medicine in sociology and sociology of health. The last perspective enables the sociologist to freely investigate both the professional and non-professional areas surrounding health and illness. Obviously, as has been said before, no less important factor accelerating inquiries into non-professional ways of help in illness (health) was the criticism of T. Parsons's classic theory, which excluded from the domain of the subdiscipline such crucial research fields as non-professionals' healing activities and the subjective (everyday) meaning attributed to health and illness. It is only the construction of the foundations of 'theoretical alternative' that has made it possible to conduct analyses concerned mainly with patients' specific experiences in contact with non-conventional therapists. In Poland this type of research enabled us *inter alia* to describe everyday interpretations of the Kashpirovsky phenomenon (characteristics of psychophysical sensations felt during teletherapy, presentation of one's own subjective interpretations of changes in health and illness, and of assumed cause-and-effect relations between the fact of occurrence of one's own illness and diverse etiological factors, etc.) (Piątkowski et al. 1993; Sokołowska 1969; Bejnarowicz Ibid: 251-268).

The views on health and illness formulated within the conception of symbolic interactionism open promising opportunities for conceptualization of sociological studies on non-medical healing systems. Symbolic interactionism may provide inspiration in investigating everyday attitudes and behaviors surrounding the concepts of health and illness. This trend emphasizes the importance of symbols in social life and describes the process of their subjective reception. The researcher is interested here in the art of interpreting symbols of collective life (Chicago School and Iowa School). It also stresses the ability to understand the daily, commonsense art of interpretation of events and behaviors. Symbolic interactionism fits in the sociological interpretive paradigm constructed in opposition to the classic normative one (e.g. T. Parsons's structural-functional theory). The basic applied analytical category is the term 'interactions', denoting social activity, in which individual persons interact with one another via mutual communication, modifying one another's social behaviors and actions. In this interpretation, communication is an exchange of meaningful symbols by verbal and non-verbal means (words, gestures, etc.). Participants in collective life alternate their roles as senders and receivers of social messages: as a result, the consensus of interaction is either maintained or breaks down (Blumer 1969; Hałas 1987; 1998, I: 353-357; 2000: 14).

Like phenomenology and ethnomethodolgy, symbolic interactionism is a research directive used in analyses in the sociology of health, illness and medicine. Classic studies of this kind conducted in the early 1960 were concerned *inter alia* with the doctor-patient interaction (J. Emerson 1970), the social context of establishing medical diagnosis (T. Scheff 1968), and sociothanatology

(B. Glaser and A. Strauss 1965). From this perspective we can distinguish two vital research directives in sociomedical projects:

- the need to take into account the viewpoints of subjects/actors of collective life (the acting person and his/her system of commonsense knowledge);
- the necessity of utilizing, among the research techniques applied, the analysis of personal documents permitting us to discover the subjective world of sensations, experiences and actions of ordinary people. At the same time, according to symbolic interactionists, a desirable source of information can be participant observation (e.g. covert)

The analysis of the process of communication between the subjects of a social relationship (e.g. patient-healer) accurately shows benefits from symbolic interactionism. Both sides interact with each other and modify mutual actions, giving each other advice and instructions. This serves to maintain order and harmony in the relationship, the point of view of the relationship's participants being important. In our study of non-medical healing systems we seek to understand the patients' motives for choosing 'other medicine', which is why we apply the analysis of personal documents as a source of data and attempt to interpret them from the standpoint of lay people (Scambler 2000: 16-19).

Symbols and their attributed meanings, and ways of their interpretation play a special role in the field defined by the concepts of health-illness-medicine (or non-medical healthcare). Symbolic elements are also observable in modern-day patterns of doctor-patient relationship, in patient-healer (especially spiritual healer) interaction or patient-folk doctor/therapist (Penkala-Gawęcka 19991, 74: 43-54). A singular role is played here by the ability to 'read symbols', for example by the patient in his/her contact with the healer (folk therapist), and the ability to invest them with a meaning appropriate to a situation. Symbols and the meanings ascribed to them, and the ability to use and read them correctly are the elements that strengthen the social bond during the healing process; they reinforce faith, hope and the client's trust in the healer, which is often a necessary condition for regaining health both in its objective and subjective dimensions. This specific intersubjective communication is the result of consent to communicate at the same emotional level; it also facilitates adopting the patterns of social roles (expected by the partner), thus enabling close cooperation in achieving objectives (strengthening, regaining or maintaining health) and quick adaptation and adjustment of own behaviors towards behaviors of other persons, for example the healer or folk doctor, etc. (Uramowska-Żyto 1992; Twaddle and Hessler 1977; Cockerham 2004; 15-17). We should observe that just as symbolic interactionists point out that in the doctor-patient relationship it is most often the expert (doctor) who defines the mutual situation and imposes the role, the samething also happens in the contact with the healer (folk therapist), when the process of 'ascribing meanings' almost always depends on the healer (Uramowska-Żyto 1992).

The theory of symbolic interactionism seems to be useful in one more way. It is espoused by the founders of humanistic sociology as it prefers the standpoint of the actor (subject) and demands that his everyday (commonsense) knowledge be taken into consideration .E. Hałas in his monograph on symbolic interactionism stresses the connection of this conception with the analysis of people's everyday experience of meanings. These elements are concurrent with the views of health sociologists, who try to create the model of this discipline to be consistent with the patient and his/her needs and expectations as the central point of reference. It is this purpose that the general evolution of our subdiscipline serves (from medical sociology to sociology of health) (Piątkowski and Titkow 2002). The adoption of the theory of symbolic interactionism as the theoretical point of reference should also encourage use of qualitative methods as equivalent to quantitative methods in investigating the field of health and illness as seen from the patient's perspective. That is why it is legitimate to develop this type of approach in new research projects and their conceptualizations. For several years the Polish sociology of health and illness has tried to apply, *inter alia*, new methods of analysis of personal documents (patients' letters to healers, diaries of the disabled, utterances of AIDS/HIV patients, etc.) (Libiszowska-Żółtkowska et al. 1998). Preference for the humanistic orientation in the sociology of health and medicine makes it possible, as a result, to describe the subjective, often undisclosed world of the patient's experiences in broader terms. It also permits students of the problem to gradually change the stereotyped scenario of the doctor-patient relationship, which continues to be marked by the dominance of the 'professional' viewpoint and often prevents receivers of these services from articulating their own, independent, autonomous standpoints resulting from their everyday ideas of health, illness and being ill.

Like symbolic interactionism, another theoretical orientation also appears inspiring in studying the issues of non-medical healthcare: phenomenology. We should begin with some introductory remarks. **Phenomenological theory** in its elements relating to health and illness focuses on describing and interpreting subjective human knowledge, and personal experiences of an individual who, for example, destroys his/her health or chooses a pro-health lifestyle, or experiences his/her pain, fear or hopes associated with the character of his/her disease, its course and prognosis (Zborowski 1952, 8; Mucha 2002, 4: 253; Tobiasz-Adamczyk 1999, 2: 308). This system of highly internalized feelings, experiences and behavioral patterns allows one to ascribe a subjective sense to the concepts of pain, illness, health, recovery, wellbeing, deterioration of health, etc. (Schuetz 1962 and 1964). The adoption of this perspective and its application to the Polish realities may bring us closer to answering a number of questions of a highly heuristic value and great practical importance, for example:

1. Why do the Poles, while rating health as highly important, neglect it in everyday life?
2. Why do most people appreciate the value of health only after they have lost it?
3. Why does the ordinary Polish citizen consult a doctor only when he is feeling acute, long-lasting and nagging pain?
4. Why do the Poles use medicines on their own, dosing them at their own discretion, and using for example antibiotics past the expiration date to treat diseases with a viral etiology?
5. Why do patients stop treatment at the first symptoms of improvement?
6. Finally, why have many of Poland's poorest citizens, most frequently workers and farmers, for whom it should be important to maintain a fit condition and vitality necessary for doing physical work, consistently ruined their lives (with stimulants, irregular lifestyle, bad diet, absence of preventive behaviors, etc) for many years (Ostrowska 1999: 29; *Nasze zdrowie... komunikat z badań CBOS* 1993; *Leczenie się... Komunikat z badań CBOS* 1998: 1 et seq.)

Phenomenology, based on E. Husserl's philosophy, places emphasis on 'the analysis of cognitive processes' and makes 'intentionality' an important feature of human consciousness. A. Schütz asked himself a fundamental question: how do individuals 'understand their activities' in everyday life, referring *inter alia* to the interpretation of the sign system and, more broadly, to understanding other people's behaviors? Schütz's 'subjective, individualist' approach seems especially useful in getting to know the world of experiences caused by illness and it explains the personal decisions (motives) of patients going to see healers. In the same sense, this orientation enables the reconstruction of the 'world experienced' by the individual, e.g. in the context with the healer, which is frequently a reconstruction of the 'world of chronically ill people' and of subjective, personal motives for undergoing treatment outside of medical institutions (Mandes 2002: 61-65; Brener 1995). An interesting application of phenomenology to modern-day studies on health and illness was attempted by Graham Scambler (2002: 19-22) showing the vitality of this orientation, especially in research into 'the sociology of illness'.

It should stressed that phenomenology emphasizes an especially interesting area in the sociology of non-medical healthcare: the patient's (or healthy person's) everyday knowledge about the states of health and illness (Piątkowski and Titkow 2002: 17, 25). By adopting phenomenological assumptions, we can explore the area of commonsense knowledge about health, particularly views on the etiology of illnesses, diagnosis, prevention and therapeutic measures, and analyze the supposed causal relations between life events and illness (health), and the importance of thaumaturgic and religious elements that supposedly determine the spheres of health and illness; we can also examine mechanisms of taking decisions about commencement ort termination of treatment, and of regarding a particular state as health or not. Finally, we can investigate subjective criteria permitting us to recognize some symptoms as illness and determine its type (life threatening or not, advanced or not, infectious or not). All these devices aim at gathering, describing and interpreting the subjective, poorly-known world of experiences concentrated around the terms health, illness, being cured, being ill, treatment or dying. We should observe that the choice of phenomenological orientation as a research directive 'condemns' us, even more than in the case of symbolic interactionism, to choose the anthropocentric version of medical sociology as the main point of reference. The perspective of humanistic sociology provides an opportunity to present the subjective reality surrounding health and illness (Zborowski 1952, 8; and Kubiak 1998, 14). Adopting the phenomenological perspective we also fully realize how deep (and sometimes insurmountable) are the differences between the healer's or folk practitioner's and their patient's everyday knowledge and the scientistic reductionist attitude of a clinician. Illness, being ill, dying, and getting better create a characteristic, integral and important area of reality, thereby making up the world of daily life of ordinary people. Students of the traditional folk medical system realize that the intersubjective world of meanings and symbols has existed for ages, that it was cognized and defined by earlier generations; and that the key to this interpretation is given us by the process owing to socialization which we experience in our own social group (e.g. family). All this provides, among other things, a useful knowledge of how to behave in the circumstance of illnesses that we know; this is what is called health knowledge at hand (Uramowska-Żyto 1992: 133). The individual usually regards it as important because the healthy person in the modern-day world is able to achieve the most important social goals and tasks (financial success, family success, a successful sex life, attainment of high professional status, etc.). At the same time the world of everyday ideas of health and illness may prompt the individual to consider that a better way to achieve health is to use non-medical healthcare methods instead of or parallel with the ways recommended by professional medicine. We can see clearly that the character, scope and quality of 'everyday medical knowledge' impact the ways of utilization (or non-utilization) of medical institutions, and the attitude towards medical professions and non-professional therapists. The lay person (whether healthy or ill) spontaneously invests subjective meanings in everyday experiences: this is, it seems, the key to understanding specific ('strange', 'irrational', 'superstitious') attitudes towards illness. We owe the discovery of this 'non-presented world', ignored and omitted by professional doctors, to A. Schütz. That world is not only the area of human thinking and action but also the area of the human body. S. Nettleton writes in the chapter *The Sociology of the Body* (1996: 103-117) that this current, present only recently in the studies by 'phenomenologically oriented' sociologists of health and illness, is gaining in importance because of the growing health culture, the spread of popular psychotherapeutic knowledge, consumer education etc. An approach to the human body close to the phenomenological orientation is also developed by Ch. Shilling in his book *The Body and Social Theory* (Shilling 1993; recent results of studies are presented in Piątkowski and Brodniak 2005: 323-346). In light of the earlier discussion we can say that phenomenological conceptions applied to the study of non-medical healthcare make it possible to understand the areas of the subjective world produced by the fact of illness and permit us to see health and illness in their own, individual, unique, subjective context.

Another theoretical conception, which can be successfully applied both in the field of health and illness sociology and particularly in the sociology of non-medical healthcare, is **ethnomethodology**. Like phenomenology it can be successfully used to explore the area of everyday knowledge and practical measures surrounding health and illness. This approach is both a characteristic theoretical conception and a directive for practical action (Uramowska-Żyto 1992: 131-161; Garfinkel 1967; Czyżewski 1984, 8). The prefix ethno- in the name of a research trend suggests orientation towards that which is daily, general, and most frequent in social life. This research current arose in opposition to the positivist and scientistic orientation of many sociologists (especially methodologists). Harold Garfinkel, the founder of ethnomethodoly, emphasized that social life is built by people giving it their own specific, autonomous meanings. Interpretation of this world can be chaotic, changeable and inconsistent; nevertheless, those who profess the same way of thinking and acting understand one another well and cooperate (Garfinkel 2007; Olechnicki and Załęcki 1997: 59, 62, 209; Czyżewski 1998, I: 198-201). Ethnomethodologicals view stressed the active involvement of social life participants in relationships with the social world. This approach prefers interpretations not so much by expert scholars but by participants in these events. The ethnomethodologist regards the subject of action/the interaction partner as a 'practical sociologist'. This kind of perspective makes it possible to discover imperceptible mechanisms that mould everyday knowledge by means of specific interpretive procedures. Especially interesting are accounts by participants in social life. This rule shows *inter alia* the practicism of daily life and the subjectivity of its participants as well as the relativity of social concepts and norms, for example the term 'rationality'. Ethnomethodology also attaches great importance to the analysis of the contents of colloquial speech as a research method enabling reconstruction of daily knowledge about health and illness and action patterns of ordinary people. It is this inspiration that was an important methodological motive for conducting my own research, the results of which will be presented further on in the text.

The prefix ethno- symbolizes the study of 'own' 'popular' 'commonly used' meanings that ordinary people give to their social activities. Participants in the events (e.g. authors of letters to Kashpirovsky) explain the sense and motives of their social action. As in phenomenology, 'everyday knowledge and everyday experience' are categories of scientific analysis. The ethnomethodological approach, Czyżewski observes, is highly suitable for sociological investigations, for example analysis of the doctor-patient (or patient-healer) interaction. Participants the latter interaction use everyday knowledge because both are lay persons ('the healer 'acts' the role of an 'alternative doctor') (Czyżewski 1998, I: 200-201; Scambler 2002: 19-20). It is not without reason that ethnomethodological conceptions are discussed together with phenomenology and symbolic interactionism: the main reason is their interaction. The term itself, used by H. Garfinkel, directs us, as in the previous conceptions, towards the experience of daily life. Why is the ethnomethodological interest in lay people's knowledge so necessary in studies conducted as part of the sociology of non-medical healthcare? Sociologists studying for example the Polish folk medical system know very well the importance of the ethnomethodologists' postulate that knowledge about health and illness be analyzed in conformity with the rules of interpretation of the social environment by its members (participants in it). We are not able to adequately describe at least the significance of thaumaturgy in folk medical systems, or speak of 'rationality' or 'irrationality' without taking into account the character of peasant culture, the magic of place and time, the significance of religious symbols, and peasant fatalism and passivity in responding to illness situations.[41] In studying the Polish folk medical system we also adopt the ethnomethodological directive that understanding of life is shaped by the subjectivity of participants in it (Uramowska-Żyto 1992: 151). At the same time ethnomethodologists emphasize the relativity of 'rationality' and 'irrationality' norms in communities (Garfinkel 2007). Another important matter that can be used in investigations of non-medical healing systems is the conviction that social milieus assign different meanings to the same terms such as death, illness, health, disability, getting better, being ill, etc. These meanings (as is the

41 Non-material elements in modern-day folk medical systems in the US are discussed by Cockerham (2004: 175-179); for irrationalism in alternative medicine see also M. S. Goldstein, who argues that the choice of these methods in modern societies is the result of conscious decisions rather than lack of possibilities of using real medicine (2000: 295).

case with the peasant folk medical system) overlap, intermingle and function in parallel ways (Jeszke 1996: 83). Studies in modern ethnology, concerned with folk medical systems, also discover a great wealth of verbal communication associated for example with illness and being ill. Ethnomethodology with its micro-sociological attitude and emphasis on interaction sociology is, we might believe, especially attractive in exploring for example the peasant way of 'experiencing' illness (Wieruszewska 1995, 78: 104).

We can therefore say that the growing (though not sufficient) number of sociological studies on non-biomedical healthcare, being *inter alia* the result of medical sociology's evolutionary transformation into the sociology of health and medicine, reveal, among other things, everyday, 'irrational', 'illogical' knowledge about the above topics. This knowledge is in no way less important than official, (until recently) dominant well-known interpretations adopted in academic medicine. These two - professional and non-professional - systems of thinking, action, description and 'expression' of health and illness more and more often operate side by side, overlap and sometimes complement each other. The selected elements of the **conceptions of symbolic interactionism, phenomenology and ethnomethodology**, discussed in this book, can be successfully used in studies on health sociology but they also seem particularly useful if, when investigating non-medical healing systems, we choose the perspective of humanistic sociology and apply qualitative methods of description of social reality.

2.1. The Analysis of Everyday Knowledge about Health and Illness – Eliot Freidson's Approach

Eliot Freidson is one the most often quoted authors in classic medical sociology; it was he who pointed out that lay people mostly consult not with doctors about their illness but with other lay people around them or with 'paramedical' therapists. It is in this sense that Freidson created the foundations of modern-day 'sociology of illness.' Like H. Waitzkin, he also advocated a critical examination at the world of institutional systems of modern-day medicine and openly criticized many formalized structures of the medical industry. In his two studies of the early 1970s he described how 'commercial medicine' strove to secure its dominance, control and power. Freidson identified sociological mechanisms which in fact restrict the patient's free choice, as medicine uses a special mechanism of defining illness, using terms like scientific, rational, modern, which pressurizes the majority of conformist patients, 'pushing' them towards the formalized, institutionalized system of medical service (Bosk. 2000: 403-404; and Freidson 2009: 177-189).

It is Eliot Freidson's conception that changed the perspective on the reality surrounding health and illness. These views emerged in the early 1960s but the concept of lay referral system, which we will discuss here, began to function as a consistent scientific system in behavioral sciences in the early 1970s (Twaddle and Hessler 1977). Freidson's approach largely arose in opposition to Parsons' structural-functional interpretation; however, while Parsons, in accordance with the logic of functional-structural theory, considered the dominant characteristic concepts to be the notions such as 'social order', 'social harmony', 'system', 'consensus' and 'equilibrium', Freidson placed emphasis on the doctor-patient conflict, conflict of interests, difference, and clashing perspectives – lay and professional - of seeing health and illness. The founder of the conception of the lay referral system sought, for example, universal mechanisms of interpreting disease symptoms by ordinary people and attempted to describe the mechanism of exchange of information on the subject (Uramowska Żyto 1992; 95-96; Tobiasz-Adamczyk 1999: 51-59; 2005: 36; 20002; 19-130). This point of view also enabled description and comprehension of mechanisms of seeking help in illness, when an individual wishes to obtain advice and instruction from the closest circle of people around her; family and friends or colleagues, etc. By analyzing detailed behavioral patterns associated with health and illness, E. Freidson found that the more the professional (medical) and lay (commonsense) perspectives converged, the more frequently people tended to realize their health needs within academic medicine. In this approach, the lay referral system could apply both to the patient and his/her family trying to agree on the supposed diagnosis, and to the seeking of therapeutic and preventive ways as well as to specific beliefs and views on illness etiology. Freidson, as Nettleton observes, emphasized the fact of interpenetration and overlapping of lay and professional networks of help in illness, calling one the lay referral network and the other the professional referral network (Nettleton 1996).

2.1.1. Characteristics of the Lay Referral System

In his book *The Sociology of Health and Healing* M. Stacey stresses that most lay people use the informal healthcare and in this sense, due to widespread and popular self-treatment, we are all health workers. Ordinary people themselves define health/illness, determine the value of being healthy, have individual ideas on the subject and practice their own methods of prevention and therapy (Stacey 1988; Kelly and Field 2009: 261).

Sociologists seeking theoretical inspirations in studies on non-biomedical healing systems undoubtedly need to turn again to Eliot Freidson's foregoing conceptions. Two books by this author are especially relevant to our discussion: *Patients' Views of Medical Practice* (1961) and *Profession of Medicine (1*970). In the former Freidson predicts, in a sense, the expansion of non-medical healing systems; the forecast is the more accurate for being formulated in the era of triumphs of professionalization, institutionalization and formalization of healthcare systems. In the book about patients' views on the doctor's social role (1961) the author surveyed the opinions of ordinary people - workers from New York's Bronx – concerning health, illness, the process of recuperation and being ill. Freidson emphasized the importance of everyday knowledge about health and the process of patient self-identification at particular stages of being ill. It was then that the first version of the concept of lay referral system appeared, which described *inter alia* how lay people, entering in contact with other people (the healthy and the sick) sought interpretation in order to understand the essence of an illness, its symptoms, character, and prognosis. Freidson's conception explains *inter alia* the mechanism of taking a decision about who should be entrusted with healthcare in the case of one's own illness: oneself (self-treatment) or a professional. The interpretation of this range of behaviors is particularly important as most 'scenarios of behavior in illness' begin with self-treatment. It is only after these spontaneously practiced methods fail that the tendency to seek professional medical help grows. According to Freidson the crucial mechanism is that of taking health decisions, when, apart from his/her own experience, the patient refers to the knowledge of his/her family, friends, neighbors and colleagues, discussing his/her plans with them. The inclination to cooperate (work together) with a doctor may depend *inter alia* on the extent to which lay opinions concur with the doctors' opinions. Greater willingness to cooperate with professionals is determined, Freidson maintains, by 'the patient's greater cultural identification' with the views of academic medicine (Twaddle and Hessler 1977; 137-159; Cockerham 2004: 121-122; Freidson 1961; 1970).

Freidson's conceptions concerning treatment by non-professionals deserve interest not only because of their pioneering character but also because they drew attention for the first time to 'common, ordinary' knowledge about health, illness and medicine during the total domination of the system of institutionalized medicine. Freidson documented empirically in his survey of blue-collar workers that, in their health decisions, people are guided by different motives at the same time: they are guided first of all first of all by their intuition and their health culture (myths, stereotypes, actual knowledge about health and illness); only after these initial considerations, and not necessarily always, do they seek the professional physician's help. Freidson's conceptions undoubtedly enhance the status of sociological studies of non-medical healing systems and constitute their important point of reference.

To sum up, we can say that E. Freidson was the first to undermine biomedicine's omnipotence, creating the social construction of the concepts 'health and illness'. By emphasizing the asymmetrical relationship between the doctor and patient he seemed to show sick persons a way to strengthening their position and thereby the prospects for their emancipation, partial independence and autonomy. He was also the first to contrast 'formal medical knowledge' with 'daily healing experience of ordinary people'. These abilities, skills and competence had previously been omitted, belittled and marginalized (Scambler 2002: 126-127); Freidson 1975).

2.2 Everyday Knowledge about Health and Illness in Light of Results of Own Research

Everyday knowledge about health and illness is regarded by Western medical sociologists (Bird, Conrad, Fremont) as an important determinant of health consciousness, needs, attitudes and behaviors associated with decisions about commencing (or not commencing) treatment and utilization (non-utilization) of services offered by professional medicine. Popular, local medical knowledge i.e. lay views of illness tend to be contrasted with expert biomedical knowledge represented by physicians guided by evidence based medicine. The key role of lay views on health and illness is pointed out by W. C. Cockerham in his assessment of Edward A. Suchman's pioneering study of popular medical views professed by several ethnic groups in New York, surveyed by that author (1965). Heterogenic and sometimes inconsistent knowledge on this subject arises partly in conscious opposition to medicine in contacts with members of close family members, friends, neighbors, colleagues, etc. The studies and surveys conducted in New York concerned Eliot Freidson's conception (1960) in his *Client Control and Medical Practice* first published in the "American Journal of Sociology" (1960, 65) This specific system of mutual recommendations, advice and aid was especially popular in the USA among low class members having strong ethnic identification and poor education (Bird et al. 2000 145-146; Scambler 2002 115; Cockerham 2004: 121-122)

Inspired by the symbolic interactionism theory, phenomenology and ethnomethodolgy and referring to E. Freidson's already characteristic conception of the lay referral system, we carried out a qualitative pilot analysis of spontaneous utterances of 123 patients treated in 1999-2000 by selected general practitioners in healthcare centers in the Zamojski district (Lublin province). General practitioners cooperating with this author were asked to record on dictaphone or write down the most interesting excerpts from patients' utterances concerning illness etiology, symptom interpretation, assessment of diagnostic methods, preventive rules used, **home ways of treatment (self-treatment) practiced by lay people**, and assessment of the doctor-patient relationship.

2.3. Attempts to Create 'Theories of Treatment' by Non-Conventional Therapists

The earlier sections presented views on non-medical healthcare professed by representatives of natural, medical, and social sciences. We should remember, however, that non-conventional therapists can also be theorists of their own healing practices. This happens more and more often, which is why it seems justifiable to show this perspective on the basis of two selected cases: the non-conventional therapist A. M. Kashpirovsky and the bioenergy therapist S. Nardelli.

We need to stress the mass scale of the 'Kashpirovsky phenomenon', whose popularity lasted over two years (Kashpirovski's TV sessions were shown for that long). According to the OBOP figures of March 1990, 59% of adult Poles watched his programs (*Telewizyjne... Komunikat z badań OBOP* 1990). In January1991 during the conference in Kiev, at which I presented the results of my studies, A.M. Kashpirovsky, generalizing his 25 years of experience as a therapist and summing up his reflection on his treatment methods, formulated the basic principles of his own 'theory'. On the basis of his words and presented materials, we can rcduce them to the following principles:

- unquestionable dominance of practice over the elements that form the theory of treatment
- specialization in simultaneous influence on very large patient groups, directly or more often indirectly (via television)
- use of psychological measures not only for treating mental and nervous diseases but mainly somatic ones (including AIDS/HIV and cancers)
- assumption of the universal, beneficial effect of therapy on most diseases (I treat all [лечу всех])
- 'self-regulation' stimulated by a strong psychological stimulus seen as a factor able to produce positive somatic changes and improve wellbeing,
- striving for the ultimate goal: the organism will achieve the state of 'reflexive self-regulation'; stimulation of self-regulation will be effected via 'suggestion

to heal and cure' produced by psychological means; essential here are positive stimuli: the patient's faith in success increases chances of recovery,

- making no particular demands on patients apart from the duty to watch successive programs or take part in direct sessions,
- appearance of moral accents apart from health-oriented elements, reference to another person's positive features, calling for 'being good', 'doing no harm to others', etc., calling for the leading of a hygienic lifestyle. (Piątkowski et al. 1993: 7-28; Nikitin 1990: 9-33; Piątkowski 1995, 5-6: 131-133).

A.M. Kashpirovski claimed that his healing influence affects not only consciousness but also the subconscious and thereby the somatic: it is then that the organism 'restores its health matrix'. The healer maintained that each patient had 'power reserves' that should be identified, accumulated and used for healing purposes. He also asserted that his method was a kind of catalyst of biopsychic processes; he was convinced that his discovered technique of aid in illness was the world's first 'mass TV psychotherapy' (he claimed that after teletherapy sessions he received over a million letters in Russia and Ukraine alone). Kashpirovsky insisted that his original contribution to psychotherapy was to stimulate the body into spontaneous 'self-regulation of health' during which the organism is 'forced' to incite 'self-treatment' processes without the participation of doctors and medicines (Zinczenko et al., no.1, duplicated typescript). Kashpirovsky emphasized that the foundation of his 'philosophy of health' was a redefinition of the concept of illness and the use of television for simultaneous treatment of hundreds of thousands of viewers. The awareness of participating in a healing program is supposed to activate 'the biological system of self-regulating processes'; a person is able and fit when the 'self-regulation process works without reservations' The main therapeutic problem of the Kashpirovsky method is how to produce desirable reactions in people with whom there is no direct contact during a teletherapy session – the viewers have unique individual mental features, Kashpirovski's solution lies in the vagueness of his message, its very general terms; thus everyone can interpret the therapist's words in the way they consider the most suitable. A special role in this message is played by positive examples (complete recoveries from various diseases, often recognized as chronic). When self-defining his mission Kashpirovsky pointed out the importance of his own authority, prestige, competence and infallibility; he tried to be kind, warm, and compassionate. His session contained elements of overt and covert hypnosis based on the use of Erikson's technique (hypnotization by gently giving seemingly contradictory suggestions). Reconstructing his own philosophy of health Kashpirovsky stressed the importance of 'stimulating optimism', 'hope for being cured', and 'faith in the success of one's therapy': these elements were meant to be the beginning of 'healing self-regulation processes.' The healer believed that 'the human organism is susceptible to psychological control', and it should be only guided in the right direction, using appropriate stimuli: in this sense the best medicine for the sick person is another man. Kashpirovsky also contended that the evolution of his treatment method consisted in healing not only psychosomatic diseases but also endogenous conditions, previously considered incurable by academic medical therapies (Gapik 1990, 4: 12; Minakowski and Gawrońska 1992, 6: 4-5; Pisalnik 2007).

Stanisław Nardelli (1928-1985) was one of the best-known Polish bioenergy therapists. By his own accounts, he treated over two million people between 1980 and 1985. The healer emphasized that most of his patients were people whom academic medicine was unable to help (Nardelli 1986). Apart from the fact that Nardelli's popularity produced a number of mass-scale phenomena (organization of big meetings, attempts to set up institutions to investigate his phenomenon, waves of publications in the media), the reason why we are interested in the conceptions of this particular healer is that he tried to build a theory which would explain the results that he achieved. In his book *W kręgu biopola* [Within the Biofield] Nardelli repeatedly emphasizes the importance of gathering scientific documentation and developing verification methods, especially by medical doctors; finally, he often uses the term 'theory' when generalizing his achievements (Ibid: 7, 80). On the basis of the healer's many statements about his own bioenergy therapeutic properties, healing and diagnostic methods, ways of verification of the results obtained, and his models and patterns that are meant to explain 'the phenomenon of bioenergy therapeutic effect on the human organism', we can reconstruct the principal assumptions of 'clinical bioenergy therapy' and 'social bioenergy therapy' promoted by this therapist. Nardelli stresses the great importance of scientific ways of documenting and assessing the therapeutic results achieved. The crucial role will be played by the opinions of clinicians, oncologists, internists, neurologists, ophthalmologists, pediatricians, and rehabilitation specialists. Documentation of healing results should cover *inter alia* the recording of objective physiological parameters of the patient's organism during and after the procedure, and records of the subjective feelings (sensations) experienced by the sick person. Nardelli's method comprises diagnostic measures ('biodiagnosis') and treatment ('biotherapy'). According to the healer, the essence of his influence on the sick organism is the assumption that 'a person is a doctor for him/herself, therefore s/he can help him/herself by restoring the state of internal balance and homeostasis so needed by the organism' (Ibid: 62, 242-244). The organism has a definite bioenergy reserve, which it can manage; between the patient's and healer's organisms there is a specific feedback:

the weaker the healer is, the more strongly (!) he works on the patient's organism, achieving 'immediate' and 'surprising' effects (Ibid: 62). The organism's radiation can be visible as is the radiation of its 'individual organs' (65).'Improper radiation' is felt by the therapist and causes pain 'in his own organs equivalent to the patient's sore spots' (Ibid: 67). Bioenergy can be transmitted from a distance, for example via the phone and 'teleradiesthesia' (Ibid: 103). However, the principal therapeutic technique is 'bioenergy massage' (touching with fingertips or influencing with the healer's hand from a distance of 5-10 cm [2-4 inches]. Influencing with energy does not require the patient's conscious cooperation, which is why it is possible to heal unconscious persons; the essence of bioenergy transmission is feeding the patient's biofield and adjusting his/her 'energy system'.

Nardelli's theory of treatment was most influenced, as he himself said, by Rev. W. Sedlak's views presented in his work *Homo electronicus* ([Electronic Man] 1984) and in *Bioelektronika*([Bioelectronics] 1979), Father Cz. A. Klimuszko's theories of healing (*Moje widzenie świata* [My View of the World] 1978), and by L. E. Stefański's opinions. Furthermore, Nardelli referred to the views of Professors J. Aleksandrowicz and M. Sokołowska because he emphasized the need for research into non-conventional treatment methods (Ibid: 11, 202-203).

While investigating the methods of remote 'healthy flow of bioenergy' and concluding that it could be transmitted over a distance of 'thousands of miles', Nardelli developed 'models of clinical biotherapy' for over 300 illness cases and planned to compile a 'bioenergy therapeutic atlas' (Ibid: 103-105). An important element in Nardelli's theory is the conviction that bioenergy should be applied, if possible, under the supervision of and in cooperation with medical doctors in healthcare service centers; he also insisted that, among bioenergy therapists, there should be as many medical doctors as possible. Nadelli was also convinced that a great role in treatments practiced by non-physicians should be played by bioenergy therapists' ethics enabling them to help effectively and in the patient's interest, where 'the borders of medicine' end (Ibid 207: and Cockerham 2004; 171-175).

3. The Kashpirovsky Phenomenon in the Context of the Changing Society

The greater the distance between us and the commencement of studies on the 'Kashpirovsky phenomenon' (1990), the more we are confirmed in our conviction that the meteoric career of a Vinnitsa (Ukraine) psychiatrist could have happened only here and now – in the first years of the Polish systemic transformation. The figure of Kashpirovsky, a disciple of the infamous school of Soviet psychiatry, an atheist, knowing no languages, and reflecting the negative stereotype of *homo sovieticus* (the Soviet mindset), should have been in principle doomed to failure when confronted with Poles and their traditional Russophobia, fascination with the West, and their attempts to get over the period of 'compulsory Polish-Soviet friendship'. Nevertheless, it was this man who won over the hearts of millions of viewers in just a few weeks. His charismatic personality gained the high trust of a wide and diverse audience (mainly ordinary people, the then intellectual elites being critical of or indifferent to this phenomenon), his strong character won supporters among the media, and he became one of the well-known 'heroes of mass imagination', a one-man institution, who organized charity events, was awarded the Wiktor award for 'TV personality of the year" (1991), and was a private guest of the then President Lech Wałęsa of Poland, etc. This unprecedented personal (and financial) success in Poland was worth studying via sociological analyses of the case study type.[42]

A question may be asked: what elements associated with the systemic transformation then going in Poland could have had an unquestionable effect on the acceleration of the Kashpirovsky phenomenon? The crucial factor was the ability to use the uncensored commercial media. In the period 1989-1993 the Polish press from the "Polityka" weekly, "Gazeta Wyborca" daily and the "Warsaw Voice" to many women's magazines published about 220 articles, essays, interviews and analyses, whose central figure was Anatoly M. Kashpirovsky (one of the first serious texts being the essay by psychologist Professor L. Gapik- (1990, 4 (1708):12). Private profit-seeking publishing houses quickly released several books about Kashpirovsky, which were as a rule more or less successful translations of journalistic texts first published in Russia and in Ukraine. Apart from the press and radio (e.g. Kashpirovsky's participation in live night programs on Wrocław radio), he was catapulted to the peak of popularity by a series of TV

42 As part of this project, five Master's theses on different aspects of the Kashpirovsky phenomenon were defended in the UMCS Institute of Sociology's Department of Medical Sociology and Family. They were inspired and supervised by the author of the present book.

programs, in which he took part as the guest star, especially programs prepared for TV Channel II presented by H. Aczkasowa: *Wokół Kaszpirowskiego* [Around Kashpirovsky] and *Teleklinika dr Kaszpirowskiego* [Dr Kashpirovsky's Teleclinic]. Thus, the skillful use of the public media, meticulously prepared scripts of his own programs, and the telegenic personality of this 'non-conventional psychotherapist' and healer, determined Kashpirovsky's permanent presence in the Poles' social consciousness in the early 1990s. We should add that the media still remember about Kashpirovsky although the frequency of these accounts is far lower than in the period 1990-1993. In a lengthy article, the "Gazeta Wyborcza" (1994) assessed for example the healer's impact on the results of parliamentary elections in Russia through the 'use of mass-scale hypnotic session', which was allegedly to produce good results for the party on whose ticket Kashpirovsky ran for a seat in the State Duma of the Russian Federation. The effect of the successful campaign was his gaining of a parliamentary seat. In 1993-1994 the popular "Angora" weekly ran Kashpirovsky's columns, which enjoyed great popularity. In 1994 the 'Tygodnik Powszechny" weekly published a lengthy essay about Kashpirovsky on the title page - *Kaszpirowski, samodzierżawie i wielka Rosja* [Kashpirovsky, Autocracy, and Great Russia], in which W. Bereś and J. Strzałka presented the healer's huge influence on Russia's political situation in the mid-1990s. The authors maintained that the strong position of the Liberal-Democratic Party of Russia was owed largely to Kashpirovsky. His political activities were presented at length by the "Nie" weekly. The founder of teletherapy claimed that he entered active political life in order to defend his scientific discoveries (the Kashpirovsky method); he also explained that because of V. Zhirinovsky's chauvinist statements he was leaving the latter's party to be an independent State Duma deputy. In the late 1990s (1998) the press - from the "Gazeta Wyborcza" to women's weeklies - described the fate of Kashpirovski at that time, presenting him as 'the greatest magus of the century'. They wrote about his career and financial successes in the United States, where his children had already lived for a long time, his new marriage, and his plans to take part in the Russian space program. A. M. Kashpirovsky also was also a regular topic in the "Gazeta Wyborcza": when discussing a documentary by the well-known Russian director Nikita Mikhalkov, *Anna 6-18*, which was a kind of 'chronicle' of Russia's recent history, columnist Andrzej Osęka wrote that Kashpirovsky had become a symbol of Soviet transformations just like Gorbachev, Yeltsin or perestroika. Although the media now use the past tense when speaking about Kashpirovsky, he appears to have become the symbol of the first stage of Polish transformations and a constant element of social stereotypes. Agnieszka Holland, when writing the screenplay of her movie *Julia Walking Home* (2002) and making the Russian healer one of its main characters, made a conscious reference to the Polish legend of Kashpirovsky. In her press interviews Holland did not hide her great interest in bioenergy therapy.

Another factor that sustained and established Kashpirovsky's popularity was that, in pursuance of his goals, he was able to quickly enlist the support of some members of the influential Church hierarchy and church institutions, and to win the recognition of large numbers of priests, which made possible the organization of psychotherapy sessions in the largest and best-known churches in Poland (St. Mary Basilica in Gdansk, St. Florian church in Warsaw, etc.). Kashpirovsky displayed here unusual adaptive skills and admirable intuitive social engineering techniques. At the same time he was strongly affected by these kinds of meetings with masses of followers, where he learned the therapeutic power of prayers and the force of influence of the sacred sites regarded as 'the holy places'. The motivations that lay behind Kashpirovsky's decision to turn to the Church institution and clergy (intuition, calculation, accident) are not important; however, the effects of this strategy are indisputable: steadily growing social popularity, 'cultural familiarization' with the therapist, and placement in the stereotype of a positive hero.

One more element of crucial importance in building the myth was exemplary marketing and efficient running of the profitable medical services business by the therapist and his 'Kashpirovsky company' advisers. The team headed by the therapist showed economic competence and qualifications creating, for example, the business plan of the therapist's tours of larger Polish cities, attended by tens of thousands of Kashpirovsky admirers to take part in paid (expensive) mass healing sessions. According to sources close to Dr Kashpirovsky (Westa company), between 1989 and 1992 the sale of copyrighted videocassettes with recorded teletherapy programs and tickets distributed at so-called big meetings brought him about a million and a half US dollars, which was untaxed, transferred from Poland and profitably invested in the next projects in Ukraine, Russia and the US. The ability to use the rules of the health services free market and to economically exploit the free publicity he gained from participating in mass audience sessions shown on public television, and the well-publicized donations of a small portion of his money to charity were among the evidence that proved that he had mastered the rules of the economic game in the domain of health provision. Kashpirovsky and his team offered medical services at the watershed period. This stage of free market development is best characterized by the tenor of E. Freidson's conclusion that we were dealing with open competition for patients in the free market among all those wishing to sell health services. Doctors freely competed with **hypnotists** [*my emphasis* W.P.], charmers, herbalists, acupuncturists, homeopaths, and clairvoyants. Legal or other restrictions did not prohibit performing or practicing medical services, surgical or psychological. Anyone could join in the competition (Freidson 1976: 157-158; Cockerham 2004: 171-175). In light of the foregoing facts it is legitimate to say that Kashpirovsky took perfect advantage of the economic opportunities provided by economic transformations in Poland in the early 1990s, which laid the foundation for free competition in medical services in the free market of commercial medicine. To sum it up we should emphasize that the fact that Kashpirovsky enlisted the support of the re-emergent Catholic Church institutions in the 1990s, and consequently, made himself credible; he became part of the stereotype of faith healer using religious elements, and professionally utilized the commercial media to promote the chosen therapeutic method and to self-advertise. Finally, he mastered the rules of game on the emerging capitalist healthcare market. All of these elements accompanied the Polish transformation, and largely ensured Kashpirovsky's popularity, prestige, social trust, and financial success.

3.1. The Range of Public Interest

Without doubt, a first glance at the range and mass scale of social processes produced by Kashpirovsky should prompt the researcher to attempt to describe and interpret the phenomenon. Another stimulus encouraging the sociologist, especially in the early 1990s, might have been the fact that there was a risk that one of the most spectacular and mass-scale phenomena of the first stage of Polish transformation would be over before it was systematically studied. We will look at some facts defining the scale and mass character of the problem. In my conversation with him Kashpirovsky said, for example, that his archive in Kiev contained half a million letters (!) sent over the period of three years (1988-1990) by Russian and Ukrainian teletherapy participants. These materials, Kashpirovsky believed, might be an invaluable source of information for sociologists, psychologists, philosophers or physicians. An analysis of the content of this collection of personal documents would probably constitute a research project unprecedented in the history of sociological sciences (Piątkowski et al. 1993: 29-42). The scale of this phenomenon is also determined by the results of the previously-quoted sociological survey conducted by OBOP in the early 1990s on a representative sample of adult Poles. The results of the survey show that the scale of popularity of Kashpirovsky's two-year series of programs was one of the largest in the history of Polish TV (despite being shown on Channel II with a comparatively narrow reach and during a poor viewing time). The OBOP survey states that just one month after the screening of the teletherapy series, at least one of its sessions was watched by 59% (!) of those surveyed. It should be emphasized that, in standard nationwide OBOP surveys, one percent is equivalent to 280,000 adult Poles (*Telewizyjne... komunikat z badań OBOP* 1990). Another symptom of the mass scale of the phenomenon was the fact that, after an appeal by commentators and organizers of TV broadcasts (L. Gapik, W. Piątkowski, and H. Aczkasowa) we watched the influx of several thousand letters from the audience of these programs. Consequently, I was able to make a preliminary analysis of a set of 3218 letters at the UMCS Department of Medical Sociology and Family. The scale of the problem is also defined by the fact that the author of teletherapy, while touring with his healing sessions, assembled a total of at least 55 thousand people at the stadiums and large auditoriums. To sum up, we can say that, between 1989 and 1992 A. M. Kashpirovsky produced several macrosocial phenomena in Poland and left an indelible mark on the social consciousness of many Poles; he was also a specific and unique phenomenon on the emerging free market of medical services.

The continuing interest of the Poles in Kashpirovsky, called 'the famous healer' by the "Rzeczpospolita" daily (2007), is shown in an article describing his current problems: Kashpirovsky knocked down his opponent in a popular talk show, the healer sued the opponents of his methods, he criticized former President Yeltsin for issuing a decree banning mass-scale healing sessions, he reminisced that he had become the first Russian millionaire, etc. The author, A. Pisalnik, concludes that 'Kashpirovsky's supernatural abilities are not challenged by scientists'. The daily writes in conclusion: 'In the early 1990s Anatoly Kashpirovsky made an impressive career in Poland. Sessions with his participation were so popular that they were even broadcast by public television. Millions of people suffering from lesser or serious diseases spent hours looking at the therapist's rectangular face [...] He last held healing sessions in Poland in 1998. He met patients in Krakow, but the interest was smaller than he expected' (Pisalnik 2007).

3.2. The Kashpirovsky Method: Psychotherapy or Teletherapy?

We will try to determine what is and what is not the non-conventional, eclectic method(s), used by the psychiatrist Anatoly Mikhailovich Kashpirovsky. We should first refer to the description of characteristics of modern-day psychotherapy. According to Professor L. Gapik (2000) psychotherapy can be applied to treat patients suffering from some **diagnosed** [*my emphasis*, W. P.] disorders, the psychotherapeutic approach also admits the possibility of treating not only the soul but also the body. Gapik maintains that the exact definition of the psychotherapist's profession will eliminate those unlawfully using this title (e.g. bioenergy therapists), and that psychotherapeutic treatment requires long-lasting contact with the patient. The same author (1999) points out the need to base the method on reliable theoretical foundations and to integrate medical and psychological knowledge in this area to the maximum. In this approach, psychotherapeutic methods are divided into four groups: analytical psychotherapy, suggestive psychotherapy (the Kashpirovsky method being apparently close o this type), training psychotherapy, and psychological education psychotherapy. L. Gapik also contends that we must not ignore 'healing recoveries inconsistent in principle with medical knowledge', which occur extremely rarely on the peripheries of academic medicine. These cases, Gapik argues, show that there is unordered knowledge about 'special psychical stimulation which overcomes illness'. In these elements, Gapik believes, there are 'unexplored reserves of psychotherapeutic capacities that activate the human immune system' (Gapik 1999; 9-13; 2000: 9-18.).

The key question in this section can be worded like this: Does Kashpirovsky practice is psychotherapy and, if so, to what extent? Apart from differences between individual schools or variants of psychotherapy, its fundamental features are *inter alia*: reference to more or less specified theories explaining the essence of psychological influence on the organism, the striving to establish an emotional bond with the patient (therapeutic contact), the therapist's ability to distance him/herself from his/her own emotions and moral judgments – assumption of the attitude of impartial kindness, the ability to empathize with the emotional content of the patient's experience and retain the objective approach (empathy) (Aleksandrowicz and Sikora 1995: 139-146). Classic psychotherapy is most often practiced in healthcare centers, and the patient is informed about the limits of the efficacy of the method, possible contraindications and alternative therapies. Before commencing a psychotherapeutic treatment, the exact etiology and diagnosis of the condition treated should be known. Each type of psychotherapy is oriented towards a specific group of diseases and it has lower or higher efficacy within this area. Psychotherapeutic measures applied to serious somatic diseases are not an alternative to pharmacological or surgical treatment - they are only its complement. In the case of chronic diseases (tumors) it should be remembered that temporary psychotherapeutic effects, for example momentary pain relief, may prove undesirable for the patient in the long run. Before any decision to employ psychotherapy is made, the patient should also be informed about the risk of adverse effects (3-6%); finally, the therapist should know and apply in practice the rules of the Medical Deontological Code (Piątkowski 1995: 139-146).

One of the founders of European psychotherapy, Stanisław Kratochvil, when describing the methods of modern psychotherapy (1999), lists *inter alia* hypnotherapy (the approach employed by Kashpirovsky in a non-conventional form), and points out that this method uses the hypnotic state and hypnotic suggestions for therapeutic purposes. With this approach, it is possible *inter alia* to reduce pain, fear, and anti-health habits, cheer the patient up, and enhance his/her activity (Kratochvil 1999: 22-24).

To sum up L. Gapik's and S. Kratochvil's discussion we can say after Z. (1998) that the psychotherapist is defined as 'a person competent to give help (using psychological means) to individuals with functional disorders of the organism (where these functions may apply to mental processes and personality or somatic processes and functions of organs) while psychotherapy is described as a specialist treatment method consisting in correcting the organism's functional disorder by intentional application of programmed psychological measures. The aim of such measures is to improve the patient's disordered functioning and his/her relations with the environment' (Woźniak 1998: 110).

We will now discuss selected elements that make up the Kashpirovsky method. We may ask the question whether there is one particular method that this therapist uses. If we expected a presentation of a cohesive theory of treatment, our expectations would be in vain. What Kashpirovsky does consists in making not always consistent and ad hoc judgments and opinions intended to elucidate one or another therapeutic effect which Kashpirovski sometimes finds surprising. The therapist himself seems to be aware of these complications and ambiguities: for example, he is not sure which positive or negative effect described by the patient is associated with particular elements of his (Kashpirovsky's) therapy and which is consequent upon the concurrence of accidental circumstances or is the result of factors outside of the process of treatment; neither does he know why in the same patients there are alternating positive, negative or 'zero' effects. An additional complication is the fact that genuine discussion of teletherapy in terms of natural sciences is practically impossible as long as Kashpirovsky fails to show reliable documentation meeting standard requirements of medical statistics (Gryglewski 1995: 34; Misiek 1995, I, 1: 11-117; *Wielki słownik medyczny* 1996: 711; *Mała encyclopedia medycyny* 1999: 470).

We can summarize that the comparison between selected features of classic psychotherapies with diverse 'syncretic' healing methods and the techniques used by Kashprirovsky must lead us to the conclusion that what this therapist practices is not classic psychotherapy although, as we have demonstrated, it contains certain elements of it (see 2.3).

3.3. Letters to Kashpirovsky. A Methodological Challenge

Methodological questions frequently appear in this book: this author supports the idea of departing in medical sociology from the exclusive use of methods based on various questionnaire versions as the basic way of gathering information (Piątkowski 1995, 2: 288) To break the dominance of quantitative methods is especially important in the sociology of illness where it is necessary to investigate, measure and assess unique social phenomena and mental states such as dying, suffering, strong emotions accompanying being ill and recovering, experiences caused by chronic illnesses, or traumatic experiences of the dying process and the period of old age. That is why I believe that, in the subdiscipline of medical sociology, we have to attempt to introduce and promote various versions of qualitative methods and techniques: analysis of the content of personal documents, free interview, narrative techniques, participant observation etc. In the methodology of social sciences since the mid-1990s we have observed the rediscovery of the values of personal documents. As Ch. Frankfort-Nachmias and D. Nachmias maintain, it is far more difficult to gain access to personal documents than to official ones. Nevertheless, the former will be a valuable source of information to all researchers who are interested in the individual point of view of specific situations or events (Nachmias and Nachmias 338: 341). One of the typical documents of this type are letters. They contain ample factual documentation, and they are a medium that connects the sender and receiver, often showing strong links between the writers of correspondence, as well as presenting individual, unique and often thorough accounts of events in public and private life experienced by their authors. In the case of the collection of letters sent to the non-conventional therapist A. M. Kashpirovsky, the problem is not investigation of the authenticity of the message, but possible difficulties with interpretation of individual excerpts. When analyzing the content of the letters we assumed that, since it was 'technically' impossible to observe the behaviors, attitudes and needs of millions of people taking part in the therapist's sessions over several years, we could reconstruct the social elements surrounding health and illness by recording the social awareness of TV-viewers' motives and convictions on the basis of what the authors of the cited letters think. Thus, we draw the conclusions on the basis of systematically and objectively defined features of the message (Ibid: 342). We also assumed that other students of the problem would reach the same conclusions were they to repeat these procedures and study the same material. By using repeatable rules of selection, encoding, and interpretation of the selected material, we wanted to approach the desirable objectivism of analysis. We can thus study the basic indicators characterizing value hierarchies associated with health and illness, the features of health consciousness of the letter authors, attitudes towards health/illness, needs in this area, and health behaviors. In this way we followed the directives of Harold Lasswell, who recommended investigating: *Who (says) What (to) Whom (in) What Channel (with) What Effect* (Ibid). On the basis of earlier priorities, 'analysis' units were distinguished (from letters selected for the purpose) along with 'context units', i.e. larger portions of text. We were mainly interested in such elements of analysis units as 'words/terms' and 'topics' appearing in the letters. The final goal was to classify analysis units into categories (e.g. those relating to the felt effects of a non-conventional healing recovery); the formulation of categories was logically connected with the research problem defined earlier.

Using selected analysis categories we were able to establish what was said, what the message was about, and what values, goals and desires were contained in the letter author, etc. (Ibid; 347). While discussing these detailed, technical issues, we touch upon only the broader methodological problem present in modern Polish sociology, i.e. the presence and growing popularity of methods of non-survey studies. These issues are extremely varied, covering multi-aspectual discussions on the characteristics of the biographical method (J. Szczepański, M. Latoszek), description of virtues of the narrative interview (Czyżewski, Piotrowski et al.), the value of memoirs-writing (Gołębiowski), discussions on the value of content analysis (Pamuła, Kafla), the role of participant observation (Wołowik), finally the fundamentals of the methodology of 'comprehension surveys' (Siciński Wyka) that are 'outside of survey sociology' and look for models of social studies (Sułek, Nowak, Wyka,, Lutyńska) (Szczepański 1982); Latoszek 1987; Czyżewski et al; 1997; Gołebiowski 1973; Kafla 1969; Pamuła 1996; Nikodemska-Wołowiak 1999; Siciński and Wyka 1988; Sułek et al. 1989; Lutyńska 2000).

For sociologists, the letter can be a source of information that is especially rich in facts and opinions. The several thousand large letters written by the sick and the healthy formed the basis of the following remarks and comments. These are the arguments for adopting this standpoint:

- The letter provides an opportunity for a free, formally unrestricted presentation of one's own life problem and outline of the rich sociocultural background of the problem.
- This type of personal document is a special and content-rich act of social communication from which conclusions can be drawn both about the features of the letter's author and addressee, and about the social context of the events reported.
- The letter is a subjective, personal, unique communication of accounts concerning the social reality surrounding the author; it also documents man's characteristic spontaneous reactions to processes and phenomena that he

witnesses or participates in. A general value of the letter, particularly one with many topics, is its diversity, wealth and complexity in transmitting mental states, moods and other varied emotional elements.

- A special value of this interpersonal communication is the fact that not everything we can read, analyze, or interpret in the letters examined would be found in the material obtained using conventional quantitative methods.

Obviously, this kind of personal account of social facts and events and emotional states has its disadvantages, shortcomings, and limitations, resulting *inter alia* from subjective communication – the possibility of subordinating the content to the objective that one wants to achieve in the correspondence, in this case the favorable assessment of the efficacy of Kashpirovsky's treatment method, can for example be expressed in order to achieve a specific practical goal, if only to arrange an individual appointment with the therapist. A limitation of the letter material can be the letter writers' memory gaps and disorders if they are giving an account of phenomena *ex post facto*. Taking all its advantages and disadvantages into account, the letter in all its forms should be regarded as a valuable although rarely utilized source of sociological information. This is especially attractive for researchers who count on special possibilities of analyzing complex emotional states, seek descriptions of intimate, personal or even embarrassing events, or try to find characteristics of expressive elements, etc. Talking about one's own disease, pain, disability, physical or mental handicaps is often impossible for the suffering persons (even in a terminal condition), hence the questionnaire method has its limitations because respondents in this category refuse to be interviewed in a sociological survey or to participate in any other form of recording their opinions. A letter to someone particularly trusted (A. M. Kashpirovsky was one) can sometimes be shockingly honest, true and moving. It very often contains the most truth about oneself, the experienced stages of one's illness, and the social background of these events.

We should emphasize once again that the letter is always a subjective 'portrait of its author' and his/her own interpretation of the social reality. However, if we analyze a collection of several thousand letters on many subjects we obtain a broader, more objective, more accurate and less distorted insight into the studied reality associated with people's health consciousness, attitudes, needs and behavior in the states of health and illness.

Conclusions

My reason for writing the book, in which I adopted the perspective of the sociology of health, illness and medicine was my intention to complement and enrich the knowledge about Polish society with information on certain detailed ways of taking care of health and coping with illness. The characteristic of these increasingly popular methods and, in general, of the approach to health is the well-established conviction that responsibility for the functioning of our organism can be taken 'into our own hands'. Under such circumstances, the sick person who is not a physician inclines towards the view that s/he has sufficient information on the etiology of illness, methods of diagnosing it, and its prevention and treatment, and the knowledge of how to use these in practice in order to independently take care of his/her own health or that of his/her family. In oversimplified terms, this is the character of **self-treatment**, one of the three forms of non-medical healing/healthcare described above. It also turned out that some people are convinced that they have such considerable competence in the matters of treatment (knowledge and instrumental skills) that they themselves attempt to help in illness, offering their services to all those in need, e.g. to residents of the same village. In this way, from among the members of local communities emerge folk specialists 'knowledgeable about illnesses'; these are rural folk doctors who constitute the foundations of **folk medical systems**, an integral part of folk knowledge and, more broadly, of the characteristic peasant culture. In the late nineteenth century when 'dissident orientations' appeared within the academic medicine of the time, there was a growing popularity of the authors of 'medical heresies', which ultimately took the form of the doctrine of mesmerism and homeopathy. At present these orientations and the therapists/healers who practice them constitute the system of **therapeutic practices of healers** within complementary and alternative medicine (CAM): this is the third of the three practices which make up the system of non-medical healthcare.

The book presents my own taxonomic conception permitting a description of the relevant area of sociomedical studies, it characterizes the internal structure of non-biomedicla healthcare, discusses its features and specificity and emphasizes qualitative differences between lay, non-scientific knowledge of health and illness together with the resultant treatment techniques, and the model of evidence based medicine (EBM). Thus, the area defined by my term 'sociology of non-medical healing systems or healthcare' was described using my own terminology and names. The results of my own studies were referred to and compared with the analogous achievements of the Polish and Western sociology of health, illness, and medicine. The study described the historical evolution of the oldest ways of coping with illness - in Poland these took the form of self-treatment or folk medical systems; it described Polish characteristic sociocultural factors affecting the features and character of the two modes. All three forms of help in health and illness, especially self-treatment and practices of modern-day healers, began to develop intensively in Poland after 1990 because the emerging society - capitalist, democratic, pluralist, civic and liberally-oriented - created new, previously non-existent opportunities for the development of 'other medicine'. Therefore, the social range of the phenomenon in question and its complex causes are also the object of the author's interest.

This study has been written by a health and illness sociologist and, as the analysis of the literature shows, it is part of the classic, mainstream studies conducted by the European medical sociology[43]. We should emphasize that, since, 1990 there have been no scientific monographs concerned with the subject of this study. This applies not only to the research field of the Polish sociology of health, illness and medicine but also to anthropology (the book by D. Penkala-Gawęcka about healthcare in Kazakhstan, cited and discussed here), psychology and clinical medicine. Nor can we easily find a comparable study in European literature; therefore we can conclude that this completed research project is a pioneering one. The author's natural frame of reference is his original subdiscipline - the sociology of health, illness and medicine - but the general background of this discussion is obviously general sociology Similarly, most of the literature utilized and cited consists of sociomedical items but the interdisciplinary nature of the problems analyzed makes numerous references to medical anthropology, ethnology, medical history and clinical sciences entirely natural.

To discover the everyday, 'handy' knowledge about health and illness, often used by lay people, and the practical actions resulting from having it is one of the research priorities in the European sociology of health and illness (Prior 2003, 25: 42). For the purpose of these studies, in this book I adapt E. Freidson's classic sociological conception of lay referral system. I also discuss pilot surveys inspired by this approach. Like Freidson's conception, the elements of sociological theories, especially symbolic interactionism, phenomenology and ethnomethodology, are especially useful in relevant analyses, which was justified in my book. Such points of reference seem helpful in the description, characteristics and interpretation of subjective, emotional, 'irrational' lay knowledge about health and illness, and of behaviors resulting from the possession of this knowledge (Lawton 2003, 25: 23-40).

43 The founder of British sociology of health and illness emphasizes the importance of studies on 'alternative forms of healthcare' Nettleton (2007, 65: 2409-2412) Cf. also Bury and Gabe 2009: 9..

My own studies also covered the analysis, classification and interpretation of the unique collection, which I have gathered, of 1311 letters sent by TV-viewers to the Polish TV company , addressed to the non-conventional therapist A. M. Kashpirovsky. We can say with full conviction that these kinds of personal documents are a rich and inspiring source of poorly explored knowledge about a specific 'non-presented world'. It shows unknown emotions, value hierarchies, kinds of health consciousness, attitude, needs and behaviors towards health and illness represented by lay people. We should note that these types of lay knowledge, beliefs and stereotypes directly or indirectly affect decisions concerning the ways and form of treatment. On the basis of such grounds people choose a partner in their struggle against an illness. This can be a physician, a healer or, as my own studies show, both of them (see also Doktór and Koseła 1989, 3: 189-193). The knowledge provided by my investigations not only has the form of 'pure science' but, when properly used, can also have diagnostic and social engineering values. It can enhance the efficacy of therapeutic and preventive measures taken by physicians by improving their relationship with patients and strategies for health (social) policy. The latter has so far ignored the existence and growing popularity of non-medical (non-conventional) healthcare and the fact that this domain is not only the object of interest on the part of millions of Poles but also significantly and permanently affects their behavior and attitudes towards health and illness.

Bibliography

Albrecht M. 2002. „Badania kliniczne w homeopatii - ocena krytyczna". *Homeopatia Polska.* 2.

Albrecht P., W. Chrząstowski-Ostoja, A. Horwath. 2001. „Jatrogenny zespół rzekomego guza mózgu jako skutek niekonwencjonalnej metody leczenia kadmem." *Pediatria Polska.* 4.

Albrecht G.L., R. Fitzpatrick, S.C. Scrimshaw (ed.). 2003. *The Handbook of Social Studies in Health and Medicine,* Sage Publ., London.

Armstrong D. 2003. *Social Theorizing about Health and Illness* in G.L. Albrecht, R. Fitzpatrick, S.G. Scrimshaw (eds.), *Social Studies in Health and Medicine.* London: Sage Publ.

Aleksandrowicz J., G. Sikora. 1995. „Psychoterapia - nauka czy sztuka?" in K. Imieliński (ed.). *Medycyna u progu XXI wieku. Sztuka leczenia.* Warszawa: PAM.

Amsterdamski S. 1999. „Science". Z. Bokszański et al. (eds.). *Encyklopedia socjologii.* T. 2, Warszawa: Oficyna Naukowa.

Babbie E. 2003. *Badania społeczne w praktyce* (transl. W. Betkiewicz et al.). A. Kłoskowska-Dudzińska (ed.). Warszawa: PWN.

Baer H.A. 2010. *Complementary and Alternative Medicine: Processes of Legitimation, Professionalization, and Cooption.* in W.C. Cockerham. (ed.) *The New Blackwell Companion to Medical Sociology.* Oxford: Wiley-Blackwell.

Baer H.A. C. Jen, L.M. Tanassi, C. Tsia, H. Wahbeh. 1998. "The drive for professinalization in acupuncture. A preliminary view from San Francisco Bay Area". *Social Science and Medicine.* 46.

Bąjka J., Z. Bajka. 1996. "Health Problems in Polish Paramedical Periodicals". in *Health and Social Change in the Integration of Europe. ESHMS. 6th Biennal Conlerence. Budapest.*

Baranowski Z. 2005. "Inwazja magii". *Nasz Dziennik* . 23.04.2005.

Barański J., W. Piątkowski (eds.). 2002. *Zdrowie i choroba. Wybrane problemy socjologii medycyny.* Wrocław: Wrocławskie Wyd. Oświatowe.

Barczyński M., J. Bogusz (eds.). 1993. "Medicine". *Medyczny słownik encyklopedyczny.* Kraków: Oficyna Wydawnicza Agora.

Bauman Z. 1995. *Ciało i przemoc w obliczu ponowoczesności. Wykłady Kopernikańskie w Humanistyce.* Toruń: Wyd. Uniwersytetu Mikołaja Kopernika.

Bejnarowicz J. 1969. *Wiedza medyczna ludności wsi podhalańskiej.* in M. Sokołowska (ed.). *Badania socjologiczne w medycynie.* Warszawa: KiW.

Bernstein J.H., J.T. Shuval. 1997. "Nonconventional Medicine in Israel. Consultation Patterns of the Israeli Population and Attitudes oj Primary Care Physicians. *Social Science and Medicine.* 44.

Bird C., P. Conrad, A. Fremont (eds.). 2000. *Handbook of Medical Sociology.* Upper Saddle River: Prentice Hall.

Blumer H., 1969. *Symbolic interactionism. Perspective and method.* Englewood Cliffs: Pretince Hall.

Boisset M. 1994. "Alternative Medicine Used by Rheumatology Patient in a Universal Health Care Setting". *Journal of Rheumatology*. 21.

Bokszański Z., et al. (eds.). 1998*Encyklopedia socjologii.* T.1. Warszawa: Oficyna Naukowa.

Bokszański Z., et al. (eds.). 1999*Encyklopedia socjologii.* T.2. Warszawa: Oficyna Naukowa.

Bokszański Z., et al. (eds.). 2000*Encyklopedia socjologii.* T.3. Warszawa: Oficyna Naukowa.

Bokszański Z., et al. (eds.). 2002*Encyklopedia socjologii.* T.4. Warszawa: Oficyna Naukowa.

Borkowski T. 1980. *Lek zatruty, fałszowany, omyłkowo sporządzony i znachorski,* Wrocław: Ossolineum.

Boström H., S. Rosner. 1992. "Quality of Alternative Medicine". *Qualitative Assurance of Health Care*. No. 2.

Bożyk Z. 2004. "Podstawy teoretyczne homeopatii". *Homeopatia Polska.* 2.

Bradby H. 2009. *Medical Sociology: An Introduction*. London: Sage.

Brown P. (ed.). 2000. *Perspectives in Medical Sociology. 3rd ed.,* Long Grave: Waveland Press.

Brody H., J.M. Rygwelski, M.D. Fetters. 2000. *Etyka we wzajemnym oddziaływaniu medycyny konwencjonalnej i komplementarnej.* in W.B. Jonas, J.S. Levin (eds.). *Podstawy medycyny komplementarnej i alternatywnej.* Kraków: Wyd. Universitas.

Brylak M. 1970. *Medycyna ludowa.* in R. Reinfuss (ed.). *Monografia powiatu myślenickiego.* T.2. Kraków: Wydawnictwo Literackie.

Brzeziński T. 1996. „Karta Praw Pacjenta – spodziewane korzyści i niebezpieczeństwa". *Pro Medico. Biuletyn Okręgowej Izby Lekarskiej w Katowicach*listopad. numer specjalny, etyka.

Brzeziński T. (ed.). 2000. *Historia medycyny, 2nd* ed. Warszawa: PZWL.

Budak L., K. Lampek, T. Tahin. 1996. "Alternative Medicine, Attitudes, Health-Beliefs and Value Preferences". in *Health and Medicine in the New Europe. ESHMS. 6th Biennal Conference, Budapest.*

Bujak F. 2001. *Wyznaczniki zdrowia psychicznego ludności wiejskiej.* in F. Bujak, J. Zagórski (eds.). *Obciążenia fizyczne i psychiczne pracą w rolnictw*Lublin: Instytut Medycyny Wsi.

Bujak F. 2003. „Opinie uczniów kończących szkoły rolnicze o życiu na wsi i zagrożeniach zdrowia fizycznego i psychicznego rolników". *Medycyna Ogólna*. 9.

Burszta J. (ed.). 1967. *Kultura ludowa Wielkopolski.* T.3. Poznań: Wyd. Poznańskie.

Bursztа J. 1967. *Lecznictwo ludowe.* in *Kultura ludowa Wielkopolski.* T.3. Poznań: Wyd. Poznańskie.

Bury M., J. Gabe. 2009. General Introduction. in M. Bury, J. Gabe. (eds.). in M. Bury, J. Gabe. (eds.). *The Sociology of Health and Illness. A Reader*. London, New York: Routledge.

Busby H., G. Williams, A. Rogers. 1997. *Sociology of Scientific Knowledge and the Sociology of Health and Illnes.* in M.A. Elston (ed.). *The Sociology of Medical Science and Technology*. Oxford: Blackwell.

Butrym Z. 1976. „Lekarze ośrodków zdrowia o swojej sytuacji po ubezpieczeniu rolników". *Wieś Współczesna*. 10.

Bystroń J.S. 1947. *Etnografia Polski.* Warszawa: Czytelnik.

Bystroń J.S. 1947. *Kultura ludowa.* Warszawa: Wyd. Trzaska, Evert i Michalski.

Cant S., U. Sharma. 2003. *Alternative Health Practices and Systems.* in G.L. Albrecht, R. Fitzpatrick, S.C. Scrimshaw (eds.), *The Handbook of Social Studies in Health and Medicine,* London: Sage Publ.

Chałasiński J. 1938*Młode pokolenie chłopów*T.3. Warszawa: Państwowy InstytutKultury Wsi.

Chałasiński J. 1968. *Młode pokolenie wsi Polski Ludowej.* T.5. Warszawa: LSW.

Chodak S. 1999. „Jan Stanisław Bystroń jako prekursor socjologii historycznej". *Annales UMCS.* sectio I. vol. XXIV.

Chorąży M. 1998. „Medycyna paranormalna. Manipulacja umęczoną duszą". *Polityka.* 3.

Giarelli G. 2006. "The Ambivalent Pluralism. The Role of unconventional Medicine in Italian, HNS. in *European Health. Old and New Challanges. Tackling Health Inequalities. ESHMS. 11th International Congress, Kraków.*

Cockerham W.C. (ed.). 2004. *Medical Sociology.* 9th ed. Upper Saddle Rivier: Pearson.

Cockerham W.C., Glasser M. (eds.). 2001. *Readings in Medical Sociology,* Upper Saddle Rivier: Prentice Hall.

Cockerham W.C., G. Scambler. 2010. *Medical Sociology and Sociological Theory.* in W.C. Cockerham. (ed.) *The New Blackwell Companion to Medical Sociology.* Oxford: Wiley-Blackwell.

Coe R.M. 1970. *Sociology of Medicine.* New York: Mc Graw Hill.

Colt G.H. 1996. "The Healing Revolution". *Life Magazine*, September.

Connor L. 2004. "Relief, risk and renewal, mixed therapy regiments in an Australian suburb". *Social Science and Medicine.* 59.

Conrad P. 2000. *Medicalization, genetics and human problems.* in Ch.E. Bird, P. Conrad. A.M. Fremont (eds.). *Handbook of Medical Sociology. 5th ed.* Saddle Upper River: Prentice Hall.

Corin E. 1995. *The Cultural Frame: Contex and Meaning in the Construction of Health.* in B.C. Amick, S. Levine, A.R. Tarlov, D. Chapman-Walsh. *Society and Health.* New York, NY: Oxford University Press.

"Co robi chory Polak. Raport z badań". 1996. Warszawa: OBOP.

Cousins N. 1976. "Anatomy of Illness, As perceived by the Patient". *New England Journal of Medicine.* 295, 26.

Csorba H. 1966. *Szpital – pacjent. System społeczny kliniki internistycznej.* Wrocław: Ossolineum.

„Cuda dzisiaj. Arka Noego". *Gazeta Wyborcza* suplement. 9-10.09.1994.

Czaczkowska E.K. 2004. „Demon wyjawił swe imię. Rozmowa z ks. E. Szaniawskim". *Rzeczpospolita* z dnia 28 07 2004.

Czarnowski S. 1995. *Powstanie i społeczne funkcje historii.* in J. Szacki (ed.). *Sto lat socjologii polskiej. Od Supińskiego do Szczepańskiego.* Warszawa: PWN.

„Czy Polacy są przesądni? Komunikat z badań". 2006. Warszawa: CBOS.

Czyż L.M. 1989. *Ziołolecznictwo Lasowiaków, Rzeszowiaków i Podgórzan na podstawie materiałów Muzeum Okręgowego w Rzeszowie* in B. Kuźnicka (ed.). *Historia leków naturalnych.* Warszawa: IHNOiT PAN.

Czyżewski M. 1984. „Socjologia a życie potoczne. Studium z etnometodologii i współczesnej socjologii interakcji". *Acta Univ. Lodziensis. Folia Sociologica.* 8.

Czyżewski M. 1998. „Ethnomethodology". Z. Bokszański et al. (eds.), *Encyklopedia socjologii.* T. l. Warszawa: Oficyna Naukowa.

Danilkiewicz W.C. 1993. *Samoleczenie jako zachowanie w chorobie dorosłych mieszkańców wsi.* Unpublished doctoral dissertation. Lublin: Instytut Medycyny Wsi.

Delvecchio-Good M.J., B.J. Good. 2000. *"Paralel Sisters", Medical Anthropology and Medical Sociology.* in Ch.E. Bird, P. Conrad, A.M. Fremont (eds.), *Handbook of Medical Sociology.* Upper Saddle River: Prentice Hall.

Dew K. 2000. "Deviant insiders, medical acupuncturists in New Zealand". *Social Science and Medicine.* 50.

The paper Published by Senate of Republic of Poland. No. 19. 05.08.1998. <http//www.senat.gov.pl>.

Dobrowolski K. 1966. *Studia nad żvciem społecznym i kulturą.* Wrocław-Warszawa-Kraków: Ossolineum.

Doktór T. 1989. *Ucieczka czy innowacja.* in T. Doktór, K. Koseła (eds.). *Ruchy pogranicza religii i nauki jako zjawisko socjopsychologiczne.* T. 3.Warszawa: Wyd. Uniwersytetu Warszawskiego.

The paper Published by Central Council of Phisicians. 05.11.2000. <http.//www.nil.org.pl>

Domański H., A. Rychard, P. Śpiewak. 2005. *Polska jedna czy wiele?* Warszawa: Wyd. Trio.

Dulczewski Z. 1975. *Florian Znaniecki jako twórca metody autobiograficznej w socjologii.* in A. Kwilecki (ed.). *Florian Znaniecki i jego rola w socjologii,* Poznań: Wyd. UAM.

Dyczewski L. 1983. *Ten który rozdał życie. Wstęp, biografia św. Maksymiliana i wybór tekstów.* Warszawa: Wyd. Kurii Prowincjalnej oo. Franciszkanów.

Dyczewski L. 1995. *Kultura polska* w *procesie przemian,* Lublin: Wyd. Towarzystwo Naukowe KUL.

Dyjak A. 2005. „Żywienie a zdrowie i rozwój dzieci wiejskich. Zarys problematyki". *Zdrowie Publiczne.* 115 (1).

Dziadosz R., A. Wiśniewska. B. Skrętowicz. 1970. „Stopień korzystania z opieki zdrowotnej przez mieszkańców jednej wsi w zależności od zatrudnienia (w rolnictwie i poza rolnictwem)". *Medycyna Wiejska.* T. V. nr 1-2.

Dziadul J. 1993. „Lekarski desant ze Wschodu". *Polityka.* 14.08.1993.

„Dzialalność paramedyczna a Kodeks Etyki Lekarskiej". 2001. *Medicus - pismo Okręgowej Izby Lekarskiej w Lublinie.*

Dzun. W. 1989. „Przemiany społecznej struktury wsi w Polsce Ludowej*Wieś Współczesna* Nr 6.

Easthope G., B. Tranterr, G. Gili. 2000. "General practitioners attitudes towards complementary therapies". *Social Science and Medicine*. 51.

Eildermann H. 1953. *Społeczeństwo pierwotne jego ustrój i religia.* Warszawa KiW.

Elling R. 1981. "Political economy, cultural hegemony and mixes or traditional and modern medicine". *Social Science and Medicine.* 2.

Emerson J. "Behaviour in Private Places. Sustaining Definitions of Reality in Gynecological Examinations". *Recent Sociology.* 2.

Ezzy D. 2000. "Illness narratives, time, hope and HIV". *Social Science and Medicine*. 50.

Ferguson M. 1993. *Na rozdrożu. Przemiana ludzi.* in P. Macura (ed.). *New Age.* Kraków: Nakład Wyd. Nomos.

Filip R., R. Lenart. 2007. „Promocja zdrowia ze szczególnym uwzględnieniem profilaktyki chorób układu sercowo-naczyniowego wśród populacji wiejskiej w Polsce". *Zdrowie Publiczne.* 117 (1).

Firkowska-Mankiewicz A. 1990. *Reorientacja badań nad zdrowiem i chorobą – społeczny model choroby.* in A. Firkowska-Mankiewicz (ed.). Rodzina a problemy zdrowia i choroby. Warszawa: PBP 09.02.

Firkowska-Mankiewicz A. 1994. *Psychospołeczny kontekst odwrotu od medycyny konwencjonalnej.* in K. Imieliński (ed.). *Medycyna u progu XXI wieku. Filozofia i technika leczenia.* Warszawa: PAM.

Frankowska J. 2008. „Szepty na biesy. Na własne oczy". *Polityka.* 4.

Florek M. 2006. „Pacjent wiejskiego ośrodka zdrowia wobec zachowań zdrowotnych. I. Edukacja i profilaktyka zdrowotna a pacjent wiejskiego ośrodka zdrowia". *Zdrowie Publiczne.* 116 (2)

Fox R.C. 1989. *The Sociology of Medicine: A Participant* Observer's View. Upper Saddle River: Prentice Hall.

Freidson E. 1970. *Patients Views of Medical Practice.* New York: Russel Sage Foundation.

Freidson E. 1970. *Profession of the Medicine. A study of the Sociology of Applied Knowledge.* New York: Doold, Mead.

Freidson E. 1970. *Professional Dominance. The Social Structure of Medical Care.* New York: Artherton Press.

Freidson E. 1976. *Zastosowanie teorii organizacji. Modele organizacji i usług w opiece zdrowotnej.* in M. Sokołowska, I. Hołówka, A. Ostrowska (eds.). *Socjologia a zdrowie.* Warszawa: PWN.

Freidson E. 2004. *The Social Organisation if Illness.* in M. Bury, J. Gabe. (eds.). *The Sociology of Health and Illness. A Reader.* London, New York: Routledge.

Gabe J., M. Bury, M.A. Iston. 2006. *Key Concepts in Medical Sociology*. London: Sage.

Gajdziński P. 1992. „Gastarbeiterzy". *Wprost.* 01.11.1992.

Gapik L. 1990. „Fenomen Kaszpirowskiego". *Polityka.* (1708). 4.

Garfinkel H. 1967. *Studies in Ethnometodology,* Engelwood Cliffs: Prentice Hall.

Garfinkel H. 2007. *Studia z etnometodologii.* H. Szulżycka (transl.). Warszawa: PWN.

Garnuszewski Z. 1996. *Akupunktura we wspólczesnej medycynie,* Warszawa: Wyd. Amber.

Gazeta Kielecka. 1993. 10.02.

Gazeta Lekarska. 1994, 5, The statement of senator Zbigniew Kułak on Senate Meeting 30.03.1994.

Gazeta Lekarska. 1994, 9.

Gazeta Lekarska. 1997. 3.

Gazeta o Pracy. Gazeta Wyborcza suplement. 1995.03.04.

Gazeta Prawna. Gazeta Wyborcza supplement. 1995.25.01.

Giarelli G. 2006. *The ambivalent pluralism. The role of unconventional medicine in the Italian HNS.* in *XI European Congress of European Society for Health and Medical Sociology.*

Giddens A. 2004. *Socjologia,* Warszawa: PWN..

Gillert P. 2006. „Prawo pacjenta: Lekarstwo Abrahama". *Rzeczpospolita.* 29-30.07.

Gniazdowski A. 1990. *Wprowadzenie,* in A. Gniazdowski (ed.). *Zachowania zdrowotne.* Łódź Wyd. Instytutu Medycyny Pracy im. Prof. J.Nofera.

Glaser B., A. Strauss. 1965. *Awareness of dying.* Chicago Aldine Publ.

Gliński P. 1998. *Dylematy tożsamości ruchu ekologicznego,* in A. Sułek. M.S. Szczepański (eds.). *Śląsk–Polska-Europa. Zmieniające się społeczeństwo w perspektywie lokalnej i globalnej. Xięga X Ogólnopolskiego Zjazdu Socjologicznego.* Katowice: Wyd. Uniwersytetu Śląskiego.

Goldstein M.S. 2000. *Alternative medicine and medical sociology.* in C. Bird, P. Conrad, A. Fremont (eds.). *Handbook of Medical Sociology.* Upper Saddle Rivier: Prentice Hall.

Goldstein M.S. 2000. *Emergence of alternative medicine.* in P. Brown (ed.). *Perspectives in Medical Sociology.* Long Grove: Waveland Press.

Goldstein M.S. 2000. *The growing acceptance of complementmy and alternative medicine,* in Ch.E. Bird, P. Conrad, A. Fremont (eds.). *Handbook of Medical Sociology.* Upper Saddle Rivier: Prentice Hall.

Gottschalk-Olsen K. 1990. *The Encyclopedia of Alternative Health Care.* New York: Simon and Schuster.

Grossinger R. 1980. *Planet Medicine, From the Stone Age Shamanism to Post-industrial Healing.* New York: Anchor Books.

Górski P. 1996. „Niekonwencjonalne metody w alergologii". *Alergia, Astma, Immunologia.* 1(3).

Graham S. 1974. "The Sociological Approach to Epidemiology", *American Journal of Public Health*. Vol. 64. no. 11.

Gregosiewicz A. 2002. „Świeckie uzdrawianie całego człowieka". *Gazeta Lekarska.*

Grun J., I. Sadowska, D. Romanowska. 1993. „Adin, dwa, tri ...". *Wprost*". 14.02.1993.

Gryglewski R.J. 1995. *Medycyna - ile w niej nauki, ile w niej sztuki?* In K. Imieliński (ed.). *Medycyna XXI wieku. Sztuka leczenia.* Warszawa: PAM.

Gumuła W. 2002. „Socio-economic and political transformation". in Z. Bokszański et al. (eds.). *Encyklopedia socjologii.* T. 4, Warszawa: Oficyna Naukowa.

Gutkowska K. 2003. *Diagnoza fumkcjonowania wiejskich gospodarstw domowych na przełomie wieków.* Warszawa: Wyd. SGGW.

Guttman K., „Szamani w kolizji z prawem", *Nasz Dziennik* z dnia 02. 11.2000.

Hałas E. 1987. *Społeczny kontekst znaczeń w teorii symbolicznego interakcjonizmu.* Lublin: Wyd. KUL.

Hałas E. 1998. "Symbolic interactionism". in Z. Bokszański et al. (eds.). *Encyklopedia socjologii.* T. 1. Warszawa: Oficyna Naukowa.

Hałas E. 2006. *Interakcjonizm symboliczny. Społeczny kontekst znaczeń.* Warszawa: PWN.

Hirschkorn K.A. 2006. "Exclusive verus everyday forms of professional knowledge, legitimacy claims in conventional and alternative medicine". *Sociology of Health and Illness.* 28. 5.

Idler E.L. 2010. *Health and Religion.* in W.C. Cockerham. (ed.) *The New Blackwell Companion to Medical Sociology.* Oxford: Wiley-Blackwell.

Imieliński K. 1994. (ed.). *Medycyna u progu XXI wieku. Filozofia i techniki leczenia.* Warszawa: PAM.

Imieliński K. (ed.). 1995. *Medycyna u progu XXI wieku. Sztuka leczenia.* Warszawa: PAM.

Jagiełłowicz A.B. 2002. *Pole oddziaływania medycyny konwencjonalnej i medycyny komplementarnej jako zmienna układu społeczno-kulturowego naszych czasów.* in B. Płonka-Syroka (ed.). *Studia z dziejów kultury medycznej.* T.V: *Społeczno-ideowe aspekty medycyny i nauk przyrodniczych XVIII-XX wieku.* Wrocław: Wyd. Arboretum.

Jaguś I. 2002. *Lecznictwo ludowe w Królestwie Polskim na przełomie XIX i XX wieku.* Kielce: Kieleckie Towarzystwo Naukowe.

Jakubczak F. 1976. *Być w środku życia. Wspomnienia kobiet wiejskich.* T.3. Warszawa: KiW.

Jarvis D.C. 1989. *Folk medicine. A New England almanac of natural health care from noted Vermont country doctor.* New York: Fawcett Crest.

Jastrzębska J. (ed.). 2003. *Ubezpieczenia społeczne i zdrowotne w rolnictwie.* Lublin: Instytut Medycyny Wsi.

Jawłowska A. 1995. *Ład czy rozpad? Zmiany w sferze aksjonormatywnej.* in A. Sułek, J. Styk (eds.). *Ludzie i instytucje. Stawanie się ładu społecznego. Pamiętnik IX Ogólnopolskiego Zjazdu Socjologicznego.* T. 2. Lublin: Wyd. UMCS.

Jaźwiecka-Bujalska D. 2000. Między magią a religią, czyli zabobony i przesądy wśród duchowieństwa katolickiego we współczesnej Polsce. Kraków: Wyd. Universitas.

Jedynak W. 1995. „Duchowe oszustwa". Niedziela. nr 29.

Jeszke J. 1996. *Lecznictwo ludowe w Wielkopolsce w XIX i XX wieku. Czynniki i kierunki przemian*. Wrocław: Wyd. Arboretum.

Jeszke J. 1998. *Historyczne źródła współczesnych nurtów lecznictwa niemedycznego i ich społecznej akceptacji*. in M. Libiszowska-Żółtkowska, M. Ogryzko-Wiewiórowska, W. Piątkowski (eds.). *Szkice z socjologii medycyny*. Lublin: Wyd. UMCS.

Jütte R. 2001. *Historia medycyny alternatywnej. Od magii do naturalnych metod leczenia*. Warszawa: Wyd. WAB.

Kaja J. 1976. „Kierunki i etapy rozwoju polityki zdrowotnej Polski Ludowej". *Studia Nauk Politycznych*. nr. 1.

Kakai H., G. Maskarinec, D.M. Shumay, Y. Tatsumura, K. Tasaki. 2003. "Ethnic differences in choices of health information by cancer patients using complementary and alternative medicine. An exploratary study with corespondence analysis". *Social Science and Medicine*. 56.

Kaliszuk W. 1999. „Funkcjonowanie instytucji medycznej w świetle wyników obserwacji uczestniczącej". *Promocja Zdrowia. Nauki Społeczne i Medycyna*. nr 17.

Kamiński S. 2000. „Magiczny doktor". *Medicus - pismo Okręgowej Izby Lekarskiej w Lublinie*. 5.

Kański M., S. Wasilewski. 1981. „Clive Harris jako zjawisko spoleczne (próba opisu). *Studia Socjologiczne*. 3 (82).

Kapuściński R. 1997. „Lapidarium III". *Gazeta Wyborcza. Magazyn* (suplement). 4.04.1997.

Katechizm Kościoła Katolickiego. 1994. Poznań: Wyd. Pallottinum.

Karski J.B. Z. Słońska, B. Wasilewski. (ed.). 1994. *Promocja zdrowia. Wprowadzenie do zagadnień krzewienia zdrowia*, Warszawa: Sanmedia.

Kawczyńska-Butrym Z. 1990. „Socjologia rodziny i socjologia zdrowia - wiedza komplementarna". *Roczniki Socjologii Rodziny*. (90). T. II.

Kawczyńska-Butrym Z. 2002. *Zdrowie i choroba jako kategoria opisu położenia społecznego*. in W. Piątkowski, A. Titkow (ed.). W stronę socjologii zdrowia., Lublin: Wyd. UMCS.

Kelly M.P., D. Field. 2004. *Medical Sociology, Chronic Illness and the Body*. in M. Bury, J. Gabe. (eds.). *The Sociology of Health and Illness. A Reader*. London, New York: Routledge.

Kelner M., B. Wellman. 1997. "Health Care and Consumer Choice, Medical and Alternative Therapies". *Social Science and Medicine*. 45.

Kempny M. 1993. *O potrzebie analizy kulturowej w czasach przełomu*, in A. Jawłowska, M. Kempny, E. Tarnowska. (eds.). *Kulturowy wymiar przemian społecznych*. Warszawa: IFiS PAN.

Klamut M.K. 1996. „Od biotechnicznego do holistycznego modelu medycyny". *Alma Mater*. nr 4.

Klemens W. 1993. „Jak polscy lekarze walczyli ze znachorami w Gdańsku, wywiad z dr W. Grabą, wiceprzewodniczącym Okręgowej Izby Lekarskiej w Gdańsku". *Medyk* . 10.

Kocik L. 2001. *Trauma i eurosceptycyzm polskiej wsi*. Kraków: Wyd. Universitas.

Kodeks Etyki Lekarskiej. 1994. Warszawa: Oficyna Wydawnicza Naczelnej Izby Lekarskiej.

Komunikat Prezydium Rady Naukowej przy Ministrze Zdrowia i Opieki Społecznej. (The Paper Published by Ministry of Health and Social Welfare, 29.03.1983).

Konarska I. 2002. „Złote czasy uzdrowicieli". *Przegląd*. 18.

Konarska I. 2006. „Doktor blagier". *Wprost*. 19.02.2006.

Konecki K. 2000. *Techniki badań jakościowych*. in K. Konecki. *Studia z metodologii badań jakościowych. Teoria Ugruntowana*. Warszawa: PWN.

Kopaliński W. 1968. *Słownik wyrazów obcych i zwrotów obcojęzyc:nych*. Warszawa: Wyd. Wiedza Powszechna.

Kosiński S., S. Tokarski. 1987. *Ochrona zdrowia ludności wiejskiej*. Warszawa: PWN.

Kosiński S. 1983. *Społeczno-kulturowe i strukturalne przemiany warunków zdrowotnych polskiej wsi (1864-1980)*. Lublin: Wyd. UMCS.

Kościelak L. J. 2004. *Kwestia zmian instytucjonalnych w ubezpieczeniach zdrowotnych*. in W. Piątkowski (ed.). *Zdrowie-choroba-społeczeństwo. Studia z socjologii medycyny*. Lublin: Wyd. UMCS.

Kość K. 2004. „Na pograniczu magii i nauki. Rozważania o współczesnym wróżbiarstwie". *Literatura Ludowa*. 2 (48).

Kowalczewska A. 2001. *Ezoteryka na sprzedaż*. Warszawa: Wyd. Akademickie Dialog.

Krasnodębski Z. 1996. *Postmodernistyczne rozterki kultury*. Warszawa: Oficyna Wydawnicza.

Krasnowska V. 1994. „Z procesu Julka Czarodzieja". *Medicus - Pismo Okręgowej Izby Lekarskiej w Lublinie*. 45/40.

Krasuska M.E., A. Stanisławek, M. Mazurkiewicz. 2003. „Complementary and alternative care within cancer care". *Annales UMCS. sectio D*. Vol. L VIII, 2.

Kraszewski W. 2003. „Science". in *Wielka Encyklopedia PWN*. T.18. Warszawa: PWN.

Kronenfeld J.J. 2011. *Health Care Policy and Medical Sociology*. in B.A. Pescosolido, J.K. Martin, J.D. McLeod, A. Rogers. (eds.). *Handbook of the Sociology of Health, Illness and Healing. A Blueprint for the 21st Century*. New York: Springer.

Kruczek G., J. Majter, Łozowski S. 2001. *Sięgnij po zdrowie*. Bielsko Biała: (Typescript).

Kobielski W. 2003. *Kierunki zmian w systemie ubezpieczenia rolników*. in J. Jastrzębska (ed.). *Ubezpieczenia społeczne i zdrowotne w rolnictwie*. Lublin: Instytut Medycyny Wsi.

Kubiak A.E. 1998. „Kosmologia i antropologia uzdrawiania". *Promocja Zdrowia. Nauki Społeczne i Medycyna*. 14.

Kubiak A.E .1999. *O ponowoczesności New Age raz jeszcze*. in M. Kempny, G. Woroniecka (eds.). *Religia i kultura w globalizującym się świecie*. Kraków: Wyd. Nomos.

Kubiak A.E. 2005. *Jednak New Age*. Warszawa: Jacek Santorski & Co. Agencja Wydawnicza.

Kubiak H., K. Slany. 1999. "migrations". in Z. Bokszański et al. (eds.). *Encyklopedia socjologii*. T. 2. Warszawa: Oficyna Naukowa.

Kukiz T. 1974. „Chorzy na oddziale Chorób Wewnętrznych pochodzący z rejonu działania oddziału". *Zdrowie Publiczne*. nr. 10. T. 85.

Kutrzeba-Pojnarowa A. 1977. *Kultura ludowa i jej badanie. Mit i rzeczywistość*. Warszawa: Lud. Spół. Wyd.

Kuźnicka B. (ed.). 1989. *Historia leków naturalnych*, T. II.. Warszawa: IHNOiT PAN.

Kuźnicka B. (ed.). 1993. *Historia leków naturalnych*. T. III. Warszawa: IHNOiT PAN.

Lachowski S. 2001. „Dbałość rodziców o zdrowie dzieci w rodzinach mieszkających na wsi". *Medycyna Ogólna*. 7.

Lahelma E. 2010. *Health and Social Stratification*. in W.C. Cockerham. (ed.) *The New Blackwell Companion to Medical Sociology*. Oxford: Wiley-Blackwell.

Latoszek M. 1993. *Zachowania i postawy wobec przemian ochrony zdrowia*. Gdańsk: Wyd. AM.

Lata, listy, ludzie. Adresat M.F. Rakowski. 1993. Warszawa: Polska Oficyna Wyd. BGW.

Lawton J. 2003. "Lay experiences of health and illness, past research and future agendas". *Sociology of Health and Illness*. Vol. 25.

Leczenie się domowymi sposobami. Komunikat z badań CBOS. 1998. Warszawa: CBOS.

Leczyć mogą tylko lekarze. 1985. „Służba Zdrowia". 13/1942. 31.03.1985.

Lewczuk K. 1989. *Zachowania w chorobie ludności wiejskiej w okresie międzywojennym w Pamiętnikach chlopów i w Pamiętnikach lekarzy*. (Unpublished typescript). Lublin: Wydz. Pielęgniarski AM.

Lewonowska E., D. Czapska, J. Ustymowicz. 1989. „Ocena stanu sanitarno-higienicznego gospodarstw w rejonie gmin Jeleniewo, Rutka, Tartak i Szypliszki". *Medycyna Wiejska*. XXIV, nr 2.

Libera Z. 1989. *Magiczne sposoby pozyskiwania roślin*. in B. Kuźnicka (ed.). *Historia leków naturalnych*, T. II. Warszawa: IHNOiT PAN.

Libera Z. 2003. *Znachor w tradycjach ludowych i popularnych XIX-XX wieku*. Wrocław: Wyd. Tow. Przyjaciół Ossolineum.

Libiszowska-Żółtkowska M., M. Ogryzko-Wiewiórowska, W. Piątkowski. (eds.). 1998. *Szkice z socjologii medycyny*. Lublin: Wyd. UMCS.

Libiszowska-Żółtkowska M. 1998. Religia w trosce o zdrowie. Wybrane zagadnienia z pogranicza socjologii medycyny i socjologii religii, in Libiszowska-M. Żółtkowska, M. Ogryzko-Wiewiórowska, W. Piątkowski. (ed.). Szkice z socjologii medycyny. Lublin: Wyd. UMCS.

Linde K., W.B. Jonas. 2000. *Ocena medycyny komplementarnej i alternatywnej. Rzetelność naukowa a pragmatyzm terapeutyczny*. in W.B. Jonas, J.S. Levin. (eds.). *Podstawy medycyny komplementarnej i alternatywnej*. Kraków: Wyd. Universitas.

Linde K., Jonas W.B. 2000. *Postępowanie naukowe w medycynie*. in W.B. Jonas, J.S. Levin. (eds.). *Podstawy medycyny komplementarnej i alternatywnej*. Kraków: Wydawnictwo Universitas.

Lisowska M. 1995. „Polskie Towarzystwo Medycyny Naturalnej". *Pielęgniarka i Położna* 10.

Letter to Ministry of Justice, Prof. Lech Kaczyński from 05.11.2000. <http://www.nil.org.pl>.

Listy do Bobera. Nie tylko o gospodarce. 1992. Warszawa: Nowe Wyd. Polskie.

Listy do Rzecznika Praw Obywatelskich Tadeusza Zielińskiego. 1994 Warszawa: Wyd. Biuro Rzecznika Praw Obywatelskich.

Litwin F. 1945. *Dziennik Zdrowia*. nr 1.

Łazowski J. 2005. „WHO a medycyna niekonwencjonalna". *Sztuka Leczenia*. T. XI. nr 1-2.

Mackiewicz M., A. Wiśniewska, R. Dziadosz, A. Rotter. 1970. „Z badań nad zgłaszalnością i chorobowością ludności wsi". *Zdrowie Publiczne*. nr 8.

Mac Lachlan M. 1997. *Culture and Health*. Chichester, NY: John Wiley and Sons Publ.

Mach Z. 1998. "Antropologia a socjologia". in Z. Bokszański et al. (eds.). Encyklopedia socjologii. T. 1, Warszawa: Oficyna Naukowa.

Macura P. (ed.). 1993. *New Age*. Kraków: Zakład Wyd. Nomos.

Mała encyklopedia medycyny PWN. 1999. Warszawa: PWN.

Małkowska M. 2005. „Nie zapomniał ale lekceważy". *Rzeczpospolita*. 27.12.2005.

Mariański J. 2005. Religijność w społeczeństwie polskim w perspektywie zsekularyzowanej Europy. in W. Wesołowski, J. Wlodarek (eds.). Kręgi integracji i rodzaje tożsamości. Polska, Europa, Świat. Warszawa: Scholar.

Marlicz K. 2003. „Alternative medicine in the contemporary clinical oncology". *Gastroenterologia Polska*. 10.

Marody M. (ed.). 2004. *Wymiary życia społecznego. Polska na przełomie XX i XXI wieku*. Warszawa: Wyd. Scholar.

Marston R. 2000. *Wstęp*. in W.B. Jonas, J.S. Levin. (eds.). *Podstawy medycyny komplementarnej i alternatywnej*. Kraków: Wyd. Universitas.

Matlęga M. 1989. „Życie i zdrowie starych, samotnych rolników. *Wieś Współczesna*. nr 1.

Mądel K. 1995. *Wartości ogólnoludzkie i chrześcijańskie w listach Vincenta van Gogha do brata i przyjaciół w latach 1872-1880*. Warszawa: Wyd. Bobolanum.

McKinlay J. 2006. *When there is no doctor: reasons for the disappearance of primary care during the early 21st century*. Plenary lecture at Eleventh International Congress of the European Society for Health and Medical Sociology. Cracow.

Meek G.W. (ed.). 1979. *Healers and the Healing Process*, Wheaton: Theosophical Pub House.

Mechanic D. 1968. *Medical Sociology. A selective view*. New Yourk: The Free Press.

Meschig R., H. Schadewaldt. 1982. „Trepanacje czaszki we wschodniej Afryce". *Hexagon Roche*. nr 4.

"Miesięcznik informacyjny AM we Wrocławiu". 2003. IX, nr 4 (74) <http://www.gazeta.am.wroc.pl/gazeta74.html#3>

Miles M.B., A.M. Huberman. 2000. *Analiza danych jakościowych*. S. Zabielski (transl.). Białystok: Wyd. Trans Humana.

Misiek J. 1995. „Czy medycyna jest nauką?". *Sztuka Leczenia*. T. 1. nr l.

Morgan H.L. 1887. *Społeczeństwa pierwotne czyli badanie kolei ludzkiego rozwoju od dzikości poprzez barbarzyństwo do cywilizacyi*. Warszawa: Wyd. Prawda.

Moszczeńska W. 1968. *Metodologii historii zarys krytyczny*, Warszawa: PWN.

Mrozowska M. 2003. "Kolejny bubel legislacyjny". *Homeopatia Polska*. 3.

Mucha J. 1995. Kultura dominująca jako kultura obca. Mniejszości kulturowe a grupa dominująca we współczesnej Polsce. in A. Sułek, J. Styk (eds.). *Ludzie i instytucje. Stawanie się ładu społecznego. Pamiętnik IX Ogólnopolskiego Zjazdu Socjologicznego*. T. 2. Lublin: Wyd. UMCS.

„Na czarno i legalnie". *Gazeta w Lublinie – Gazeta Wyborcza suplement*. 22.07.1994.

Nardelli S. 1986. *W kręgu biopola*. Katowice: Wyd. KAW.

Nasz Dziennik. 2000.17.07.

Nasz Dziennik. 2003.02.04.

Nasze zdrowie i zdrowy styl życia. Komunikat z badań CBOS. 1993. Warszawa: CBOS.

Nettleton S. 1996. *A Sociology of Health and Illness*, Cambridge: Polity Press.

Nettleton S. 2007. "Retaining the sociology in medical sociology". *Social Science and Medicine*. 65.

Nettleton S. 2009. The Sociology of Health and Illnes. 2nd Edition. Cambridge: Polity Press.

Nestorowicz M. 2004. *Prawo medyczne. Wyd. VI, uaktualnione i rozszerzone*. Toruń: Wyd. "Dom Organizatora" TNOiK.

Nikitin L. 1990. Spotkania z doktorem Kaszpirowskim. T. Rychlewska. (transl.). Warszawa: Wyd. Omega.

Nowak J. (ed.). 2005. *Maria Konopnicka. Listy do Ignacego Wasilewskiego*. Warszawa: Inst. Badań Literackich PAN.

Nowak P. 1989/1990. „Jerzy Szacki i Piotr Sztompka. Dwa spojrzenia na relację socjologia a historia". *Annales UMCS. Sectio I*. Vol. XIV/XV.

Odonus B. 1993. „Perspektywa perlistego uśmiechu". *Gazeta Wyborcza*. 06.12.1993.

Olechnicki K. P. Załęcki. 1997. *Słownik socjologiczny*. Toruń: Wyd. Graffiti. Operacz M. 1997. *Leczenie akupunkturą*. Warszawa: PZWL.

Opinia publiczna o medycynie niekonwencjonalnej. Komunikat z badań CBOS. 1991. Warszawa: CBOS.

O niektórych aspektach świadomości końca wieku. Komunikat z badań CBOS. 1997. Warszawa: CBOS.

Oojendijk J., J.P. Mackenbach. 1981. "What is Better?" *The Netherlands Institute of Preventive Medicine*. Vol. 4.

Ostrowska A. 1981. „Rola pacjenta i lekarza, zmiany w scenariuszu". *Studia Socjologiczne.* 3 (82).

Ostrowska A. 1990. „Chory w rodzinie - implikacje praktyczne płynące z teorii socjologicznych". *Roczniki Socjologii Rodziny.* T.II.

Ostrowska A. 1999. *Styl życia a zdrowie.* Warszawa: Wyd. IFiS PAN.

Ostrowska A. 2004. *Polska socjologia medycyny na tle zachodniej.* in W. Piątkowski (ed.). *Zdrowie, choroba, społeczeństwo. Studia z socjologii medycyny.* Lublin: Wyd. UMCS.

Ostrowski K. 1954. *O czasach, znachorach i lecznictwie.* Warszawa: Wiedza Powszechna.

Ostrowski L. 1989. „Mieszkańcy wsi starsi wiekiem żyjący w' niedostatku". *Wieś Współczesna.* nr 11.

Palska H. 1999. *Badacz społeczny wobec tekstu. Niektóre problemy analizy jakościowej w socjologii i teoria literatury.* in H. Romański, K. Latyńska, A. Rostocki. (eds.). *Spojrzenie na metodę. Studia z metodologii badań socjologicznych.* Warszawa: Wyd. IFiS PAN.

Paluch A. 1989. *Zerwij ziele z dziewięciu miedz. Ziołolecznictwo ludowe w Polsce w XiX i początku XX wieku.* Wrocław: Wyd. Pol. Tow. Ludoznawczego.

Paluch A. 1998. „Etnologia wobec zagadnień medycyny jako obszaru penetracji badawczych". *Medycyna Nowożytna.* T. 5.

Pamiętniki chłopów. 1935. Warszawa: IGS

Pamiętniki chłopów. 1936. Seria druga, Warszawa: IGS

Pamiętniki lekarzy. 1939. Warszawa: Wydawnictwo Zakładu Ubezpieczeń Społecznych.

Pamiętniki lekarzy. 1964. Warszawa: Czytelnik.

Parsons T. 1951. *The social system.* New York: The Free Press.

Parsons T. 1969. *Struktura społeczna a osobowść.* Warszawa: PWE 1969.

Pawlicki M. 1997. „Rola 'leczenia niekonwencjonalnego' w onkologii. Próba oceny". *Farmacja Polska. 1.*

Pawlicki M. 1999. Bariery postępu w leczeniu nowotworów złośliwych. *Gazeta Lekarska.* 1.

Pawlicki M., B. Rysz-Postawa. 2001. „Delays in the commencement ol cancer treatment". *Nowotwory – Journal of Oncology.* 5.

Pawlicki M., B. Żuchowska-Vogelgesang, et al. 1999. „Wyniki badań nad przyczynami opóźnień w leczeniu chorych na raka piersi z próbą oceny czynników psychologicznych". *Współczesna Onkologia.* 6.

Pawluch D., R. Cain, J. Gillett. 2000. "Lay construction of HIV and complementary therapy use." *Social Science and Medicine*. 51.

Penkala-Gawęcka D. 1991. „Medycyna komplementarna w Polsce i jej badanie". *Lud*. T. 74.

Penkala-Gawęcka D. 1995. „Medycyna ludowa i komplementarna w polskich badaniach etnologicznych". *Lud*. T. 78.

Penkala-Gawęcka D. 1996. „Ethnopharmalogical Aspects of Complementary Medicine". in *Medicament et Aliments*, Metz 1996.

Penkala-Gawęcka D. 2006. „Polska droga do antropologii medycznej - wkład środowiska wrocławskiego". *Zeszyty Etnologii Wrocławskiej*. 1 (8).

Penkala-Gawęcka D. 2006. *Medycyna komplementarna w Kazachstanie. Siła tradycji i presja globalizacji*. Poznań: Wyd. UAM.

Penkala-Gawęcka D. 2008. *Antropologia medyczna dzisiaj, kontynuacje, nowe nurty, perspektywy badawcze*. in W. Piątkowski, B. Płonka-Syroka. (eds.). *Socjologia i antropologia medycyny w działaniu*. Wrocław: Wyd. Arboretum.

Pescosolido B.A. 2011. *Taking "The Promise" Seriously: Medical Sociology's Role in Health, Illness, and Healing in a Time of Social Change*. in B.A. Pescosolido, J.K. Martin, J.D. McLeod, A. Rogers. (eds.). *Handbook of the Sociology of Health, Illness and Healing. A Blueprint for the 21st Century*. New York: Springer.

Pędich W. 2004. *Zróżnicowanie warunków życia i sytuacji socjalnej ludzi starych na wsi*. in L. Solecki (ed.). *Problemy ludzi starszych i niepelnosprawnych w rolnictwie*. Lublin: Instytut Medycyny Wsi.

Pfeil M. 1994. "Role of Nursing in Promoting Complementary Therapies". *British Journal of Nursing*. No. 3.

Piątkowski W. 1981. „Medycyna naukowa wobec naturalnych sposobów leczenia. Konwergencja czy konfrontacja?". *Studia Socjologiczne*. 3 (82).

Piątkowski W. 1984. *Naturalne sposoby leczenia*. Wrocław: Ossolineum.

Piątkowski W. 1987. „Wywiad z Prof. J. Aleksandrowiczem". *Kamena*. September.

Piątkowski W. 1988. *Lecznictwo niemedyczne w Polsce w XX wieku*. Wrocław: Ossolineum.

Piątkowski W. 1990. *Spotkania z inną medycyną*. Lublin: Wyd. Lubelskie.

Piątkowski W. 1990. *Zdrowie i choroba w rodzinach chłopskich*. in A. Firkowska-Mankiewicz. (ed.). *Rodzina a problemy zdrowia i choroby*. Warszawa: CPBP 09.02.

Piątkowski W. 1991. *Zachowania w chorobie w rodzinie chlopskiej (głos w dyskusji)*. in Z. Tyszka (ed.). *Stan i przeobrażenia wspólczesnych rodzin chłopskich*. Poznań: CPBP 09.02.

Piątkowski W. 1992. *Problemy rodzinne dzieci chorych na hemofilię*. in R. Rokicka-Milewska (ed.). *Hemofilia u dzieci*. Warszawa: PZWL.

Piątkowski W. 1994. "Complementary Medicine in Poland. Sociological Approach. in *Health and Medieine in the New Europe. ESHMS. 5th Biennal Conference, Vienna.*

Piątkowski W. 1995. Lecznictwo niemedyczne w euroamerykańskim kręgu kulturowym. Przyczyny społecznego zainteresowania. in K. Imieliński (ed.). Medycyna u progu XXI wieku. Sztuka leczenia. Warszawa: PAM.

Piątkowski W. 1996. "Polish Complementary Medicine. Selected Results of Qualitative Analysis". in *Health and Social Change in the Integration of Europe. ESHMS. 6th Biennal Conference. Budapest.*

Piątkowski W. 1998. O potrzebie badań socjologicznych nad nieprofesjonalnymi sposobami realizacji potrzeb zdrowotnych w społeczeństwie pluralistycznym. in A. Snłek, M. Szczepański. (eds.). Śląsk-Polska-Europa. Zmieniające się społeczeństwo w perspektywie lokalnej i globalnej, Księga X Ogólnopolskiego Zjazdu Socjologicznego. Katowice: Wyd. Uniwersytetu Śląskiego.

Piątkowski W. 1998. *W stronę socjologii lecznictwa niemedycznego.* in M. Libiszowska-Żółtkowska, M. Ogryzko-Wiewiórowska, W. Piątkowski (eds.). *Szkice z socjologii medycyny.* Lublin: Wyd. UMCS.

Piątkowski W. 1999. „Lecznictwo niemedyczne jako sposób interpretacji kultury". *Annales UMCS. Sectio L.* Vol. XXIV.

Piątkowski W. 1999. Stosowanie niekonwencjonalnych metod leczenia w świetle badań socjologicznych. Analiza wybranych dylematów moralnych. in B. Płonka-Syroka. (ed.). Moralny wymiar choroby, cierpienia i śmierci. Wrocław: Arboretum.

Piątkowski W. 2000. „Lisków – fenomen rozwoju społeczności promującej zdrowie na terenach polsko-niemieckiego pogranicza (1900-1939)". *Sztuka Leczenia.* T. VI. 1.

Piątkowski W. 2000. "Patient-healer interaction. An attempt at sociological interpretation. in *Man-Medicine-Culture.West-East. 10th European Symposium of Somathotherapy. Kraków. Abstract Book.*

Piątkowski W. 2002. *Lecznictwo niemedyczne w społeczeńwtwie pluralistycznym.* in J. Barański, W. Piątkowski (eds.). *Zdrowie i choroba. Wybrane problemy socjologii medycyny.* Wrocław: Wrocławskie Wyd. Oświatowe.

Piątkowski W. (ed.). 2004. Zdrowie - choroba - społeczeństwo. Studia z socjologii medycyny. Lublin: Wyd. UMCS.

Piątkowski W., W.A. Brodniak. (eds.). 2005. *Zdrowie i choroba. Perspektywa socjologiczna.* Tyczyn: Wyd. WSSG.

Piątkowski W., J. Jezior, R. Ohme. 1993. *Listy do Kaszpirowskiego. Spojrzenie socjologiczne.* Lublin: Wyd. M. Łoś.

Piątkowski W., T. Karski. 1988. „Społeczne skutki hemofilii na podstawie materiału Kliniki Ortopedii Dziecięcej w Lublinie". *Acta Haematologica Polonica.* T. XIX. Nr 3-4.

Piątkowski W., T. Karski, T. Raganowicz. 1994. Metody usprawniania dzieci z mózgowym porażeniem dziecięcym w opiniach rodziców. in L.P. Wośko, D. Zarzycki (eds.). Wczesna diagnostyka i leczenie ortopedyczno-rehabilitacyjne dzieci z mózgowym porażeniem. Lublin: Wyd. Folium.

Piątkowski W., M. Latoszek. 1995. *O nowych sposobach badania zjawisk zdrowia i choroby.* in A. Sułek. J. Styk (eds.). *Ludzie i instytucje. Stawanie się ładu społecznego. Pamiętnik IX Ogólnopolskiego Zjazdu Socjologicznego.* T. 2. Lublin: Wyd. UMCS.

Piątkowski W., M. Latoszek. 1995. W stronę nowego paradygmatu socjologii medycyny, in A. Sułek. J. Styk (eds.). Ludzie i instytucje. Stawanie się ładu społecznego. Pamiętnik IX Ogólnopolskiego Zjazdu Socjologicznego. T. 2. Lublin: Wyd. UMCS.

Piątkowski W., A. Ostrowska. (eds.). 1994. *Niepełnosprawni na wsi.* Warszawa: IFiS PAN.

Piątkowski W., B. Płonka-Syroka (eds.). 2008. *Socjologia i antropologia medycyny w działaniu.* Wrocław: Wyd. Arboretum.

Piątkowski W., A. Titkow. (eds.). 2002. *W stronę socjologii zdrowia.* Lublin: Wyd. UMCS.

Pilecki M. 1994. „Paramedycyna - alternatywa medycyny naukowej?". *Zdrowie Publiczne.* 5.

Pilkiewicz M. 1994. *Promocja zdrowia a medycyna naturalna.* in J.B. Karski, Z. Słońska, B. Wasilewski. (eds.). *Promocja zdrowia. Wprowadzenie do zagadnień krzewienia zdrowia.* Warszawa: Sanmedia.

Pisalnik A. 2007. „Kontrowersyjny bioenergoterapeuta ukarany grzywną". *Rzeczpospolita.* 12.01.2007.

Pisalnik A. 2007. „Szkodliwy Kaszpirowski". Rzeczpospolita. 12.01.2007.

Letters from Ministry of Health and Social Welfare to Prof. A. Firkowska-Mankiewicz 28.09.1993. (Unpublished Typescricpt).

Płonka-Syroka B. 1990. *Recepcja doktryn medycznych przełomu XVIII i XIX wieku w polskich ośrodkach akademickich w latach 1784-1863.* Wrocław: Ossolineum.

Płonka-Syroka B. 1994. *Mesmeryzm od astrologii do bioenergoterapii.* Wrocław: Wyd. Arboretum.

Płonka-Syroka B. 1998. *Postawy lekarzy polskich generacji 1830-1859 wobec homeopatii i ich społeczne uwarunkowania.* in M. Libiszowska-Żółtkowska, M. Ogryzko-Wiewiórowska, W. Piątkowski (eds.). *Szkice z socjologii medycyny.* Lublin: Wyd UMCS.

Płonka-Syroka B. (ed.). 1999. *Moralny wymiar choroby, cierpienia i śmierci.* Wrocław: Wyd. Arboretum.

Płonka-Syroka B. (ed.). 2002. *Studia z dziejów kultury medycznej. T.V: Społeczno-ideowe aspekty medycyny i nauk przyrodniczych XVIII-XX wieku.* Wrocław: Wyd. Arboretum.

Płonka-Syroka B., A. Syroka (eds.). 2003. *Życie codzienne w XVIII-XX wieku i jego wpływ na stan zdrowia ludności.* Wrocław: Wyd. Arboretum.

Płonka-Syroka B. 2007. *Mesmeryzm. Od astrologii do bioenergoterapii. Wyd. III, poprawione i uzupełnione.* Wrocław: Wyd. Arboretum.

Płonka-Syroka B. 2008. Medycyna alternatywna w perspektywie antropologii historycznej. in W. Piątkowski, B. Płonka-Syroka (eds.). *Socjologia i antropologia medycyny w działaniu.* Wrocław: Wyd. Arboretum.

Popielski B. 1993. „Paramedycyna w Polsce". *Sztuka i Medycyna.* 3.

„Poszukać prawdy o zdrowiu i chorobie". 1989. *Express - Magazyn Ilustrowany.* Wyd. specjalne. 2.

Prior L. 2003. "Belief, knowledge and expertise, the emergence of lay expert in medical sociology". *Sociology of Health and Illness.* Vol. 25.

Puchalski K. 1990. *Zachowania związane ze zdrowiem i chorobą jako przedmiot nauk socjologicznych. Uwagi wokół pojęcia.* in A. Gniazdowski. (ed.). *Zachowania zdrowotne.* Łódź: Wyd. Inst. Medycyny Pracy im. Prof. J. Nofera.

Puchalski K., E. Korzeniowska. 2004. *Dlaczego nie dbamy o zdrowie? Rola potocznych racjonalizacji w wyjaśnianiu aktywności prozdrowotnej.* in W. Piątkowski (ed.). *Zdrowie - choroba - społeczeństwo. Studia z socjologii medycyny.* Lublin: Wyd. UMCS.

„Pytanie o uzdrowicieli". 2000. *Gazeta Wyborcza.* 02.11.2000.

Radzicki J. 1960. Znachorstwo w aspekcie medyczno-sądowym, prawnym i społecznym. Warszawa: Wyd. IW PAX.

Rafalski H. 1961. „Stan zdrowotności ludności wiejskiej a działalność służby zdrowia". *Wieś Współczesna.* No. 11.

Randi J. 1995. *Däniken, Tajemnica Syriusza i inne trele morele.* Łódź: Wyd. Pandora.

„Raport. Leczenie jemiołą chorób nowotworowych". 2004. *Homeopatia Polska.* 3.

„Raporty o stanie zdrowia ludności wiejskiej". 1982. Lublin: Instytut Medycyny Pracy i Higieny Wsi.

Riley D., et. al. 2001. „Homeopatia i medycyna konwencjonalna. Wyniki badania porównawczego skuteczności w podstawowej opiece zdrowotnej". *Homeopatia Polska.* 4.

Robinson D., S. Henry. 1977. *Self-help and Health. Mutual aid for modern problems.* London: Martin Robertson Publ.

„Rocznik Statystyczny GUS". 1997. Warszawa: GUS.

Rokicka-Milewska R. (ed.). 1992. *Hemofilia u dzieci.* Warszawa: PZWL.

Rudziński Z., S. Tokarski. 1972. „Zgłaszalność ludności wiejskiej do zakładów społecznej służby zdrowia w świetle powszechnego ubezpieczenia rolników". *Medycyna Wiejska.* no 4.

Rutkiewicz A. 1994. „Prawa cudzoziemców - temat wstydliwy". *Prawo co Dnia. Gazeta Wyborcza* suplement. 28.01.1994.

Rutkowska E., S. Kamiński, A. Kucharczyk. 2000. „Alternatywne sposoby leczenia bólów lędźwiowych. *Medicus - pismo Okręgowej Izby Lekarskiej w Lublinie.* 8/9.

Rutkowska E., J. Kulesza, W. Janusz. 2000. „Przyczyny niepowodzeń terapii manualnej w leczeniu dyskopatii lędźwiowej. *Postępy Rehabilitacji.* 14 (1).

Saldak B. 1964. „Opieka zdrowotna na wsi w okresie XX-lecia PRL". *Zdrowie Publiczne.* No. 7.

Scambler G. 2002. *Health and Social Change. A Critical Theory.* Buchingham: Open University Press.

Schepers R.M.I., H.E.G.M. Hermans. 1999. "The medical profession and alternative medicine in the Netherlands, its history and recent developments". *Social Science and Medicine*. 48.

Scimeca D. 2004. „Homeopatia jutro". *Homeopatia Polska*. 4.

Sciupokas A. 1996. "Alternative Health Care, Prospects of Integration in Lithuania. in *Health and Social Change in the Integration of Europe. ESHMS. 6th Biennal Conference. Budapest.*

Senior M., B. Viveash. 1998. *Health and Illness*. New York: Palgrave Macmillan.

Seyda B. 1962. *Dzieje medycyny w zarysie*. Warszawa: PZWL

Sharma U. 1996. *Using Complementary Therapies: a Challenge to Orthodox Medicine*. in *Modern Medicine Lay Perspective and Experiences*. London: UCL Press.

Shilling C. 1993. *The Body and Social Theory*. London: Sage.

Shuval J. 1992. *Social Dimensions of Health*. London: Praeger Publ.

Shuval J. 1998. "Complementary medicine and biomedicine. Patterns of Pragmatic Collaboration and coexistence". in *The Making of Health Policies in Europe. ESHMS. 7th Biennal Conference, Rennes*.

Shuval J. 2006. *Cohabitation or true marriage? Integration of bio and alternative health care*. in XI International Congress of the European Society for Health and Medical Sociology. Cracow.

Siciński A. 2002. *Styl życia - Kultura - Wybór. Szkice*. Warszawa: Wyd. IFiS PAN.

Siekierski S. 2003. *Codzienne troski kobiet w świetle listów do „Poradnika Domowego"*. in R. Sulima (ed.). *Życie codzienne Polaków na przełomie XX i XXI wieku*. Łomża: Oficyna Wydawnicza „Stopka".

Sikorski R. et al. 1964. *Dalsze badania nad stanem zdrowia kobiet wiejskich*. Lublin: Wyd. AM.

Silverman D. 2008. *Interpretacja danych jakościowych*. KT. Konecki (ed.). I. Ostrowska (transl.). Warszawa: PWN.

Sitek W. 2002. „Florian Znaniecki". in *Encyklopedia socjologii*. T.4. Warszawa: Oficyna Naukowa.

Skrętowicz B., R. Gorczyca. 2005. Percepcja funkcjonowania systemu opieki zdrowotnej w środowisku wiejskim w okresie reform. in W. Piątkowski, W.A. Brodniak. (eds.). *Zdrowie i choroba. Perspektywa socjologiczna*. Tyczyn: Wyd. WSSG w Tyczynie.

Skrzypek E. 2006. „Rozmowa pióra". Interview with G. Posłuszejko. *Nasz Dziennik*. 02.01.2006.

Skrzypek M. 2004. *Status socjoekonomiczny (SES) jako podstawowa kategoria socjomedyczna w badaniach nad chorobą wieńcową z perspektywy stanu zdrowia społeczeństwa*. in W. Piątkowski (ed.). *Zdrowie – choroba – społeczeństwo.Studia z socjologii medycyny*. Lublin: Wyd. UMCS.

Słońska Z. Misiuna M. 1993. *Promocja zdrowia. Słownik podstawowych terminów*. Warszawa: Agencja PromoLider.

Sokołowska M. 1980. *Interpretacja socjologiczna zjawiska Clive 'a Harrisa*. in *Człowiek, jego ból, cierpienie i prawo do szczęścia*. II Krajowa Konferencja lekarzy i humanistów. Gdańsk 11-12 grudnia 1978. Gdańsk: Krajowa Agencja Wydawnicza.

Sokołowska M. 1980. *Granice medycyny*. Warszawa: Wiedza Powszechna.

Sokołowska M. 1987. „Medycyna alternatywna". *Problemy*. 1.

Sokołowska M., A. Sarapata, B. Nowakowski. 1965. *Lekarze przemysłowi - wybór prac konkursowych lekarzy przemysłowych*. Warszawa: Ossolineum.

Sokołowska M. (ed.). 1969. *Badania socjologiczne w medycynie*. Warszawa: KiW.

Sokołowska M., L. Hołówka, A. Ostrowska A. (eds.). 1976. *Socjologia a zdrowie*. Warszawa: PWN.

Solarz I. 1937. *Historia powstania spółdzielni zdrowia w Markowej*. Warszawa.

Stacey M. 1988. *The Sociology of Health and Healing*. London: Unwin, Heyman Ed.

Stanway A. 1982. *Alternative medicine. A guide to natural therapies*. Harmondsworth: Penguin Books.

Starowolski Sz. 1606. *Votum o naprawie Rzeczpospolitej*.

Sterkowicz S. 1995. „Listy do Kaszpirowskiego. Spojrzenie socjologiczne". *Promocja Zdrowia, Nauki Społeczne i Medycyna*. No 5/6.

Sterkowicz S. 2002. *Mundus vult decipi*. "Gabinet Prywatny". 9.

Sterkowicz S. 2004. „Zdelegalizować paramedycynę". Służba zdrowia. No. 9-12.(3309-3312).15-16.02.2004. <http://www.sluzbazdrowia.com.pl>

Stevenson F.A., N. Britten, C. Barry, C.P. Bradley, N. Barber. 2003. "Self-treatment and its discussion in medical consultations, how is medical pluralism managed in practice?". *Social Science and Medicine*. 57.

Stomma L. 1986. *Antropologia kultury wsi polskiej XIX wieku*. Warszawa: Inst. Wyd. PAX.

Stopka A. 1995. (ed.). Letters to the Pope, about book *Przekroczyć próg nadziei*. – Readers of „Gość Niedzielny" Katowice: Wyd. Drukarnia Archidiecezjalna w Katowicach.

Strauss A. 1972. *Chronic illness and the quality of life*. St.Louis: C.V.Mosby.

Styk J. 1988. „Przeobrażenia roli wartości religijnych w życiu chłopa", *Chrześcijanin w Świecie*. 20. No. 7,

Styk J. 1993. *Chłopski świat wartości. Studium socjologiczne*. Włocławek: Wyd. Duszpasterstwa Rolników.

Sułek A., J. Styk. (eds.). 1995. *Ludzie i instytucje. Stawanie się ładu społecznego. Pamiętnik IX Ogólnopolskiego Zjazdu Socjologicznego*. T. 1 i 2, Lublin: Wyd. UMCS.

Sułek A., M. Szczepański. (eds.). 1998. *Śląsk-Polska-Europa. Zmieniające się społeczeństwo w perspektywie lokalnej i globalnej*. Księga X Ogólnopolskiego Zjazdu Socjologicznego. Katowice: Wyd. Uniwersytetu Śląskiego.

Sułkowski H. 2003. „Rozważania o medycynie nie tylko klinicznej". *Sztuka Leczenia*. T. IX. No. 3-4.

Sułkowski H. 2007. „Co z legalizacją homeopatii". *Homeopatia Polska*. 13.

Szacki J. 1981. *Historia myśli socjologicznej*. T. I i II. Warszawa: PWN.

Szacka B. 2003. *Wprowadzenie do socjologii*. Warszawa: Oficyna Naukowa.

Szaro J. *Znachorzy*. in M. Sokołowska, J. Hołówka, A. Ostrowska. (eds.). *Socjologia a zdrowie*. Warszawa: PWN.

Szczepański J. 1967. *Socjologia. Rozwój problematyki i metod*. Warszawa: PWN.

Szczepański J. 1973. *Odmiany czasu teraźniejszego*. Wyd. II poszerzone. Warszawa: KiW.

Sztompka P. 2003. *Trauma kulturowa. Druga strona zmiany społecznej*. in A. Kojder, K. Sowa (eds.). *Los i wybór. Dziedzictwo i perspektywy społeczeństwa polskiego*. Pamiętnik XI Ogólnopolskiego Zjazdu Socjologicznego. Rzeszów: Wyd. Uniwersytetu Rzeszowskiego.

Sztompka P. 2002. *Socjologia. Analiza spoleczeństwa*. Kraków: Wyd. Znak. Kraków.

Sztompka P. 1986. „Socjologia jako nauka historyczna". *Studia Socjologiczne*. 2.

Sztumski J. 1999. *Wstęp do metod i technik badań społecznych*. Katowice: Wyd. Śląsk.

Szumowski W. 1935. *Historia medycyny filozoficznie ujęta*. Kraków: Wyd. Gebethner i Wolff.

Śliwińska S. 1974. *Zdrowie kobiet gospodyń wiejskich na tle warunków ekonomiczno-społecznych, odżywiania i pracy zawodowej*, Warszawa: Wyd. PAN.

Śliwiński P.L. OFM Cap. 2004. *Miejska mistyka instant na przykładzie Festiwali Medycyny Naturalnej w Krakowie*. in A. Koseski, A. Stawarz (eds.). *Sfera sacrum i profanum w kulturze współczesnych miast Europy Środkowej*. Warszawa, PTEM - Pułtusk. WSH im. A. Gieysztora.

Świątoniowski G., T. Kłaniewski, et al. 2002. „Ocena zasięgu stosowania niekonwencjonalnych metod leczenia przez chorych na wybrane porównywalne rokowania, jednostki onkologiczne i kardiologiczne". *Onkologia Polska*. 5. 2.

Świderska-Możdżan T., K. Możdżan. 1979. „Opieka zdrowotna Gminnego Ośrodka Zdrowia przed i po wprowadzeniu powszechnego ubezpieczenia rolników". *Zdrowie Publiczne*. T. 90. no 2.

Taylor J. 1990. *Nauka i zjawiska paranormalne*. Warszawa: PiW.

Telewizyjne spotkania z A. Kaszpirawskim. Komunikat z badań. 1990. Warszawa: OBOP.

The Wall Street Journal – Polska.2007.11.16.

Thomas R.K. 2003. *Society and Health Sociology for Health Professionals*. New York, Boston: Kluwer Academic.

Thomas W.L., F. Znaniecki. 1976. *Chłop polski w Europie i Ameryce*. T. 1-5, Warszawa: Ludowa Spółdzielnia Wydawnicza.

Titkow A. 1983. *Zachowania i postawy wobec zdrowia i choroby*. Warszawa: PWN.

Tobiasz-Adamczyk B. 1998. „Szkice z socjologii medycyny". *Sztuka Leczenia*. 4.

Tobiasz-Adamczyk B. 1999. "medical sciences". in Z. Bokszański et al. (eds.). *Encyklopedia socjologii*. T.2. Warszawa: Oficyna Naukowa.

Tobiasz-Adamczyk B. 2002. *Relacje lekarz - pacjent w perspektywie socjologii medycyny*. Kraków: Wyd. Uniw. Jagiellońskiego.

Tobiasz-Adamczyk B. 2005. *Kilka uwag o socjologii choroby*. in W. Piątkowski, W.A. Brodniak (eds.). *Zdrowie i choroba. Perspektywa socjologiczna*. Tyczyn: WSSG.

Tobiasz-Adamczyk B., K. Szafraniec, J. Bajka. (eds.). 1999. *Zachowania w chorobie. Opis przebiegu choroby z perspektywy pacjenta*. Kraków: Wyd. Coll. Medicum UJ.

Tokarski S. 1992. *Choroby społeczne mieszkańców polskiej wsi XX wieku. Analiza socjomedyczna*. Lublin: IMW.

Tovey P., J. Adams. 2003. "Nostalgic and nastophobic referencing and the authentication of nurses use of complementary therapies". *Social Science and Medicine*. 56.

Tomaszewska A. 2004. „Fenomen medycyny naturalnej". *Okolice - Kwartalnik Etnologiczny*. 1/2.

Tomaszewski W. 1999. „Niekonwencjonalne metody leczenia w medycynie sportowej - akupunktura". *Medycyna Sportowa*. 94.

Trotter R.T. 2003. Etnography and Network Analysis, The Study of Social Context in Cultures and Societies. in G.L. Albrecht, R. Fitzpatrick, S. Scrimshaw (eds.). The Handbook of Social Studies in Health and Medicine. London: Sage Publ.

Tryfan B. 1988. *Znaczenie badań nad rodziną wiejską dla polityki społecznej na wsi*. in Z. Tyszka (ed.). *Badania nad rodziną a praktyka spoleczna*. Bydgoszcz: Wyd. Pomorze.

Tryfan B. 1992. „Wiejska starość w perspektywie międzynarodowej". *Roczniki Socjologii Wsi*. T. IV. Trevelyan J., B. Booth. 1998. *Medycyna niekonwencjonalna. Prawda i mity*. Warszawa: PZWL.

Tulli R. 1983. *Zdrowie i tycie jako wartości w kulturze wsi polskiej*, Warszawa (typescript).

Tulli R. 1990. *Rozwój koncepcji zdrowia, choroby i leczenia*. in A. Ostrowska (ed.). *Wstęp do socjologii medycyny*. Warszawa: Wyd. IFiS PAN.

Tuszkiewicz A. (ed.). 1968. *Przyczyny zaniedbań i opńinień w leczeniu ludności wiejskiej województwa lubelskiego*. Lublin: Wyd. AM.

Twaddle A.C., R. M. Hessler. 1977. *A Sociology of Health*. St. Louis: Mosby.

Tylkowa D. 1989. *Medycyna ludowa w kulturze wsi Karpat polskich*. Wrocław: Ossolineum.

Tyszka Z. (ed.). 1988. *Badania nad rodziną a praktyka społeczna*. Bydgoszcz: Wyd. Pomorze.

Tyszka Z. (ed.). 1991. *Rodziny polskie o rótnym statusie społecznym i środowiskowym*. Poznań: CPBP 09.02.

Tyszka Z. (ed.). *Stan i przeobrażenia współczesnych rodzin polskich*. Poznań: CPBP 09.02.

Uramowska-Żyto B. 1976. *Polskie piśmiennictwo w dziedzinie socjologii medycyny w latach 1969-1974. Wybrane pozycje.* in M. Sokołowska, J. Hołówka, A. Ostrowska (eds.). *Socjologia a zdrowie*. Warszawa: PWN.

Uramowska-Żyto B. 1992. *Zdrowie i choroba w świetle wybranych teorii socjologicznych.* Warszawa: IFiS PAN.

Uzdrawiacz. 2005. 7 (176).

Uzdrawiacz. 2006. 1 (182).

Uzdrawiacz. 2006a. 2 (183).

Uzdrawiacz. 2006b. 3 (184).

Verhoff M., L.R. Sutherland. 1995. „General practitioners's assessment of and interest in alternative medicine in Canada". *Social Science and Medicine.* 41.

Villanueva-Russell Y. 2005. "Evidence based medicine and its implications for the profession of chiropractic". *Social Science and Medicine.* 60.

Waitzkin H. 2000. *Changing Patient-Physician relationship in the Changing Health Policy Environment.* in Ch.E. Bird, P. Conrad, A.M. Fremont (eds.). *Handbook of Medical Sociology. 5th ed.* Upper Saddle River: Prentice Hall.

Walewski P. 2001. "Przychodzi chora do znachora". *Polityka.* 18.

Walsh N. 1993. "Does a Highly Diluted Homeopatic Drug Acts as Placebo in Healthy Volunteers?" *Journal of Psychosomatic Research.* 37.

Wąsik M. 1997. „Julek Czarodziej przed Sądem Najwyższym". *Medicus - Pismo Okręgowej Izby Lekarskiej w Lublinie.* 2 (73).

Wdowiak L., S. Kurzeja, K. Siwńska. 1980. „Postawy wobec zdrowia ludności w wieku produkcyjnym mieszkającej na wsi". *Medycyna Wiejska.* T. XV. No. 4.

Weiss G.L. L.E. Lonnquist. 2006. *The Sociology of Health, Healing and Illness.* 5th. Upper Saddle River: Prentice Hall.

Wielka encyklopedia medycyny. 2003. "unconventional medicine". Warszawa: PWN. T. XVII.

Wielki słownik medyczny. 1996. Warszawa: PZWL.

Wielosz-Tokarzewska E., L. Szczepański. 2002. „Alternatywne metody zwalczania bólu". *Reumatologia.* 4.

Wieruszewska M. 1995. „Wieś polska w perspektywie badań etnologicznych i socjologicznych". *Lud.* T. 78.

Wieruszewska M. 2006. *Tożsamość wsi w perspektywie ponowoczesności.* in J. Styk, M. Łacek, D. Niczyporuk (eds.). *Endogeniczne czynniki rozwoju obszarów wiejskich.* T.6. Lublin: Wyd. UMCS.

Więckowska E. 1994. „Kilka uwag o lecznictwie niemedycznym". *Przegląd Lekarski.* 51/12.

Więckowska E. 2002. Błąd lekarski. Błąd medyczny. Odpowiedzialność prawna i zawodowa lekarza. in J. Barański, W. Piątkowski (eds.). Zdrowie i choroba. Wybrane problemy socjologii medycyny. Wrocław: Wrocławskie Wydawnictwo Oświatowe.

Woźniak Z. 1991. *Socjomedyczne aspekty funkcjonowania rodzin w różnych środowiskach*. in Z. Tyszka (ed.). *Rodziny polskie o różnym statusie społecznym i środowiskowym*, Poznań: CPBP 09.02.

Woźniak Z. 1991. „Zdrowie-choroba-niepełnosprawność a rodzina. Relacje wzajemne w perspektywie teoretvczno-metodologicznęj". *Roczniki Socjologii Rodziny*. T. III.

Witos W. 1978. *Moje wspomnienia*. Warszawa: LSW.

Wróblewski A.K. 1990. *Wstęp*. in J. Taylor. *Nauka i zjawiska paranormalne*. Warszawa: PiW.

Wyka A. 1993. *Badacz społeczny wobec doświadczenia*. Warszawa: Wyd. IFiS PAN.

Youngson R.M. 1997. „medicine". *Collins. Slownik encyklopedyczny – medycyna*. Warszawa: Wydawnictwo RTW.

Youngson R.M. 1997. „alternative medicine". *Collins. Słownik encyklopedyczny - medycyna*. Warszawa: Wydawnictwo RTW.

Zamorski K. 1998. „history". in Z. Bokszański et al. (eds.). *Encyklopedia socjologii*. T.1. Warszawa: Oficyna Naukowa.

Zarządzenie Ministra Zdrowia w sprawie powolania Rady do Spraw Niekonwencjonalnych Metod Terapii z dnia 25 czerwca 2002 roku, "Dziennik Urzędowy Ministerstwa Zdrowia" No 03.02.09.

Zborowski M. 1952. „Cultural components in Responses to Pain". *Journal of Social Issues*. 8.

Zieleniewski M. 1845. *O przesądach lekarskich ludu naszego*. (doctoral dissertation). Kraków: Wyd. UJ.

Zinczenko E.A., L.M. Szwąjdak. 1991. *Biuletyn Informacyjny*. Kiev.

Żukowska D. 2001. „Znachorzy XXI wieku". Interview with M. Gajewski. *Nasz Dziennik*". 13.02.2001.

Index

D

E

F

G

H

I

J

K

Y

Z